Dental
Morphology
and
Evolution

Dental Morphology and Evolution

EDITED BY
ALBERT A. DAHLBERG

The University of Chicago Press
Chicago and London

International Standard Book Number: 0–226–13481–4
Library of Congress Catalog Card Number: 73–158726
The University of Chicago Press, Chicago 60637
The University of Chicago Press, Ltd., London
© 1971 by The University of Chicago
All rights reserved. Published 1971
Printed in the United States of America

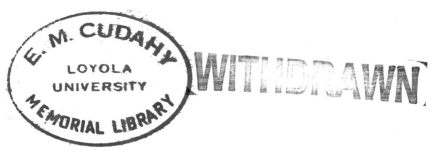

Contents

Preface

The purpose of symposia on dental morphology is to promote the exchange of ideas about dentition—specifically tooth form—by anatomists, paleontologists, embryologists, anthropologists, and odontologists. The First International Symposium on Dental Morphology was held in Fredensborg, Denmark, in 1965. The papers presented were published in one volume that was welcomed by students working in related scientific areas. The Second International Symposium on Dental Morphology was held in 1968 at Royal Holloway College in England. The sessions were designed to treat phylogeny, ontogeny, and morphology on three separate days. This publication of the papers presented at the symposium is in response to the reception received by the publication of the papers of the first symposium.

These international symposia are not the sole attempts toward communication and synthesis of ideas among the many disciplines. Scientific societies, aware of the difficulty of assessing the reports of studies in numerous journals, in many languages, have arranged meetings to accommodate individuals working on dentition in its many aspects. The American Association of Physical Anthropologists has consistently planned sessions of a half day or longer for papers and symposia on dentition. In 1962 the Society for the Study of Human Biology held meetings in the British Museum (Natural History), London, which were devoted to papers and discussions about teeth. These papers were published in a volume entitled *Dental Anthropology,* edited by D. R. Brothwell.

The members of the organizing committee for the First International Symposium were P. O. Pedersen and Verner Alexandersen of Copenhagen and Albert A. Dahlberg of Chicago. The meeting was held in Fredensborg, Denmark, 27–29 September 1965. There were sixty-five participants. These papers covered phylogenetic, ontogenetic, genetic, and morphological aspects of dentition, and there was a special session on field problems. The papers were published as a supplement volume of the *Journal of Dental Research,* September–October 1967, volume 46, number 5, pp. 769–992.

The Second International Symposium was held at Royal Holloway College, Englefield Green, Surrey, on 28–30 September 1968. Professor Percy Butler, with assistance from many colleagues in different countries and in different disciplines, arranged the meeting.

The editor wishes to thank his colleagues who contributed, his supporting editorial staff—Coenraad F. A. Moorrees of Boston, Philip Hershkovitz of Chicago, Percy Butler and K. A. Joysey of England—and the University of Chicago Press.

Albert A. Dahlberg

Introduction

Concepts and information relating to tooth morphology were updated at the 1968 Second International Symposium on Dental Morphology at Royal Holloway College, England. Professor Butler was mainly responsible for the fine collection of materials and organization of the program.

Several of the papers presented have been expanded for this volume and are classics in their fields. Two especially deserve this comment: The treatment of occlusal surface cusp evolution by Hershkovitz, and Turnbull's clarification of the marsupial dentition problems.

Alan Boyde's electron microscopic studies of the histology of mammalian teeth are a landmark in the actual viewing of their physical structures.

Some revealing factors affecting the final tooth form are to be found in the papers on ontogeny. Butler discusses the growth elements of the developing tooth germ and points to the determination of tooth size and form by the limiting effect of the calcified bridges that result when the different calcification processes extend to finally meet and join. Different gradients of growth and timing can thereby alter the proportions of a tooth. The presentation by Kollar and Baird complements Butler's observations. By adding an amino acid analogue to the nutrient environments of early developing tooth germs they demonstrated the retardation and final cessation of growth in the teeth. Subsequent washing and removal of this animo acid was followed by a return of the growth activity which had been temporarily interrupted. Kollar and Baird also show that the mesodermal tissues are the determinants of the final tooth form, regardless of the original donor site of the ectodermal elements. Further, they report success in the mesodermal tissues' inducing the tooth germ formation process in ectoderm from the lip furrow. Miller has done impressive tissue culturing of tooth germs and reports some differences in results. Tonge added substance to the dental tissue studies in culture at early stages. At the meeting Shirley Glasstone presented her evidence concerning differentiation factors in her cultures of early mandibular joint tissues in 13-day-old mouse embryos. She concluded that "formation of a mandibular joint in tissue culture indicates that the factors promoting joint formation are not necessarily the function of those operating in the intact developing embryo but are intrinsic to a particular region of explanted 13 day mouse embryo maxillary and mandibular mesenchyme." Stack approaches growth studies in a different manner, with chemical analysis and weighing of very early developmental levels.

It was appropriate at the symposium that Poole give an introductory résumé background of the phylogeny of dental tissues. This prepared the way for Boyde's comparative histology, Crompton's report on early mammalian tooth patterns, and Clemens's mesozoic tribosphenic dentitions.

Simons's presentation of recent advances in fossil hominoid dentitions brings these exciting materials up to date.

A final group of papers dealt with dentitions of modern hominids in various aspects. Goose presents his discussion of inheritance of tooth size in a family study. Dahlberg discusses the elusive aspects of dental traits in respect to their penetrance and expressivity. Brabant describes the teeth of Megalithic man and Beynon those of Afghan Tajik individuals. In an outstanding new presentation, Kovacs crystallizes some proposals for study of the roots of teeth to supplement the knowledge of the well-studied crowns.

One paper, by Hiiemae and Crompton, deals with the aspect of function of the temporomandibular joint by the use of radiological techniques.

In the background of these many studies are a number of biological principles which govern the developmental processes. The concepts of variability and embryology and the evidences of phylogeny are foremost among these.

The observation of gradations in degree and extent of occurrence of characterizations of repeated biological structures has contributed much toward comprehending the processes involved in trait production in teeth. Study of the range of forms of the many morphological units gives insight into the developmental process itself. Limitation or intensification of cell activity by the timing and extent of biochemical activity is evident. The interruptions in sequences or exceptions to the rule, such as the missing hypoconulid in some lower second molars, are clues to what occurs.

Finally, study of the finished forms in their great variety and range in the phylogenetic picture is brought to bear on the discussion and results of ontogenetic study. As Gregory and others have stated, phylogenetic events are seen as significant signposts in much of the ontogenetic process, but the purpose of all development is not to review the past but rather to produce the best organism. In doing this ontogeny does not necessarily have to recapitulate phylogeny, but compatible changes in sequence or pathways of development of advantage to the future organism are possible and are subject to selective pressures at any time from the very earliest periods of development.

The papers assembled in this book are a summary and exposition of the recent and present work of scientists from various fields attacking the problem of teeth in form, substance, and structure.

Part I

Ontogeny

1   Growth of Human Tooth Germs

P. M. Butler   *Royal Holloway College, Englefield Green,
Surrey, England*

At the previous symposium I discussed some problems of the morphological development of teeth, with particular emphasis on the differences between the teeth of the same individual (Butler 1967*b*). That discussion was based essentially upon qualitative description, because at the time quantitative data on tooth development were very limited. Two of the contributions to the previous symposium illustrate the main methods available: Gaunt's work (1967) was based on measurement of serial sections and Stack's (1967) on weights and measurements of the calcified parts of teeth. A third method, the direct measurement of extracted soft tooth germs, was first applied by Kraus and Jordan (1965) in their book *The Human Dentition before Birth,* which appeared just before the 1965 symposium. This method has an advantage over the study of sections in that it is possible to measure a much larger number of individuals and so obtain statistically more significant results; moreover, it is possible to combine measurements of the calcified parts of teeth with those of the soft parts. Immediately after the 1965 symposium I spent a year in Dr. Kraus's laboratory examining his collection of extracted tooth germs, and my purpose today is to summarize the results of this work.

    The method is not without its difficulties. As is always true when dealing with embryonic material which has been fixed post-mortem, the specimens are subject to shrinkage and distortion, and the process of dissecting them out involves a further risk of damage. For these reasons many of the specimens had to be rejected, and in the sample on which the investigations were based the number of teeth ranged from 39 in the case of M^1 to 99 in the case of dm_2. Another difficulty was measurement. Camera lucida drawings were made of each speci-

3

men from a number of standard directions, at a known magnification, and measurements were made on the drawings. This was found just as accurate as the use of a micrometer eyepiece and more convenient. The main source of inaccuracy is orientation. The tooth was examined in a petri dish in 40% glycerin, and it was supported by cotton wool in what was judged to be the correct position. No rigorous attempt has been made to separate errors due to measurement from those due to the variability of the material, but by repetition of the process of measurement on a number of specimens the measurement error did not exceed ±4%. The observed variability, after elimination of the effect of tooth size, is much greater than this; in the case of dm_2, deviation from regression when measurements are plotted against the mesiodistal length may amount to about ±15% in overall width measurements and ±20% in intercuspal distances and cuspal heights. As this variability is not appreciably less in the later stages of development when the crown is largely calcified, the effect of shrinkage appears to be small in comparison with the inherent variability of the material. The collection came from a wide area of the United States and it is racially and sexually heterogeneous, though white males predominate. Moreover, it was derived mainly from abortions and stillbirths, and might be expected to contain a relatively large proportion of abnormal specimens. Nevertheless, it has proved possible to use the collection to make certain deductions about the growth of teeth.

Growth may be considered from two aspects: increase of size with time, or change of shape with time; in the second case one speaks of relative growth. In most rapidly growing embryonic structures growth accelerates, in such a way that if the logarithm of the measurement of size is plotted against time a straight line is obtained. This means that the growth is of the exponential or compound-interest type, and it may be explained by supposing that the new material added at each stage can itself grow in subsequent stages, so that the growing stock continually increases. Likewise, in relative growth, if the logarithms of two measurements are plotted against each other a straight line is obtained, and the growth is described as allometric.

Sooner or later, however, the growth ceases to accelerate and begins to decelerate. This decrease of growth rate has been explained in various ways, as for example, the using up of a stock of essential material, the accumulation of inhibiting substances, the slowing down of cell division as a result of histological differentiation. Whatever the explanation, growth gradually slows down and eventually ceases when the organ attains its full size. During the phase of deceleration, allometry may still hold if the growth of the two measurements compared is decelerating at the same rate.

Sometimes, instead of the accelerating, compound-interest type of growth you get a simple-interest type, in which size increases in a straight line when plotted against time. In such instances one can imagine a growing stock which is producing new material that does not itself grow, but differentiates histologically and adds to the formed part of the organ. Such a situation occurs, for example, in the cambium of a tree and in the growth zone between the epiphysis and diaphysis of a long bone. On general grounds one would expect a tooth to show this type of growth, at least in the later stages when growth is confined to a basal zone after the more occlusal parts have already calcified.

If a measurement of tooth size is plotted against age it is seen that there is an early period of rapid growth, in the deciduous molars up to about 20 wk fetal age, followed by a period of gradual decline of growth rate (fig. 1). My data

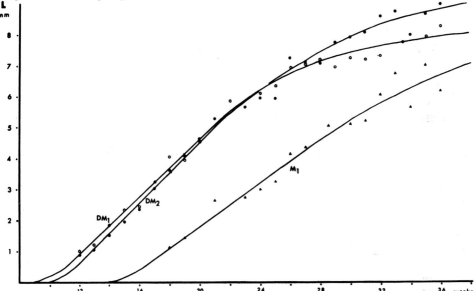

Fig. 1. Growth curves of mesiodistal length of dm_1, dm_2, and M_1. Mean values of available specimens, incorporating data from Kraus and Jordan (1965).

are insufficient to decide whether growth during the early period is constant or accelerating. Kraus and Jordan (1965) published measurements of the mesiodistal lengths of 37 American Indian fetuses and 36 American Negro fetuses of known age, and calculated the regression of length against age for each tooth. In the case of dm^1 they found a significant difference between the two races, but they did not take into account the slowing down of growth after 20 wk. If specimens aged more than 20 wk are excluded, the racial difference disappears, and moreover the growth rate agrees with that calculated from my own data, based mainly on fetuses of European descent. The three sets of data were therefore combined to give about 100 specimens of each tooth over an age range of

12–20 wk. The result is very close to a straight line, the deciduous molars growing in length at a rate of between 0.4 and 0.5 mm/wk. The first permanent molars, of course, start much later, and their growth begins to slow down at about 27 wk. Using about 20 specimens of each permanent molar, no curvilinearity can be detected over the range 18–27 wk, but the rate of growth is less than that of the deciduous molars: 0.28 and 0.35 for M^1 and M_1 respectively.

It was not possible to obtain reliable measurements of teeth much less than 1 mm in length, and some acceleration at this very early stage might be expected. However, differentiation, with cessation of mitosis, can be detected even in the bud stage, when growth is confined to the peripheral portion of the enamel organ. In the graphs I have assumed that some acceleration takes place in the very early stages, but if it occurs it is unlikely that growth is fully exponential.

The slowing down of growth of the deciduous molars after about 20 wk and the first permanent molars after about 27 wk was recognized by Moss and Chase (1966), using the data of Kraus and Jordan. They interpreted it as an interphase, a critical stage in the development of the tooth. In their graphs the suddenness of the break is exaggerated by converting the lengths to logarithms. I came to a similar conclusion in a study of the growth of the first upper molar, again using a logarithmic conversion (Butler 1967*d*). Such a logarithmic conversion is, however, justifiable only when growth is exponential, when the accelerating curve is transformed into a straight line. If growth of the tooth is additive, length should be plotted directly against time, and then it is seen that deceleration sets in gradually and continues over a long period, from 20 wk till after birth.

Moss and Chase ascribed the interphase to the initiation of calcification. My studies do not confirm this. Dm_1 begins to show calcification on the protoconid at 14–16 wk, well before deceleration begins: on dm_2 calcification starts at 18–20 wk, just before deceleration; M_1 begins to calcify at 29–32 wk, after the beginning of deceleration. Growth and calcification seem to be independent processes. This is what one would expect if growth is thought of as confined to the most basal level of the tooth whereas calcification takes place at a more occlusal level. For much of the development of the tooth the height of the uncalcified zone at the base of a cusp remains nearly constant, the rate of calcification equaling the rate of growth. Within the uncalcified zone one can imagine a zone of intensive growth at the base, and above it a zone where growth is giving place to differentiation (fig 2). For reasons that are not clear the height of the uncalcified zone differs from tooth to tooth: it is much greater on the first permanent molar than on the first milk molar. The effect of this is that the permanent molar reaches a greater size before calcification begins (fig. 3).

Before the calcification of a cusp its tip undergoes a characteristic series of

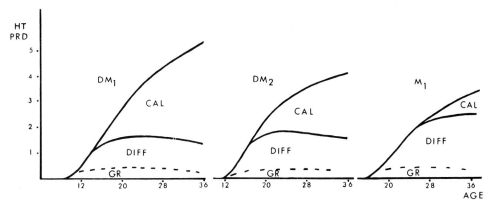

Fig. 2. Growth in height of protoconid of three lower teeth. The height is divided into the height of the calcified cap (*CAL*) and that of the uncalcified zone, which remains nearly constant but differs from tooth to tooth. The uncalcified zone is interpreted as containing a growth zone (*GR*) and a zone of differentiation (*DIFF*).

changes (Butler 1967c). Beginning as a flat area of the inner enamel epithelium, it becomes a rounded dome which increases in height and develops a point, which becomes more acute as development proceeds (fig. 4). This process, as pointed out by Turner (1963), is accompanied by a differentiation of the odontoblast layer, and it presumably involves an interaction between the ameloblasts and the odontoblasts. A similar process takes place along ridges, which also become sharpened before calcification. I have called the process maturation of the pattern (Butler 1967a), and it may be regarded as an indication of histological differentiation in the uncalcified zone. On the permanent molar pattern maturation proceeds more slowly, in relation to growth of the tooth, than on the milk molars. This would mean that differentiation in the uncalcified zone is slower, and thus the cells are farther removed from the base of the tooth before they form dentin and enamel.

I turn now to relative growth. Teeth change their shape as they develop: the cusps are formed in a definite order, and there are changes of proportion; for example, the talonids of the lower molars increase in width in comparison with the trigonids. It is natural to think of allometry in this connection, and to try to fit straight lines of the form $\log Y = b \log X + a$ to the data. When this was done for dm^2 and dm_2 it was found necessary in most cases to fit different regression lines to the data from the earlier and later phases of development. At first I thought that this implied a change in the pattern of growth at the interphase (Butler 1967a), but there is a simpler explanation: the regression of $\log Y$ on $\log X$ is not a straight line but a curved one. To get a straight line it is necessary to plot Y against X without conversion to logarithms; then there is no change of slope at the interphase (Butler 1968), but the entire period of

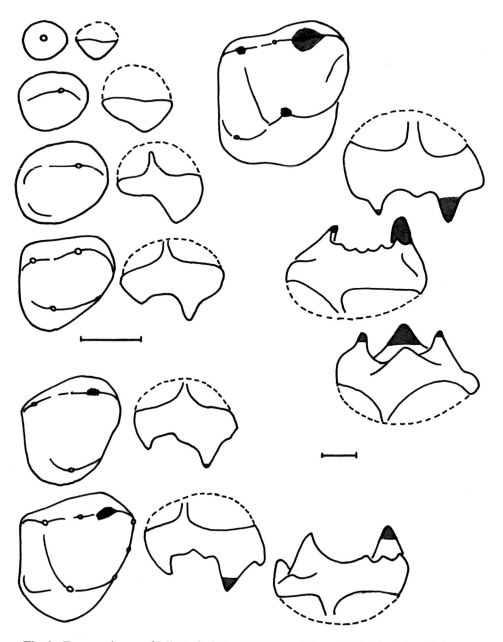

Fig. 3. *Top*, specimens of M[1], dm[2], dm[1] and cd from different individuals but of the same length, to show different degrees of calcification.

2d row, the same teeth in buccal view.

3d row, specimens of these four teeth from different individuals, showing the differing sizes at which calcification commences.

4th row, a seres of M[1]–cd from one individual to show size relations of completed teeth.

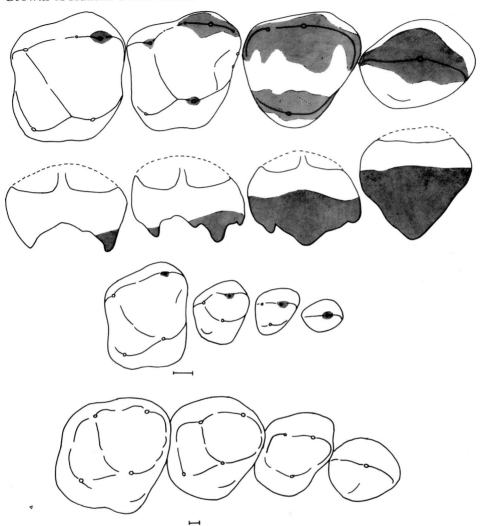

Fig. 4. Camera lucida drawings of specimens of dm² at various stages of development. The scale lines represent 1 mm. The four younger specimens are drawn at a larger scale than the remainder. All specimens seen in occlusal and buccal views; the specimen at the bottom of the figure also in mesial view, and the oldest specimen, on the right, in mesial and disto-lingual views. Calcification shaded.

growth can be represented by a single straight line, of the form $Y = BX + A$. This is what one would expect if the growth of Y and X were additive, such that the growth rate is independent of the size attained. The slope of the line, B, is the ratio of the growth rate of Y to that of X, and the fact that there is no change of direction despite the considerable decline of growth rate in the period after 20 wk indicates that this decline affects the tooth as a whole, and not just individual dimensions. Changes of shape are due to the line's not passing through the origin (fig. 5). For instance, in dm₂ and M₁ the talonid seems to start growing at a later age than the trigonid, so that at first it is proportionately

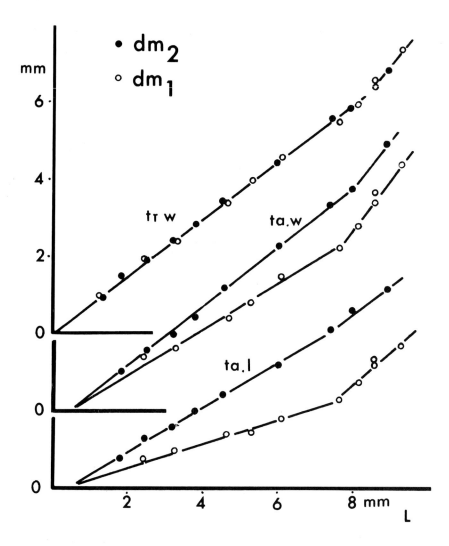

Fig. 5. Growth of trigonid width (*tr.w*), talonid width (*ta.w*) and talonid length (*ta.l*) relative to mesiodistal length, in dm₂ and dm₁.

small; but owing to its greater growth rate it eventually equals or exceeds the trigonid in length and width. In dm₁ the talonid also starts late, but its growth rate is less and it remains proportionately small in the completed tooth, despite the fact that the talonid continues to grow rapidly after growth of the trigonid has slowed down.

In dm$_2$, when the heights of the cusps are plotted against the mesiodistal length of the tooth they follow a series of parallel straight lines: they all grow at the same rate but start at different times (Butler 1968). Toward the end, growth in height continues after growth in length ceases, and the lines are bent upward (fig. 6). In dm$_1$ the cusps do not grow in height at the same rate; the protoconid grows proportionately more rapidly and the entoconid more slowly.

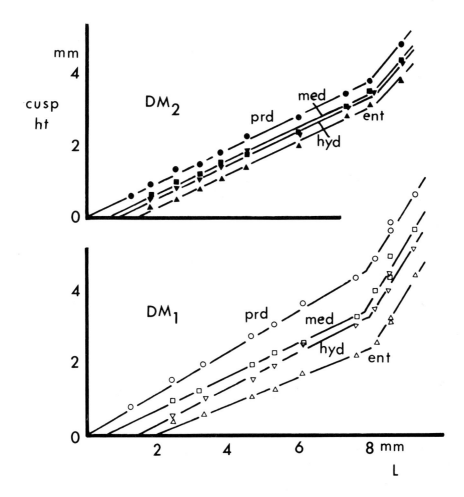

Fig. 6. Growth in height of the four main cusps, relative to mesiodistal length, in dm$_2$ and dm$_1$.

This results in a greater predominance of the trigonid, and especially of the protoconid, on the completed tooth.

By extrapolating the growth lines to zero, one can estimate the tooth length at which the various elements of the pattern start. Trigonid width and protoconid height may be regarded as starting to grow with the tooth. The metaconid differentiates later: its height can be considered as starting to grow when the tooth length is between 0.4 and 0.5 mm in dm_1, dm_2, and M_1. The talonid appears shortly after the metaconid, when the tooth length is about 0.6 mm. Of the talonid cusps, the hypoconid starts before the entoconid: in dm_2 and M_1 the hypoconid starts at a length of about 0.6 mm, the entoconid at a length of about 1.4 mm; in dm_1 these cusps start somewhat later, at about 1.7 and 2.0 mm respectively. It is interesting that the order of starting is the same as that postulated in the tritubercular theory.

One more aspect remains to be considered. The intercuspal distances, measured horizontally between the tips of the cusps, behave in an unusual manner. During the early period of rapid growth they increase nearly in proportion to tooth length, but at a later stage the cusps begin to tilt apart. Their tips separate at a greater rate than can be accounted for by growth of the base on which they stand (Butler 1967d); as the crown expands the cusps remain near the edge, so that the trigon and talonid basins occupy a progressively larger proportion of the area of the crown. This process must be due to growth in the uncalcified areas between the cusps, and it comes to an end when the calcified areas of the cusps unite. The degree to which spreading of the cusps can take place depends upon the incidence of calcification. In dm_1 calcification takes place at a smaller tooth size than in dm_2, and the spreading process is abbreviated compared with dm_2. Within dm_2, the entoconid remains separate from the metaconid and hypoconid for some time after the other cusps have united, and in the later stages the talonid basin enlarges by displacement of the entoconid alone. Thus the order of union of the cusps plays a part in determining the final pattern.

We may therefore summarize the developmental history of the tooth as follows: (1) There is an early formative period in which major new elements of the pattern make their appearance in a certain order. (2) This is followed by a period of steady growth, at constant rate; during this time the growth rates may differ from tooth to tooth, resulting in differences of proportion between each tooth and its neighbor. (3) About 7 wk later, growth of the tooth as a whole begins to slow down, but the growth rates of its various dimensions keep in the same proportion as in stage 2. During stage 3 the cusps begin to tilt apart. Superimposed on this sequence, and to some extent independent of it, is the process of histological differentiation leading to calcification. On dm_1 calcification begins midway through stage 2, in dm_2 near its end, and in M_1 early in stage 3. Calcification eventually brings the process of growth to an end, but not everywhere at once: growth in height continues after growth in length ceases; the distance between two adjacent cusps goes on increasing until their calcified caps unite.

REFERENCES

Butler, P. M. 1967a. Comparison of the development of the second deciduous molar and first permanent molar in man. *Arch. Oral Biol.* 12:1245–60.

———. 1967b. Dental merism and tooth development. *J. Dent. Res.* 46:845–50.

———. 1967c. The prenatal development of the human first upper permanent molar. *Arch. Oral Biol.* 12:551–63.

———. 1967d. Relative growth within the human first upper permanent molar during the prenatal period. *Arch. Oral Biol.* 12:983–92.

———. 1968. Growth of the human second lower deciduous molar. *Arch. Oral Biol.* 13:671–82.

Gaunt, W. A. 1967. Quantitative aspects of the developing tooth germ. *J. Dent. Res.* 46:851–57.

Kraus, B. S., and Jordan, R. E. 1965. *The human dentition before birth.* Philadelphia: Lea and Febiger.

Moss, M. L., and Chase, P. B. 1966. Morphology of Liberian Negro deciduous teeth. I. Odontometry. *Amer. J. Phys. Anthrop.,* n.s. 24:215–29.

Stack, M. V. 1967. Vertical growth rates of the deciduous teeth. *J. Dent. Res.* 46:879–82.

Turner, E. P. 1963. Crown development in human deciduous molar teeth. *Arch. Oral Biol.* 8:523–40.

2 Tissue Interactions in Developing Mouse Tooth Germs

E. J. Kollar

Department of Anatomy,
The University of Chicago

G. R. Baird

Zoller Dental Clinic,
The University of Chicago

The orderly sequences of morphological and biochemical events that culminate in the formation of the adult tooth are the product of tissue interactions that occur throughout the developmental history of the tooth. Certainly the classic paper of Huggins, McCarroll, and Dahlberg (1934) clearly illustrates this notion. In that study canine teeth, as well as isolated enamel organs and dental pulp, were transplanted heterotopically. The conclusion was clear; both epithelial and mesodermal components must be present for tooth formation to continue or for differentiated tissue states to be maintained. More recently, Koch (1967) and Kollar and Baird (1969) demonstrated that in embryonic mouse tooth germs separation of the epithelial and mesodermal components stops further development in each component. Koch further demonstrated that physical contact was not necessary and, indeed, that extracellular matrices indicative of and requisite for enamel and dentin formation were laid down despite separation of the two components by a Millipore filter. Thus, it is clear that throughout the history of the tooth both components must be present and in communication if normal development is to proceed. Although these data are in themselves interesting, the demonstration that tissue interactions are operative in the developing tooth germ implies a great deal more to the developmental biologist.

A growing number of similar tissue interactions between an epithelium and a mesodermally derived component are being examined (Grobstein 1967; Hilfer 1968; Wessells 1967). The conclusions from these studies have important bearing on the developmental process at large as well as providing specific insights into the particular organ system under investigation. These studies indicate that such epitheliomesenchymal interactions are inductive systems. In addition, it is the mesoderm that provides the inductive cue (Cairns and Saunders 1954; Rawles 1963) to a responsive epithelium. Moreover, the structural specificities for the resultant complex structure can be shown, in many instances, to reside in the mesoderm (Cairns and Saunders 1954; Kollar and Baird 1969). As a consequence, conclusions about the properties of epitheliomesenchymal interaction often may be inferred from the demonstration that a given structure is the product of an embryonic tissue interaction.

The wealth of data that demonstrates these concepts cannot be discussed here; the area has been reviewed a number of times in recent years (Billingham and Silvers 1963; Gaunt and Miles 1967; Sengel 1963; Wessels 1967). Instead, our recent studies on vibrissae development illustrate these concepts and are relevant to some of the conclusions about tooth germ development that will be discussed later.

The vibrissae primordia begin as thickenings of the snout epithelium in association with condensations of the mesenchyme (Kollar 1966). These primordia occur in rows along the snout and several rows appear as development proceeds. In addition, within each row the vibrissae appear sequentially, so that advanced stages as well as the earliest stages may be examined within each row. Of interest to us is the observation that the vibrissae are associated at an early stage in their history with branches of the trigeminal innervation to the snout.

Downgrowths of the snout epithelium are associated with condensations of mesenchyme that will become the future dermal papillae of the vibrissal follicles. It had been generally assumed that, like the feather dermal papillae, these condensations of mesodermal cells provide the inductive cue to the epithelium, thereby evoking the epithelial specialization necessary for hair-follicle formation (Chase 1954; Oliver 1968; Wessells and Roessner 1965). However, the origin, mode of action, and developmental properties of these cells in the mouse are not clearly established.

It is imperative to establish unequivocally that the papilla is the inductive agent. Embryonic skin can be easily separated into the epithelial and mesodermal components if subjected to cold trypsinization (Garber, Kollar, and Moscona 1968; Kollar 1966, 1970; Rawles 1963). Snout skin was treated and clean sheets of epithelium free of mesodermal contamination were prepared. Similarly, the plantar surfaces of embryonic foot plates were stripped and the snout and foot components were reciprocally exchanged. Thus, vibrissae follicle bearing snout epithelium was confronted with foot mesoderm; conversely, snout mesoderm with its resident dermal papillae was confronted with the normally hairless plantar epithelium. Vibrissal follicles develop only in those combinations of *snout mesoderm* and plantar epithelium. Thus, the mesoderm can elicit new developmental pathways from this ectopic epithelium. In short, vibrissae follicles were induced by the dermal papillae (Kollar 1970).

Because the mesenchyme of the head is generally thought to be derived from the ectomesenchyme of the cranial neural crest, it seemed reasonable to attempt disruption of vibrissal development with an agent previously shown to selectively impair the developmental performance of ectomesenchyme in the Amphibia (Wilde 1955). This agent is beta-2-thienylalanine (B2T), an analogue of phenylalanine. Low concentration of B2T (1–2 mM/L) added to our culture medium inhibits follicle formation in explants of snout skin from 11- and 12-day mouse embryos (Kollar 1968). Follicles do not develop in such explants after 6 days in culture. Significantly, equimolar concentrations of phenylalanine and the analogue applied simultaneously in no way impair follicle development. Such control cultures are essentially identical to explants grown on medium without any additive. Thus, B2T competitively inhibits some element in the system that is sensitive to phenylalanine concentration. We suggested from this work that B2T was incorporated into some enzymatic or structural protein and, in this fashion, disrupted inductive interactions taking place at this time (Kollar 1968).

The similarities between the early stages of vibrissae-follicle and tooth-germ development, the similar innervation, and the presumed neural crest origin of the dental papilla made the tooth germ a logical choice for extension of these studies of B2T inhibition of epidermal derivatives. We reported earlier in detail (Kollar and Baird 1968) that tooth germs are sensitive to this analogue. Tooth germs from 13- to 15-day-old embryos were cultured on agar-solidified Eagle's medium containing 1 or 2 mM/L of phenylalanine, 1 or 2 mM/L of B2T, or equimolar concentrations of the amino acid and the analogue. The presence of phenylalanine or equimolar concentrations of the amino acid and analogue did not affect the cultures and were equivalent to control cultures (fig. 1). After 6 days in culture advanced cytodifferentiation of the ameloblasts and odontoblasts was seen.

However, when B2T was added to the medium development was suppressed. There was no recognizable tooth structure in treated explants of 13-day embryonic tooth germs (fig. 2). The epithelium was present and had stratified and keratinized. It is important to mention that the explants were not suppressed because of a generalized cytotoxicity. Many mitotic figures were present in both the epithelium and the mesenchymal portions of these explants. In addition, bone continued to develop despite the marked suppression of the tooth germ rudiment. The relationship of Meckel's cartilage, the blood elements, and the developing bone provided morphological landmarks in many of these explants which confirmed their source. It was clear that the dental components of the

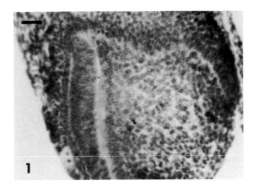

Fig. 1. After 4 days in culture in the presence of equimolar concentrations of phenyla-lanine and beta-2-thienylalanine, this explanted 15-day embryonic incisor germ displays normal morphogenesis. × 430. (Scales indicate 50 μ except in figs. 3 and 10, in which the scales equal 1 mm.)

mandible had been explanted and that tooth germ development was suppressed.

The data from cultures of 15-day-old tooth germs were especially instructive. The 15-day tooth germs are advanced in their development and are nearing recognizable cytodifferentiation of the epithelial and mesenchymal components. In these explants treated with 1 mM/L of the analogue, the tooth germ was easily identified in the treated cultures after 6 days in vitro. However, cytodif-ferentiation had not occurred. Indeed, the enamel organ appeared hyperplastic and ruffled with heightened mitotic activity along the inner enamel epithelium. When the concentration of the analogue was increased to 2 mM/L similar re-sults were noticed after two days in vitro followed by regression of the epithe-lium during subsequent days of culture.

It is clear that B2T, at the concentrations used in this study, does not kill the explants; rather, it specifically disrupts tooth germ development. Moreover, the

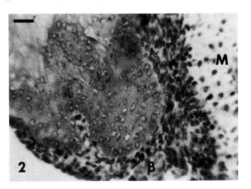

Fig. 2. An explant of a 13-day embryonic incisor tooth germ treated for 6 days with beta-2-thienylalanine. Note Meckel's cartilage (M) and blood cells (B). × 430.

analogue appears to be a competitive inhibitor of phenylalanine; other data (Caviness 1966a, b) confirm this and demonstrate that B2T does not inhibit protein or nucleic-acid synthesis and is incorporated into protein to about 40% of the control phenylalanine content.

In view of data that demonstrate that this analogue inhibits the unpigmented ectomesenchymal neural crest in the Amphibia (Wilde 1955) and that appearance of the mammalian dental papilla can be correlated with the presence of trigeminal neural crest (Milaire 1959; Pourtois 1964), we entertained the speculation that the dental papilla may well be the site of action of this inhibitor. Furthermore, we noticed that at elevated levels of inhibitor, the dental papilla exhibits a sensitivity to the analogue; evidence of cytotoxicity appears in the papilla without obvious signs of damage elsewhere in the explants. It may be of interest to recall that Cohen (1958) noticed that sympathetic ganglia (another neural crest derivative) do not grow in media containing P-fluoro-phenylalanine. However, the site of action of B2T remains unknown.

Our experiments to localize the incorporation of this analogue with radioactive tracers have begun, but it is too early to comment on these data. What has become clear is that the action of this inhibitor is reversible. If cultures are treated with the analogue for short periods and give evidence of inhibition and are then moved to a control medium, development proceeds in an orderly fashion. These data demonstrate the reversibility of this inhibition and lead us to suspect that the inhibition that we see is due to the incorporation of the analogue into the protein (enzymatic or structural) of the cells in our cultures. We are working on the assumption that an as yet undetermined factor essential for the induction or maintenance of the embryonic tooth germ is severely but reversibly disrupted by this amino acid analogue. Koch (1968) recently showed for the tooth germs, as did Grobstein and Cohen (1965) for salivary gland rudiments, that collagenase disrupts the normal tissue configurations in explants of these tissues. Thus, the modification of a single protein may severely disrupt the developmental sequence. Unfortunately, there are no data concerning the cellular or molecular incorporation of B2T. Nevertheless, the inhibition of tooth germ development by B2T offers a biochemical tool with which to study the intimate tissue interactions responsible for tooth development.

This work raised anew the questions of the developmental potentialities of the dental papilla cell population and its relationship to the epithelium. Because the mesoderm imparts local specificity for the type of skin derivative (e.g., feather, vibrissae, scales) in other developmental systems, we have examined the role of the dental mesenchyme in the ontogeny of tooth shape (Caviness 1966a; Gaunt and Miles 1967). Molar and incisor tooth germs from 12- to 16-day embryos were excised and treated with trypsin to facilitate

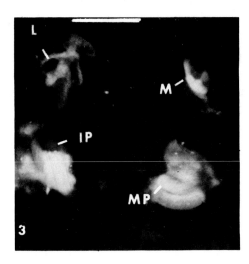

Fig. 3. Isolated epithelial and mesodermal components of 15-day embryonic incisor and molar rudiments. Note the lip furrow epithelium (*L*) associated with the incisor enamel organ, the incisor papilla (*IP*), the molar enamel organ (*M*), and the molar papilla (*MP*). × 20.

separation of the enamel organs and dental papillae of these germs. As we demonstrated earlier for snout skin, this procedure permits confident isolation of the epithelial and mesodermal components (fig. 3). Homologous, that is, control, recombinants were reconstructed consisting of enamel organs and dental papillae from the same mandibular segment. The recombinations were not adversely affected by the stripping procedures and type-specific tooth germs were produced after six days of culturing (fig. 4).

The reciprocal exchanges were of great interest. Heterologous, that is, experimental, exchanges of incisor enamel organs with dental papillae from molars and vice versa were prepared for each of the developmental stages considered. In this portion of our work we used a double scoring standard wherever possi-

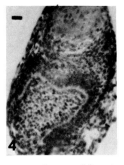

Fig. 4. After 6 days in culture, the control recombinant of 15-day-old molar enamel organ and papilla gives clear evidence of normal morphogenesis. × 100.

ble. The generalized incisiform and molariform pattern was used as a criterion; in addition, the differential pattern of cytodifferentiation along the labial surface of the mouse incisor was used to confirm our scoring of these experimental recombinants.

In all combinations of the tooth germ elements in which the site of origin, age of the components, or both parameters varied, the data consistently indicated a strong influence of the dental papilla on the emerging shape of the tooth germ. Thus, when molar epithelium from a 14-day-old embryo was confronted with the heterologous and isochronal incisor papilla from a 14-day embryo, the result was clearly an incisiform tooth germ. Similarly, in the heterologous and heterochronal combination of incisor epithelium from a 15-day embryo confronted with molar mesoderm from a 14-day-old embryo, a typically molariform germ was observed (fig. 5).

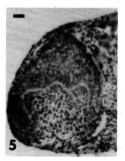

Fig. 5. An experimental combination of 14-day embryonic molar mesoderm and 15-day embryonic incisor epithelium. Note the molariform shape of this germ. × 100.

Despite wide variation in age, the papillar influence was strongly impressed on the epithelium. For example, when incisor epithelium from a 13-day-old embryo was confronted with a molar papilla from a 16-day-old embryo, the resulting tooth germ was clearly molariform (fig. 6). Such a recombinant represents an extreme case of a recombinant heterologous with reference to the spatial origin of the components and heterochronal with respect to the temporal development of the tooth germs.

These data are consistent with the conclusions from investigations on a number of integumental derivatives. That is, the structural specificity for the three-dimensional shape of the structure resides in the mesoderm. However, we are aware that these data do not shed light on possible initial interactions which may impose this regional specificity in the mesoderm of the developing mandible. Certainly, the preliminary results of Dryburgh (1967) and Miller (1969) suggest that the presumptive incisor and molar epithelia of the mandible may influence the mandibular mesoderm. Epithelium younger than 13 days of

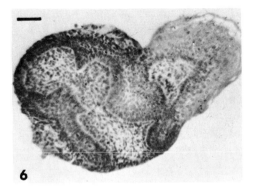

6

Fig. 6. An experimental confrontation of 13-day embryonic incisor epithelium and 16-day molar mesenchyme. Note the molariform shape of this germ. × 250.

gestation might impose specificity on the undetermined and plastic mesoderm. This possibility notwithstanding, it appears that once the local mesodermal specificities are established, they remain stable and are capable of influencing epithelial differentiation through the beginning stages of cytodifferentiation in 16-day-old tooth germs.

The execution of these experiments introduced another facet of importance to the investigation of the factors that control the emergence of tooth shape. The delicate and collapsed enamel organ could not be oriented with certainty on the dental papilla; shifting of the epithelium is inevitable during the early hours of culture. In addition, folding of the epithelium resulted in the random placing of the various parts of the enamel organ on the mesodermal component. Despite these variables, the subsequent development of recognizable tooth germs suggests that the epithelium retains sufficient plasticity to respond to the organizing influence of the papilla. Certainly, this notion was forecast by the work of Glasstone (1952) that showed that bisected rabbit molars display remarkable developmental plasticity and form two harmonious molars.

However, our experiments differ from those of Glasstone in that epithelium and mesoderm do not maintain previously established tissue interfaces; the epithelial and mesodermal components have been physically separated. Moreover, it is likely that after separation, folding, and random placement on the mesoderm, entirely new portions of the enamel organ are confronted by the dental papillar cells. These observations provoke some interesting questions. Do the entire enamel organs of older, and presumably stable, tooth germs reorganize into new structural patterns? Do the dental papillae from 13- to 16-day embryonic tooth germs induce the complete reorganization of all portions of the enamel organ, or does some unspecialized cell population in this epithelial structure reconstitute the tooth germ? Is the cervical loop portion of the enamel organ the source of such unspecialized cells?

We found these questions particularly intriguing not only from the viewpoint of tooth development but from the viewpoint of epitheliomesenchymal interactions as a whole. We undertook a series of experiments to test the various possibilities. Incisor enamel organs from 15- or 16-day-old embryos served as the source of the epithelial component (fig. 3). These ages were chosen because at these stages cytodifferentiation of the inner enamel epithelium is incipient or already cytologically detectable. Furthermore, isolated incisor epithelium could be divided into three areas: (1) the cervical loop area with its mitotically active and relatively unspecialized cell population; (2) the "upper half" containing the stellate reticulum and the mitotically quiescent and developmentally advanced inner enamel epithelium; and (3) the lip furrow band that is closely associated with the incisor rudiments at this stage. These epithelial fragments were then confronted with incisor and molar papillae from 14-, 15-, and 16-day embryos.

As we expected, the cervical loop region was capable of reconstructing a tooth germ (fig. 7). Needless to say, these tooth germs were diminutive and

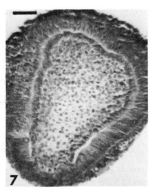

Fig. 7. An experimental recombinant of the cervical loop epithelium and the papilla from a 16-day embryonic incisor germ. After 6 days in culture, this explant has reestablished the normal histotypic relationship between these two components. × 250.

negative results were obtained when the epithelium failed to make intimate contact with the mesoderm. Nonetheless, enough cases were obtained to confirm our suspicion that the cervical loop epithelium was able to reorganize and perhaps provide a source of cellular material for tooth reconstruction. As might be expected, the epithelium derived from the 15-day incisor enamel organs responded significantly better and gave a higher yield of positive cases.

Surprisingly, when the "upper half" portions of the enamel organ containing the more advanced inner enamel epithelium were combined with mesoderm, recognizable, although distorted, tooth elements were observed (fig. 8). As before, the 15-day-old enamel organs were more likely to respond to the presence of the papilla. Although we scored many of these explants as negative because after 6 days in culture such combinations failed to produce recognizable tooth germs, the association of epithelium and mesoderm was sufficiently well established to indicate a loss of the original organizations and the beginnings of new histotypic patterns.

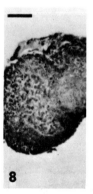

Fig. 8. An experimental confrontation between "upper half" incisor enamel organ epithelium and a molar papilla. Both components were derived from 15-day embryonic tooth germs. Note the site of tissue interaction and the suggestive molariform shape. × 250.

The most astonishing data, however, were obtained when the lip furrow band was associated with papillar mesoderm. These recombinations often displayed areas of tissue interaction suggesting early stages of tooth formation (fig. 9). Although we were compelled to score such suggestive tissue arrangements as negative, these results did imply the possibility that the lip furrow

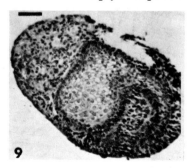

Fig. 9. This explant was composed of lip furrow epithelium and molar mesoderm from 15-day embryonic tooth germs. Note the suggestive tissue arrangements seen after 6 days in organ culture. × 250.

band was indeed capable of participating in the reconstruction of tooth germs in such experimental confrontations.

At least two factors apply to the interpretation of these results. First, the nutritional requirements of embryonic mouse tissue must be considered when the tissue is subjected to severe experimental traumata such as those inflicted in these studies. Negative results with one set of culture conditions must not be relied upon until confirmation under improved culture conditions. Second, and this may be related to the first factor, Grobstein and Zwilling (1959) demonstrated the phenomenon of critical mass in tissue associations. That is, minimal amounts of tissue must be present before recognizable differentiation can take place. By reducing the amount of epithelium we may have been adversely biasing the success of our experimental explants. Glasstone (1952) similarly reported that in the bisected rabbit molar germs, fragments smaller than one-half of the germ failed to regulate into harmonious molars.

These considerations prompted us to repeat these experiments. We made recombinations in the same manner as described earlier and allowed the tissue components to cohere for one or two days in organ culture. The recombinations were then grafted to the CAM or to the anterior chamber of the eyes of homologous hosts. The results confirmed our original observations.

Despite the double scoring criteria used in our earlier experiments, the analysis of organ cultures of experimental combinations had to be made from serial section of young tooth germs. The added advantage of long term culturing in the intraocular site provided unequivocal corroboration of our earlier results because the longer culture period permitted advanced differentiation and often allowed direct observation of the graft. For example, a combination of molar enamel organ and incisor mesenchyme from a 15-day-old embryo was allowed to grow for 5 wk in this superior explantation site (fig. 10). This particular graft was unusual in that the developing tooth "erupted" from the anterior chamber and could be photographed in situ. The explant was clearly an incisiform germ in an advanced stage of development.

Similarly, cervical loop and "upper half" combinations (figs. 11, 12) displayed perfectly formed tooth germs in this more nearly optimal in vivo transplantation site. However, the response of the lip furrow band in association with dental papillae was of greater satisfaction to us. In a more favorable culture site, these recombinants clearly showed that the lip furrow band can participate in tooth formation under these experimental conditions (figs. 13, 14). Although the lip furrow band is spatially and temporally related to the enamel organ, it has not been considered to be part of the dental epithelial complex. Thus, these data take on added significance; the ability of the lip furrow band

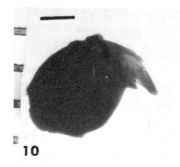

10

Fig. 10. This intraocular graft of molar enamel organ and incisor papilla was grown for 5 wk in the anterior chamber. In this photograph, the entire mouse eye is shown with an incisiform tooth growing out of the anterior chamber. × 10.

to participate in tooth formation in association with dental mesoderm is the first demonstration of tooth formation in the absence of the enamel organ.

Certainly, caution must be exercised in interpreting these results as a clear case of induction by the dental papilla. The lip furrow band is spatially and temporally related to the enamel organ and its developmental potential has not previously been tested. Moreover, the formation of dental structures from non-dental epithelium or a less closely related epithelium would provide a more stringent, and perhaps the only satisfactory, test of the inductive properties of the dental papilla.

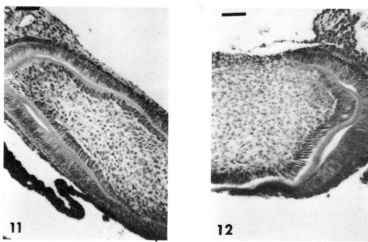

11   **12**

Fig. 11. An incisiform tooth germ developing in an explant derived from the cervical loop region and incisor papilla of a 16-day embryonic incisor germ. This explant was grown for 1 wk in the anterior chamber. × 250.

Fig. 12. An advanced tooth germ after 1 wk of intraocular growth. Incisor papilla and "upper half" epithelium taken from a 16-day embryonic incisor were the tissue sources. × 250.

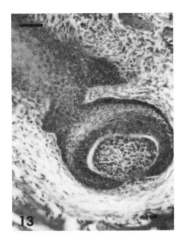
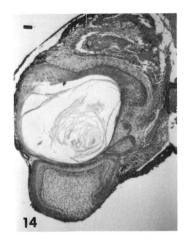

Fig. 13. A young tooth germ harvested from the CAM after 1 wk. The explant was derived from the lip furrow epithelium of a 16-day embryonic incisor germ and the molar papilla from a 14-day embryonic molar germ. Note the development of a stellate reticulum and a surfacelike epithelium in this explant. × 250.

Fig. 14. An intraocular graft grown for 1 wk. The tissue components were the lip furrow epithelium and molar papilla from 15-day tooth germs. Note the surfacelike keratinizing epithelium and the molariform tooth germ. × 100.

Although these data bring to light new facets of tooth germ development and confirm the view that as in other epitheliomesenchymal interactions it is the mesoderm that plays decisive roles in the initiation, maintenance, and structural organization of the tooth germ, the basic mechanisms that underlie these interactions are more intriguing because of these new data. The use of B2T may offer a significant new approach in unraveling the biosynthetic mechanisms involved in the enamel organ-papillar interaction. In addition, the ultrastructural organization during the emergence of three-dimensional shape of the tooth germ and the differential matrix synthesis along the enamel organ in the incisor are intriguing questions.

These data begin to define the developmental properties of the embryonic tooth germ and underscore the enormous potential of this structure as a model developmental system. The unique versatility of this epitheliomesenchymal interaction in which both components participate in the emergence of a complex structure with each component undergoing cytodifferentiation and each contributing specialized cell products offers unusual experimental possibilities. Finally, the data reviewed here bring many facets of tooth development into the perspective of other work on integumental epitheliomesenchymal interactions and may provide an opportunity for incisive attacks on some of the crucial questions of developmental biology.

ACKNOWLEDGMENTS
This work was supported in part by United States Public Health Service general
research support grant FR–5367 from the National Institutes of Health and by
American Cancer Society grant ACS–IN–41–H. We wish to thank Mrs. W.
Garner for technical assistance in some portions of this work, and we gratefully
acknowledge the generosity of Dr. B. Ginsburg, who provided us with animals
and animal-care facilities.

REFERENCES
Billingham, R. E., and Silvers, W. K. 1963. The origin and conservation of epidermal
    specificities. *New Eng. J. Med.* 268:477–80.
Cairns, J. M., and Saunders, J. W., Jr. 1954. The influence of embryonic mesoderm
    on the regional specification of epidermal derivatives in the chick. *J. Exp. Zool.*
    127:221–48.
Caviness, V. S., Jr. 1966a. The effect of beta-2-thienylalanine upon RNA synthesis
    in the macrophage. *Exp. Cell. Res.* 44:234–40.
———. 1966b. The effect of beta-2-thienylalanine upon protein synthesis in the
    macrophage. *Exp. Cell. Res.* 44:287–94.
Chase, H. B. 1954. Growth of hair. *Physiol. Rev.* 34:113–26.
Cohen, S. 1958. A nerve growth-promoting protein. In *The chemical basis of de-
    velopment,* ed. W. McElroy and B. Glass. Baltimore: Johns Hopkins Press.
Dryburgh, D. C. 1967. Epigenetics of early tooth development in the mouse. *J.
    Dent. Res.* 46:1264.
Garber, B.; Kollar, E. J.; and Moscona, A. A. 1968. Aggregation in vivo of disso-
    ciated cells. III. Effect of state of differentiation of cells on feather development
    in hybrid aggregates of embryonic mouse and chick cells. *J. Exp. Zool.* 168:455–
    71.
Gaunt, W. A., and Miles, A. E. W. 1967. Fundamental aspects of tooth morpho-
    genesis. In *Structural and chemical organization of teeth,* 1:151–97. New York
    and London: Academic Press.
Glasstone, S. 1952. The development of halved tooth germs: A study in experi-
    mental embryology. *J. Anat.* 86:12–15.
Grobstein, C. 1967. *Mechanisms of organogenetic tissue interaction.* National
    Cancer Institute Monograph no. 26.
Grobstein, C., and Cohen, J. 1965. Collagenase: Effect on the morphogenesis of
    embryonic salivary epithelium in vitro. *Science* 150:626–28.
Grobstein, C., and Zwilling, E. 1959. Modification of growth and differentiation of
    chorio-allantoic grafts of chick blastoderm pieces after cultivation at a glass-clot
    interface. *J. Exp. Zool.* 142:259–84.
Hilfer, R. S. 1968. Cellular interactions in the genesis and maintenance of thyroid
    characteristics. In *Epithelial mesenchymal interactions,* ed. R. Fleisihmajer and
    R. Billingham. Baltimore: Williams and Wilkins.

Huggins, C. B.; McCarroll, H. R.; and Dahlberg, A. A. 1934. Transplatation of tooth germ elements and the experimental heterotopic formation of dentin and enamel. *J. Exp. Med.* 60:199–210.

Koch, W. E. 1967. In vitro differentiation of tooth rudiments of embryonic mice. I. Transfilter interaction of embryonic incisor tissues. *J. Exp. Zool.* 165:155–70.

———. 1968. The effect of collagenase on embryonic mouse incisors growing in vitro. *Anat. Rec.* 160:377–78.

Kollar, E. J. 1966. An in vitro study of hair and vibrissae development in embryonic mouse skin. *J. Invest. Derm.* 46:254–62.

———. 1968. The inhibition of vibrissae development in vitro by beta-2-thienylalanine. *J. Invest. Derm.* 50:319–22.

———. 1970. The induction of hair follicles by embryonic dermal papillae. *J. Invest. Derm.* 55:374–78.

Kollar, E. J., and Baird, G. R. 1968. The effect of beta-2-thienylalanine on developing mouse tooth germs in vitro. *J. Dent. Res.* 47:433–43.

———. 1969. The influence of the dental papilla on the development of tooth shape in embryonic mouse tooth germs. *J. Embryol. Exp. Morph.* 21:131–48.

Milaire, J. 1959. Prédifférenciation cytochimique de diverses ébauches céphaliques chez l'embryon de souris. *Arch. Biol.* (Paris and Liège) 70:587–30.

Miller, W. A. 1969. Explanation of mouse dental lamina onto chorioallantois. *J. Dent. Res.* 47. Supplement to no. 6, abstract (287) of paper presented at the 46th I.A.D.R. meeting, San Francisco.

Oliver, R. F. 1968. The regeneration of vibrissae: A model for the study of dermal-epidermal interactions. In *Epithelio-mesenchymal interactions,* pp. 267–79. Baltimore: Williams and Wilkins.

Pourtois, M. 1964. Comportement en culture in vitro des ébauches dentaires de rongeurs prélevées aux stades de prédifférenciation. *J. Embryol. Exp. Morph.* 12:391–405.

Rawles, M. E. 1963. Tissue interactions in scale and feather development as studied in dermal-epidermal recombinations. *J. Embryol. Exp. Morph.* 11:765–89.

Sengel, P. 1963. The determinism of the skin and cutaneous appendages of the chick embryo. In *The epidermis,* ed. W. Montagna, pp. 15–34. New York and London: Academic Press.

Wessells, N. K. 1967. Differentiation of epidermis and epidermal derivatives. *New Eng. J. Med.* 277:21–33.

Wessells, N. K., and Roessner, K. D. 1965. Non-proliferation in dermal condensations of mouse vibrissae and pelage hairs. *Dev. Biol.* 12:419–33.

Wilde, C. E., Jr. 1955. The urodele neuroepithelium. II. The relationship between phenyl alanine metabolism and the differentiation of neural crest cells. *J. Morph.* 97:313–44.

3   Early Dental Development in Mice

William A. Miller *Department of Oral Biology,*
State University of New York at Buffalo

The experimental grafting of formed and forming tooth germs onto the chorio-allantoic membrane (CAM) of the domestic chick has been most adequately reviewed by Glasstone (1954) and the literature of the whole field of dental development by Gaunt and Miles (1967). Previous workers have been mostly concerned with the later stages of odontogenesis and with how this may be understood and modified by experimental grafting, either into another site in the same animal or into a different animal of the same or different species. Hence, similar and dissimilar ages of graft and host have been an important variable. These experiments have, however, been performed on tissue that is old enough to be already determined, in that it is certain that it will produce teeth, that enamel will be formed by the epithelial component, and that dentin and possibly cementum, will be formed from the mesodermal part.

Until relatively recently, it has been thought that the morphology of organs derived from both ectoderm and mesoderm, including teeth, was primarily determined by the ectodermal component, though both Sellman (1946) and Horstadius (1950) had demonstrated that in the Urodeles the presence of neural crest cells—ectomesenchyme—determined whether or not teeth developed in the larval forms of these animals. Sengel (1957), however, was able to demonstrate that in feather development it was the mesodermal component that initially determined feather site, and Rawles (1963) has more recently produced further evidence for this phenomenon in relation to both feather site and type. Sengel proposed three phases of interaction between the developing

The material related to the use of the chorioallantoic membrane was first presented at the Fourth International Conference in Oral Biology, Copenhagen, 1968.

embryonic tissues. First, a change in the mesoderm caused by an unknown external source; second, an interaction of mesoderm affecting overlying ectoderm; and third, a subsequent interaction of ectoderm on the subjacent mesoderm. Similar types of interaction have been demonstrated in the early development of mammalian whiskers (Wessells and Roessener 1965) and other organs derived from both embryonal layers by McLoughlin (1961). Cohen (1961) has shown evidence of similar mesodermal dependence of morphology in whiskers of adult rats and guinea pigs.

It was in 1939 that Butler first proposed that there were theoretically three fields of influence which determined the morphology of the developing teeth in mammals; an anterior incisivation field, a posterior molarization field, and an intermediate caninization field. In various mammals the three fields could be modified or suppressed; in some ungulates the upper anterior field was entirely suppressed, resulting in no upper anterior teeth, as in sheep and goats, while in the lower jaw the canine field was partially suppressed and the tooth bud influenced by the incisivation field to produce an incisiform canine tooth. In rodents, both anterior fields were modified and the canine fields suppressed while the molar and premolar fields were reduced. This resulted in the typical rodent dentition. Davis (1964), in discussing the dentition of the giant panda and its relationship to the bears, based part of his discussion on the theoretical shape of the molarization field in the species concerned.

Although there is some evidence for the morphogenic fields in mice (Glasstone 1967), there is yet little experimental evidence in mammals for the influence of mesoderm on dental ontogenesis, though the histochemical studies of Pourtois (1961, 1964) are very suggestive. Miller (1964) briefly reported on the use of the chorioallantoic membrane of the developing domestic chicken and also elder siblings as host sites in studies of early tooth development and has more recently described his findings related to the CAM in more detail (1968). Dryburg (1967) has also studied the tissue interactions in tooth development in embryo mice from 8 to 14 days post-conception using an organ culture technique, as have Kollar and Baird (1968) in their study of inhibition of tooth development in mice aged 13–15 days post-conception. Koch (1967) has studied these interactions using 0.45 μ and 0.35 μ pore size membranes in 16-day mouse embryos and was able to demonstrate transfilter induction of both the odontoblasts and preameloblasts. The CAM has also been used by Slavkin and his co-workers (Slavkin, Beierl, and Bavetta 1968; Slavkin and Bavetta 1968a, b) for studies of disaggregated ectodermal and mesodermal components of tooth germs from neonatal rabbits and as a nutrient source in the study of the growth of fetal whole teeth in rats.

Hoffman (1960) has used littermates as hosts in transplanting molar tooth germs of neonatal hamsters but not inbred strains.

The purpose of this study was to investigate the early development of the morphogenic fields in the mouse and to establish further evidence in favor of mesodermal prime induction in dental ontogenesis using both the chick chorioallantoic membrane and elder siblings as host sites.

Materials and Method

The general methodology of dating the embryos and separating and combining the tissues to be implanted onto the chorioallantoic membrane of the domestic chick has already been described (Miller 1968).

In an early series of experiments (Miller 1964) and unpublished data, jaw hemisections and separated presumptive molar and incisor areas were implanted into the cervical subcutaneous tissue of sibling mice of the same mating (fig. 1).

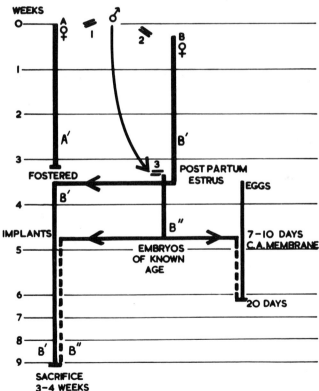

Fig. 1. Diagram of experimental design.

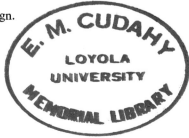

The hybrid vigor of an F1 generation from two closely inbred strains was used to ensure that both donor and host material were as homogeneous as possible. C57 and Strong A strains were used, which conveniently were of different coat color.

Experimentally, two sisters (A and B) of the Strong A strain were placed with a male of the C57 strain, and around the third day (Whitton effect [1959]) they became pregnant within 24-36 hr of each other. All this was followed by morning examination for vaginal plug and by vaginal smears. The male was left with female B, which became pregnant last. A third mating was hoped for at the postpartum estrus—usually within 24 hr after birth of litter B'. The elder litter A' was destroyed and the younger litter B' fostered to female A. At the required and precisely determined age, female B was killed and her embryos (litter B″) used as donors. Grafts from this material were either placed on the chorioallantois (Miller 1968) or into the loose connective tissue of the shoulder of the elder siblings. The latter has proved an excellent site for growth for periods of at least 6 wk, but the method was not entirely successful owing to the difficulty of locating the explants afterward.

Serial sections at $7-10\ \mu$ were cut completely through all implants recovered and alternate slides stained with hematoxylin and eosin. PAS, a three-stage Mallory connective-tissue staining technique, and the alcian-blue technique of Lison (1957) were also used.

Results

It was possible to grow tooth germs in the CAM experimental model and, on the whole, the system was relatively free from difficulties. One problem can be the failure of the graft to vascularize, often owing to movement of the chick embryo which caused the implant to wander before it could become vascularized. When this occurred only small, dried-up implants were recovered.

Many implants into the elder siblings were lost, probably owing to displacement in the loose subcutaneous connective tissue, though those recovered grew well. Crown morphology was well determined and the disturbances were slight (fig. 2). However, the rate of growth was considerably slowed (fig. 3). Because of the difficulty of locating implants and of timing the estrous cycles, this method was not used subsequently.

Consideration of the results from the eldest donor ages to the youngest shows that a pattern of change is evident.

The presumptive dental tissues removed at *13 days post-conception* were fully determined. If anterior or posterior jaw segments were implanted whole, the normal incisor and molar tooth germs developed and calcification of the

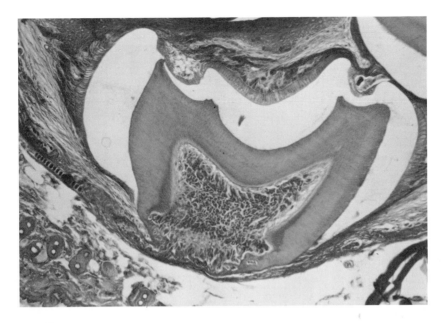

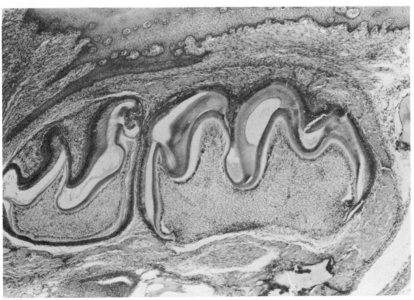

Fig. 2. First lower molar from 13-day post-conception posterior region of mandible grown for 4 wk in the subcutaneous tissue of an elder sibling. Mallory connective-tissue stain. × 100.

Fig. 3. First and second lower molars growing in situ in a 9-day post-natal mouse. Hematoxylin and eosin. × 20.

dentin, at least, and sometimes of the enamel, proceeded normally. Whiskers developed frequently in the anterior pieces and occasionally in the posterior portions and grew rather long (fig. 4.) Deranged whisker rows were sometimes observed. Glandular tissue, sometimes with a distinct capsule, was seen to develop from the posterior segments, and Meckel's cartilage was often found developing as a distinct bar of tissue (fig. 5).

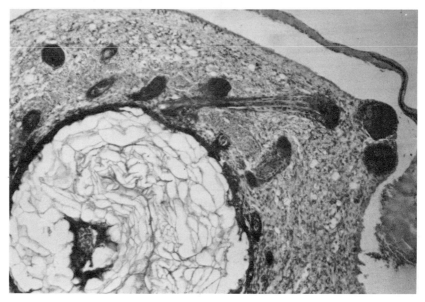

Fig. 4. Whisker germs growing on CAM in implant from anterior third of mandible. Hematoxylin and eosin. × 100.

At 12 days post-conception, growth from jaw segments produced normally shaped tooth germs, as did recombinations. The donor ectoderm determined the tooth type. The teeth were smaller than normal and did not develop as fast as in undisturbed embryos (figs. 6, 7).

By 11 days the morphogenic fields were also developed, though tooth germs themselves developed even more slowly and frequently were very distorted. Donor ectoderm again determined tooth germ morphology. In one instance a tooth "socket" was observed in a whole posterior implant to the CAM (fig. 8) in which the tooth itself was merely at the bell stage.

Tissue from *10 day post-conception* embryos produced definite but distorted molar tooth germs from the whole posterior portion. Recombinations with molar ectoderm produced distorted epithelial masses in which it was possible to see molar type morphology. In elder sibling material similar distorted molar

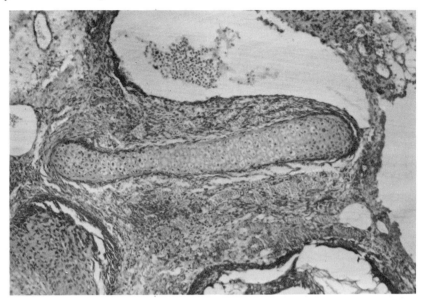

Fig. 5. Bar of Meckel's cartilage growing in posterior two-thirds fragment of mandible implanted onto the CAM. Alcian blue. × 100.

tooth germs could be seen (fig. 9). Anterior-third implants and incisor ectoderm and molar mesoderm recombinations produced epithelial masses in which it was not possible to determine morphology (fig. 10).

When mesoderm was implanted alone, the undifferentiated cells produced a ball of fibroblast type cells, and sometimes collagen fibers appeared. At the edges of the graft the cells were dispersed. Ectoderm alone frequently keratinized on the surface of the CAM or just below and, once keratinized, appeared to be in the process of exfoliation.

Around a number of the implants lymphocyte and plasma type cells were seen to have infiltrated (fig. 11). This was not a constant feature and its incidence requires further investigation.

Discussion

At the ages examined and under these experimental conditions, the morphogenic properties of the dental ectoderm of the mouse mandible seem fully determined by around 10½ days post-conception.

By 11 days post-conception the morphogenic fields are determined in both the anterior and posterior parts of the mandible, and this information resides in the ectodermal component. At 10 days it is possible that although the posterior part is completely determined, the anterior part is only partially deter-

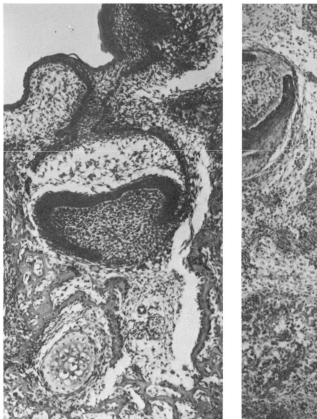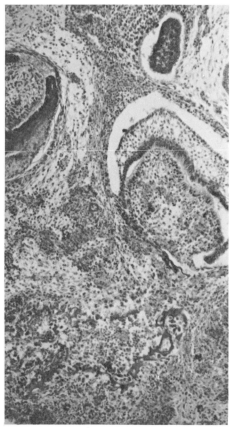

Fig. 6. Transverse section of mandible of 18-day post-conception embryo. Note the developing alveolar bone and Meckel's cartilage. Hematoxylin and eosin. × 100.

Fig. 7. Molar tooth germ from posterior jaw portion of 12-day post-conception embryo, grown for 9 days on the CAM. Compare with fig. 6. Hematoxylin and eosin. × 100.

mined. This part of the investigation should be repeated, because the anterior distortion is also related to the infiltration of inflammatory cells. The variability between anterior and posterior regions, however, fits well with the histochemical data on the migration of neural crest cells at this state of development as demonstrated by Pourtois (1964) and also agrees with the hypothesis of Sengel (1957) on the stages of interaction in the development of organs derived from both embryonal layers. The further investigation of 9-day post-conception embryos is desirable, as is the combination of heterochronous tissues to see if determination is reversible at early stages as has been reported by Kollar and Baird (1968) in later stages. The rate at which tissues already molariform

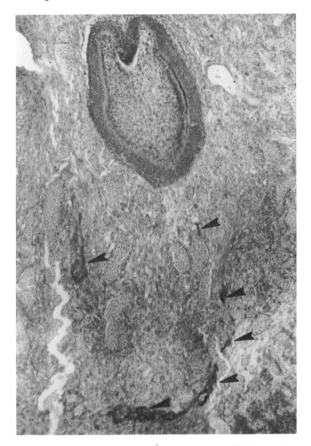

Fig. 8. Molar tooth germ from posterior two-thirds of mandible, 11 days post-conception. Note the fragments of bone which formed part of a cylinder as a socketlike structure (*arrows*) below the early molar tooth germ. Alcian blue. × 100.

change to become incisiform within 6 days of culture is remarkable in view of the general retardation of development that is normally associated with such surgical interference.

In view of Kollar and Baird's contribution to this symposium, it is also desirable that the problem of tooth germ identification in this growth site be more closely analyzed and that some form of reconstructive technique be used to determine their morphology more precisely.

It is evident that as dental development proceeds the tissues are less effected by the experimental procedures; but with earlier development, first the rate of growth and then the morphology is disturbed. The earliest ages which have been fully investigated, 10 days post-conception, appear to be an intermediate stage

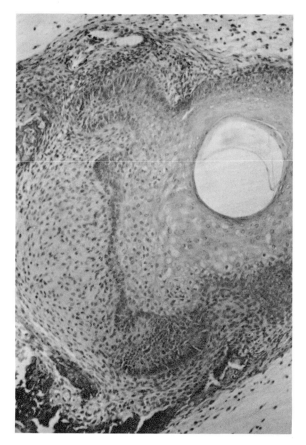

Fig. 9. Molariform tooth germ from posterior fragment of mandible of 10-day post-conception embryo grown for 1 wk in elder sibling. Hematoxylin and eosin. × 100.

in the determination of the dental morphogenic fields in the mandible of the mouse.

It has been suggested that some form of xenograft rejection phenomenon can be observed in this type of investigation using the CAM. Although several theoretical considerations make this unlikely (Ellison, personal communication) and further experiments are planned to investigate this phenomenon, it may well occur. It is conceivable that the phenomenon is also related more directly to tissue damage.

Many of the developing whiskers appeared to be pigmented when they occurred. Since pigment cells are derived from the neural crest, it will be interesting in subsequent experiments to compare the rate of migration of pigment cells in the head region and the rate of development of the morphogenic fields as described in this paper.

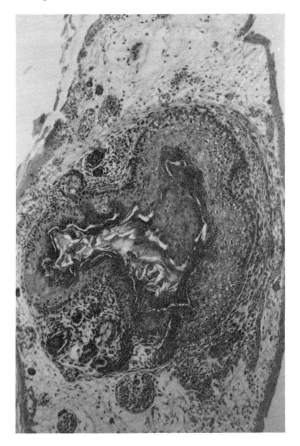

Fig. 10. Combination of 10-day post-conception molar mesoderm and incisal ectoderm. No morphology is discernable, though there is an inflammatory cell response to the graft. Hematoxylin and eosin. × 80.

Conclusion

Mouse embryos, 9–13 days post-conception as judged by vaginal plug following the use of the Whitton separation phenomenon in female mice, were removed from the gravid uterus, and the presumptive mandibular molar and incisor tooth-bearing areas were dissected out. These were separated into their mesodermal and ectodermal components by the chemoseparation technique of immersion in buffered trypsin solution at approximately 4° C.

Combinations of molar mesoderm and incisor ectoderm or of molar ectoderm with incisor ectoderm, or the correct tissue combination, were implanted onto the chick chorioallantois (CAM) for up to 13 days. Mesoderm and ectoderm were also implanted alone. Undissected presumptive tooth areas were also

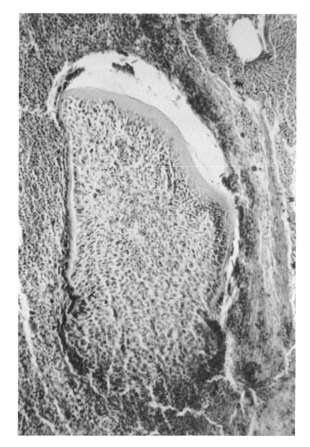

Fig. 11. Incisor tooth germ in transverse section from 13-day post-conception donor. Hematoxylin and eosin. × 100.

implanted whole onto the CAM, and a few were implanted into the subcutaneous tissues of the neck of elder siblings of the same mating.

The morphogenic field, as defined by Butler (1939), for the molars was apparently determined by 10 days post-conception and for the incisors by 10½ days. From this time on the ectodermal component of the recombinations determined tooth type. The results from younger material are equivocal.

ACKNOWLEDGMENTS

The work was supported in part by National Institutes of Health general research support grant 5–501–FR05330 to the Dental School, State University of New York at Buffalo.

REFERENCES

Butler, P. M. 1939. Studies of mammalian dentition. I. Differentiation of the post-canine dentition. *Proc. Zool. Soc. Lond. Ser. B,* 109:1–36.

Cohen, J. 1961. The transplantation of individual rat and guinea pig whisker papillae. *J. Embryol. Exp. Morph.* 9:117–27.

Davis, D. D. 1964. The giant panda: A morphological study of evolutionary mechanisms. *Fieldiana: Zoology Memoirs* 3:125–30.

Dryburg, L. C. 1967. The epigenetics of early tooth development in the mouse. *J. Dent. Res.* 46:1264 (abstr.).

Gaunt, W. A., and Miles, A. E. W. 1967. Fundamental aspects of tooth morphogenesis. In *Structural and chemical organization of teeth,* ed. A. E. W. Miles, chap. 4. New York and London: Academic Press.

Glasstone, S. 1954. The development of tooth germs on the chick chorioallantois. *J. Anat. Lond.* 70:260–66.

———. 1967. Morphodifferentiation of teeth in embryonic mandibular segments in tissue culture. *J. Dent. Res.* 46:611–14.

Hoffman, R. L. 1960. Formation of periodontal tissues around subcutaneously transplanted hamster molars. *J. Dent. Res.* 39:781.

Horstadius, S. 1950. *The neural crest.* London and New York: Oxford University Press.

Koch. W. E. 1967. *In vitro* differentiation of tooth rudiments of embryonic mice. I. Transfilter interaction of embryonic incisor tissues. *J. Exp. Zool.* 165:155–70.

Kollar, E. J., and Baird, G. R. 1968. Effect of beta-2-thienylalanine on developing mouse tooth germs in vitro. *J. Dent. Res.* 47:433–43.

Lison, L. 1957. In *Handbook of histopathological technique,* ed. C. F. A. Culling, p. 234. London: Butterworth and Company.

McLoughlin, C. B. 1961. The importance of mesenchymal factors in the differentiation of the chick epidermis. II. Modification of epidermal differentiation by contact with different types of mesenchyme. *J. Embryol. Exp. Morph.* 9:385–409.

Miller, W. A. 1964. Experimental explanation of the dental lamina in mice: Preliminary report. *J. Dent. Res.* 43:969 (abstr.).

———. 1968. Inductive changes in early tooth development. I. A study of mouse tooth development on the chick chorio-allantois. Paper read at fourth International Conference on Oral Biology, 1968.

Pourtois, M. 1961. Contribution a l'étude des bourgeons dentaires chez la souris. I. Periodes d'induction et de morphodifferenciation. *Arch. Biol. Liège.* 72:17–95.

———. 1964. Comportement en culture *in vitro* des ébauches dentaires de rongeurs prélevées aux stades de prédifférenciation. *J. Embryol. Exp. Morph.* 12:391–405.

Rawles, M. E. 1963. Tissue interactions in scale and feather development as studied in dermal-epidermal recombinations. *J. Embryol. Exp. Morph.* 11:765–89.

Sellman, S. 1946. Some experiments on the determination of the larval teeth in *Ambystoma mexicanum*. *Odont. Tidskr.* 54:1–128.

Sengel, P.H. 1957. Analyse expérimentale du dévelopement *in vitro* des germes de l'embryon de poulet. *Experimentia* 13:177–82.

Slavkin, H. C., and Bavetta, L. A., 1968a. Odontogenesis: *In vivo* and xenografts on chick chorioallantois. *Arch. Oral Biol.* 13:145–54.

———. 1968b. Organogenesis: Prolonged differentiation and growth of tooth primordia on the chick chorioallantoic membrane. *Experimentia* 24:192–94.

Slavkin, H. C.; Beierl, J.; and Bavetta, L. A. 1968. Odontogenesis: Cell-cell interactions in vitro. *Nature (Lond.)* 217:268–70.

Wessells, N. K., and Roessener, K. D. 1965. Nonproliferation in dermal condensations of mouse vibrissae and pelage hairs. *Dev. Biol.* 12:419–33.

Whitton, W. K. 1959. Occurrence of anoestrus in mice caged in groups. *J. Endocrinol.* 18:102–7.

4   The Role of Mesenchyme in Tooth Development

C. H. Tonge   *Department of Oral Anatomy, Dental School,
University of Newcastle upon Tyne, England*

Mesenchyme has a widespread role throughout the life history of tooth development and is associated with it to a varying degree in the different phases of the evolution of teeth. The source of the mesenchyme is, perhaps, the most controversial field, and its formative role in the production of dentin, pulp, and to a lesser extent, the periodontal ligament and cementum, is the most studied. Apart from this formative role, mesenchyme must also be considered to have an inductive, limiting, attachment, and reparative function in terms of the tooth. An interaction between epithelium and mesenchyme in the earlier stages of tooth induction leads to the formation of a dental papilla, and the independent status and separate identity of the tooth from the other developing structures in the oral cavity is in large measure due to the formation of the dental follicle, which is primarily a limiting capsule around the base of the dental papilla and found to extend around the tooth bud (Tonge 1967).

The mechanisms whereby specialized structures, including teeth, develop from the fertilized ovum depend upon the processes of cytodifferentiation and tissue organization, both of which are themselves the result of an inductive interaction between specific cell components or between different kinds of cells. The neural crest in different vertebrate classes shows constancy not only in its massiveness but also in the ubiquity and variety of tissues derived from it (Newth 1951). The neural crest develops from ridges at the two edges of the neural plate, the main bulk of which forms the neural tube. It is generally accepted that the ectodermal role of producing pigment cells and parts of the spinal ganglia and cranial nerve complex is reinforced by ectomesenchyme, which is more extensive in the head region than in the trunk. This ectomesenchyme not only contributes to spinal and cranial ganglia but, more significantly in amphibia, to many parts of the cartilaginous splanchnocranium and the anterior part of the trabeculae cranii (Horstadius and Sellman 1942), although this is not so in the lamprey (Newth 1951). In the amblystoma, neural crest cells were concerned in the formation of odontoblasts in addition to visceral cartilages (de Beer 1947), and the precise location of the source of the ectomesenchyme involved in tooth formation was determined by experimental extirpation and vital staining (Sellman 1946).

With regard to the source and utilization of mesenchyme in tooth development, certainly in Amphibia the role of ectomesenchyme derived from neural crest tissue has considerable support. The neural crest has been identified histochemically by its intense RNA richness and is considered to be directly concerned in inducing tooth germ formation (Pourtois 1964). More recently (Chibon 1967), through removals, grafts, and nuclear labeling of embryonic cells with tritiated thymidine in amphibians, a specific region of the neural crest has been shown to be concerned with tooth development, thus identifying a sequence in which the cells of the dental papilla and the odontoblasts derived from the neural crest later influence the formation of the enamel organ. In Mammalia, more limited evidence of tracts of ectomesenchyme in the pharyngeal region exists (Halley 1955). But the neural crest is not the only possible source of mesoderm for the head; the prechordal plate (Waddington 1956) and the notochordal derivatives might be regarded as a different system which, because of a close proximity to the endoderm, might be considered as endomesenchyme. Once the inductive mechanism has proceeded to the stage of recognition of mesenchymal sheets, clusters, or condensations, the conditions have been established for the differentiation of epithelial derivatives by a variety of epitheliomesenchymal cellular interactions. Experimental evidence (McLoughlin 1961) supports this mesenchymal role in determining the differentiation of epithelial derivatives in a wide range of embryonic organs including the limb bud, feather germs, salivary gland, preen gland, and thymus. These inductions may act through many different mechanisms, but it seems likely that the mesenchymal stimulus is relatively brief for these epithelial differentiations, and therefore the formation of odontogenic epithelium has a short time scale comparable with that in the neural plate or lens. On the other hand, a wide range of experimental evidence (McLoughlin 1961a), including the capacity of epidermis to keratinize when separated from mesenchyme and its differing reaction in different transplantation situations—keratinizing normally on limb mesenchyme, degenerating in contact with cartilage, secreting mucus and becoming ciliated if placed on gizzard mesenchyme—suggests that, apart from the brief inductions, there are more prolonged epitheliomesenchymal interactions which maintain the normal growth of differentiation of tissues throughout embryonic life and possibly into adult life.

As development proceeds, the relationship of the epithelial and mesenchymal cell layers, the type of cell aggregations, and the hormonal state of the embryo are all of significance. At a later stage, relationships exist between one differentiated epithelial mesenchymal tissue and another within the oral cavity, so that the self-determination of teeth, bone, salivary gland, cartilage, and muscle proceeds without encroachment upon the others. The mesenchymal derivatives exhibit variations in the proportion of cells, fibers, and matrix, and the mesenchymal cell and its specializations like fibroblasts are predominant, together with the intercellular tissue, in the imprecise zones between formed structures.

It would seem, therefore, that if the neural crest is accorded the role of producing ectomesenchyme concerned with tooth development, this tissue should be identifiable at an early stage not only in mammals generally but also in man. Similarly, if a more deeply mesenchymal layer is considered as being associated with intraembryonic mesoderm and of notochordal origin, there should be some relationship between the ectomesenchyme and the mesenchyme at some stage in development. In teeth, this relationship might persist until the completion of formation of a tooth and its supporting structures, since odontogenic epitheliomesenchymal relationships of an essentially embryonic character occur until early adolescence in the third permanent molar teeth in man. It may be possible, by a study of the differentiation of dentin-forming cell aggregates and those cells which limit the tooth from other tissues later becoming associated with tooth attachment, to broaden the concept of the role of mesenchyme in tooth development. Such considerations would, of course, have to be compatible with the evidence of evolution.

Materials and Methods

Most of the material is human, with a parallel study of primate and mammalian specimens. The human embryonic range covers the period from 27 to 48 days ovulation age, and the further fetal and postnatal specimens cover the time to the completion of the eruption of the permanent dentition.

Observations

For man, full descriptions of embryos (Bartelmez and Dekaban 1962; Hertig and Rock 1945, 1951; Hertig, Rock, and Adams 1956) during the first 22 days have been recorded, with the following main features. A two-cell stage exists at 1½–2½ days, a twelve-cell morula at 3 days, and a blastocyst having an eight-cell embryonic area at 4–4½ days.

By 7½ days, early endoderm has formed; an ectodermal plate is present at

9½, and a full embryonic disk at 12 days. The primitive streak forms at 15 days and completes the presomite stage. The neural fold forms at 16 days, the notochord at 18 days, and the neural groove by 19 days. At 22 days, there are seven pairs of somites, the neural tubes are closing, and the optic and otic outgrowths have become visible entities.

By 27–29 days ovulation age, not only has greater differentiation of the primitive streak and neural tube derivatives taken place, but emphasis is occurring in the establishment of the primitive vascular system, the mesenchymal aggregations in areas forming the limb buds, the intermediate cell mass and the somites. The pituitary gland is forming. The shape of the branchial area is in the process of determination, and the thyroid gland is forming as the first organ arising in the oral region.

At 31–32 days ovulation age, many examples of different inductive mechanisms can be observed. An interaction is occurring between similarly derived tissues, as seen in the development of the lens in relation to the optic cup, itself a direct outgrowth of the neural tube. Many indications of differentions occurring at different time scales in different situations can be seen; the scalp is a simple epithelium with no evidence of special structural formation, whereas an identifiable odontogenic area has become established in both jaws with, as yet, no determination morphologically as to tooth type.

By 36–38 days ovulation age, the general form of the oral cavity has taken shape; the oral floor is complete with the tongue and its musculature, the submandibular gland, and Meckel's cartilage with the mylohyoid muscle is discernible. Separate areas for individual teeth are beginning to form in the incisor area and the secondary palatal shelves are developing (fig. 1).

At 46–48 days ovulation age, the palatal shelves are fusing, facial muscles are formed, individual tooth germs are identified, and salivary glands are showing branching of their duct systems. The internal dental epithelium now has beneath it a dental papilla, the cells of which are quite distinct from those of the peripheral area forming a primitive dental follicle around the tooth germ (fig. 2). This is the earliest sign of the segregation of the tooth from adjacent structures, as this inner layer of the dental follicle separates the tooth not only from the bony alveolus but also from the vestibular sulcus which is lined only by an oral type of epithelium. This relationship of the dental follicle to the developing tooth continues throughout crown formation (fig. 3), and during root development and the beginning of the periodontal ligament differentiation.

As the bony alveolus forms around the developing tooth crown, the fibrous limiting layer of its periosteum constitutes an outer layer of the dental follicle with looser tissue between the two parts of the dental follicle. Meanwhile, the dentin-forming cells of the dental papilla become morphologically preodonto-

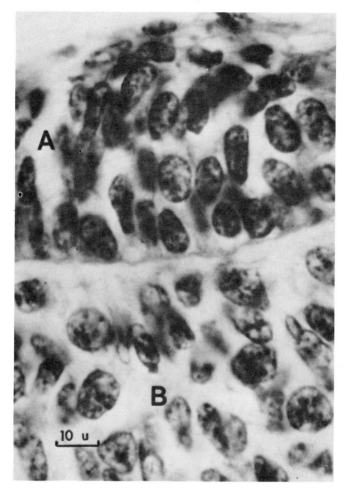

Fig. 1. The epithelial (*A*) and ectomesenchymal (*B*) area of the central incisor odontogenic region in a 15-mm crown-rump human embryo. Streeter horizon 18, 36–38 days ovulation age.

blast and pulpal in type. During the period when an active enlargement of the tooth crown is occurring, the outer layer of the dental follicle is less dense than the inner part surrounding the base of the dental papilla. As the epithelial root sheath differentiates, the space between the two layers of the dental follicle is reduced (fig. 4). Apart from collagen and reticular fibers, oxytalan fibers surround the base of the dental papilla and the cervical loop area and are a constituent part of the limiting periosteal or outer layer of the dental follicle. Previously, oxytalan fibers (Fullmer and Lillie 1958) have been observed (Beynon 1967; Goggins 1966) in relation to the periodontal ligaments of the

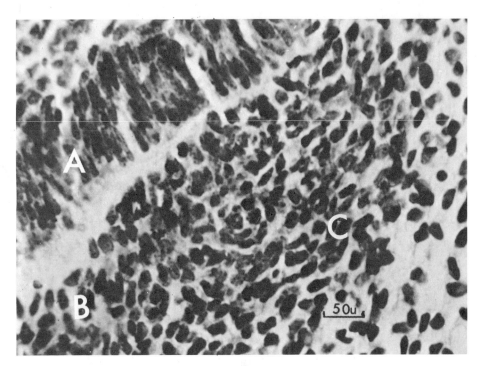

Fig. 2. The internal dental epithelium (*A*), the dental papilla (*B*), and the inner layer of the dental follicle (*C*) in a 28-mm crown-rump human embryo. Streeter horizon 23, 46–48 days ovulation age.

permanent and deciduous dentitions, as well as a general distribution to tendons, ligaments, blood vessels, and mucous connective tissues.

As root formation proceeds, the periodontal ligament forms, the limiting layer of the periosteum or outer layer of the dental follicle occupying an intermediate position owing to the growth of bone which takes place rapidly during this phase as the alveolus is modified concurrently with the eruption of the tooth (fig. 5). The mesenchymal contribution is therefore to the initial formation of the periodontal ligament on both sides of the outer layer of the dental follicle. Cementum deposition, epithelial rest formation, and the restriction of the inner layer of the dental follicle to the apical foramen occur progressively with root formation. This general attachment for the tooth is similarly arranged for mammals, primates, and man. In selachians it has basally a fibrous attachment to a continuous membrane, which lies over a cartilaginous jaw covered by a perichondrium with surface calcification. The attachment is gomphosed in

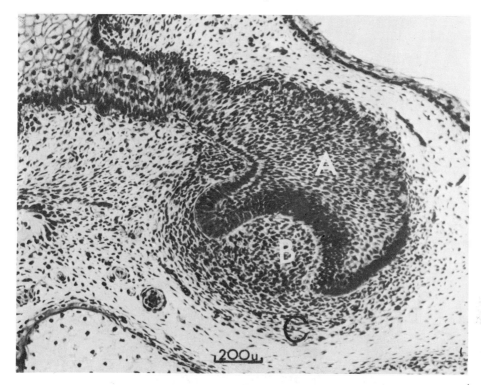

Fig. 3. The enamel organ (A), the dental papilla (B), and the inner layer of the dental follicle (C) in a human fetus of 78 days.

Pristis, Barracuda pike, and *Lepisosteus,* among others, and is hinged in the cod, hake, angler, and pike, an intervening area between the tooth and the jaw-bone being occupied by fibrous and elastic tissue or a bone of attachment or a mixture of them. In urodeles such as newts and salamander, the tooth is firmly attached to a bone of attachment at its base, forming a group classified as having an acrodont attachment. In Reptilia attachment is usually by anchylosis, forming in crocodiles the thecodont type of socket for the teeth which is used again by the successional teeth.

Discussion

Throughout the species examined, dentin is formed from mesenchyme, along with an attachment apparatus which includes different degrees of ankylosis, socket formation, bone of attachment, and cementum production. In all, however, the dentin-producing component is surrounded by, or embedded within, a fibrous membrane which is linked to the skeleton of the jaw. The general development (fig. 6) could, therefore, be considered to consist of an ecto-

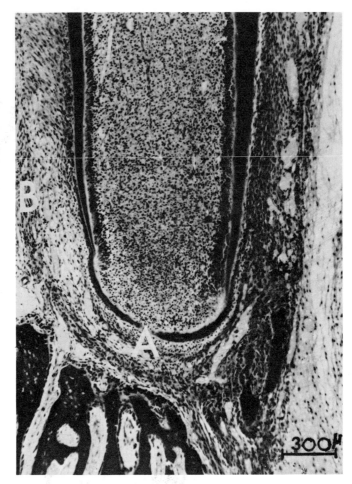

Fig. 4. The inner layer (*A*) and the outer layer (*B*) of the dental follicle in an erupting canine deciduous tooth of a cat.

dermally formed enamel organ, an ectomesenchyme of neural crest origin forming the dentin producing dental papilla, and a surrounding dental follicle which is a part of the general mesoderm of notochordal derivation. Variations in the arrangement of the latter, in the different species, account for the varieties of tooth attachment.

In an evolutionary sense, it is difficult to reconcile the hypothesis, based on paleontological data, that enamel is of mesodermal origin (Kvam 1950; Ørvig 1966) with the accepted views of mammalian and human embryologists that it is of ectodermal origin. Recently, however, the hypothesis of mesodermal enamel in fishes has been rejected (Moss 1968) on an extensive analysis of the

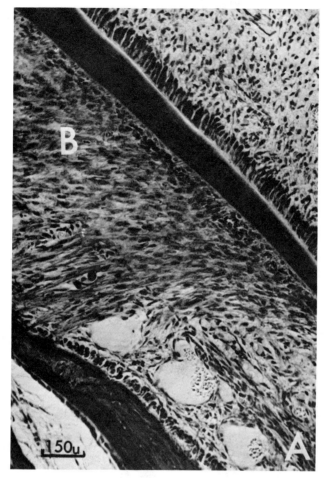

Fig. 5. The outer layer of the dental follicle (*A*), which is equivalent to the limiting layer of the periosteum and the periodontal ligament (*B*) in an erupting canine deciduous tooth of a cat.

available evidence. Whatever view is taken of the contribution of the neural crest to the mesenchyme of the head, so far as man is concerned—and the general arrangement is equally true of the mammals and primates—it occupies a restricted field which may contribute ectomesenchyme while the greater part of the mesoderm is derived from the primitive streak through the notochord and adjacent tissue (fig. 7). The concept that ectoderm, ectomesenchyme, and mesoderm are concerned with tooth formation and attachment means that there is not only an epitheliomesenchymal interaction but also an ectomesenchymal-mesodermal interaction. There certainly seems to be sufficient evidence (Glasstone 1967; Pourtois 1964) that once a specific stage in

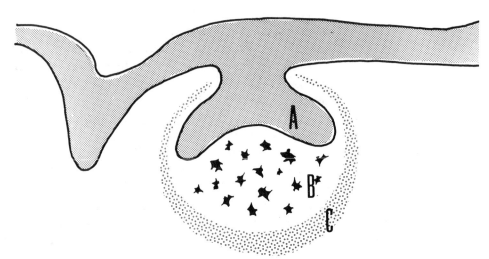

Fig. 6. Diagram showing the enamel organ (*A*), the dental papilla (*B*), and the inner layer of the dental follicle (*C*). *A* is ectoderm, *B* is ectomesenchyme, and *C* is mesoderm.

embryonic differentiation has been reached, whereby the potential epithelio-mesenchymal interaction has the capacity for permanence and progressive development, a tooth will form provided that its component layers remain in contact. The establishment of an identifiable odontogenic area results from an inductive effect of the ectomesenchyme on the epithelium. Evidence (Ørvig 1966) that tooth germ development fails to progress when the inhibitor effect of beta-2-thienylalanine upsets the inductive interaction between the epithelium and the mesenchyme points conclusively to the importance of the ectomesenchyme.

If the neural crest gives rise to ectomesenchyme which becomes closely related to the surface ectoderm, it appears possible that some similarity might be noted in the behavior of the ectomesenchyme in skin and tooth areas. Certainly the similarity of formation and reaction to suppressors in beta-2-thienyl-alanine studies of tooth germs (Kollar 1966) and vibrissae (Kollar 1966, 1968) supports this view. It also strengthens the phylogenetic link of skin and its appendages, including the teeth, and it is worth noting a further similarity in the suggestion that tooth transplantation may fail because teeth possess the same graft antigens as skin (Shulman 1964).

Now, what of the junction between ectomesenchyme and mesenchyme? It has been shown in Amphibia (Chibon 1967) that ectomesenchyme gives rise to the formation of the odontoblasts and therefore contributes to dentin. It need not give rise to the entire dentin. There are differences between mantle dentin and circumpulpal dentin, and the pulpal cells are very different from odonto-

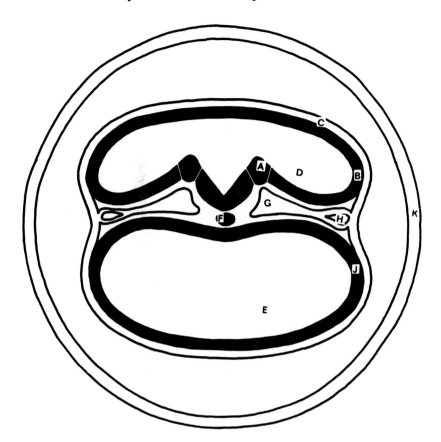

Fig. 7. Diagram showing the neural crest (*A*), ectoderm (*B*), mesoderm (*C*), amniotic cavity (*D*), yolk sac (*E*), notochord (*F*), paraxial mesoderm (*G*), intraembryonic mesoderm (*H*), endoderm (*J*), and chorion (*K*).

blasts. It is possible, therefore, that whereas odontoblasts are of ectomesenchymal origin, pulpal cells may belong to the interactive zone between ectomesenchyme and mesoderm, the inner layer of the dental follicle forming from mesoderm. The two parts of the dental follicle, one near the tooth, the other linked with the alveolus, and the loose tissue between them constitute the mesodermally derived mechanism producing cementum and bone as variants of the calcified tissues, with calcified cartilage and bone of attachment as well as collagen, reticular fibers, and elastic and oxytalan fibers present in the different species. It would not be justified to make too fine a point of possible interfaces, but it seems significant that there is a surface lining of acellular cementum upon teeth, and it might be that cellular cementum, possibly a later structure in evolution, is more linked to bone because it is laid down after the outer layer of the dental follicle (Tonge 1963), which is the limiting layer of the periosteum (figs. 4, 5), is obliterated as the periodontal ligament develops. This limiting layer of the periosteum may act as a barrier to a bone-cementum ankylosis until the orderly formation of epithelial rests and the establishment of the periodontal ligament. This is supported by the demonstration of hard-tissue ankylosis around a retained deciduous tooth, the roots of which have not undergone resorption.

In conclusion, there is some evidence, although incomplete, that the mammalian primate and human tooth has an ectomesenchymal component of neural crest origin, acting as an inductor and source of odontoblasts. The deeper layer is an interface forming the pulp, and the tissues around the base of the dental papilla, in which collagen and oxytalan fibers are demonstrable, are developed in mesoderm. The mesodermal derivatives between tooth and bone are also stratified, giving a species choice of attachment. There is a generalized delamination of these ectomesenchymal and mesodermal layers in man giving a complex of fiber systems and calcified tissue formations of dentin, bone, and cementum which bears many similarities to that postulated in relation to the dermal skeleton of fish (Holmgren 1940).

Growth and development of calcified tissues are dependent upon a hormonal system. In man between 23 and 27 days ovulation age, the pituitary, thyroid, parathyroid, and thymic glands have started to develop, and it is relevant to refer to the ultimobranchial bodies. These are present in the skink, pigeon, and chicken; they are endocrine glands producing calcitonin and are represented in mammals by the C cells of the thyroid.

Current evidence (MacIntyre 1967; Raisz and Hiemann 1967) supports the view that calcitonin is concerned in activities where large transfers of calcium take place. Since the tooth, even more than bone, is associated with calcium metabolism, the apparent lateness in embryological terms in commencing tooth development and its relatively long period of cellular interaction before morphodifferentiation may result from its dependence upon the adequate development of the hormonal system.

ACKNOWLEDGMENTS
The author thanks Mr. B. Hesselgrave for preparing the illustrations and Miss L. Noble-Nesbitt for secretarial assistance.

REFERENCES
Bartelmez, G. W., and Dekaban, A. S. 1962. The early development of the human brain. *Contrib. Embryol. Carneg. Inst.* 37:13–32.
Beer, G. R. de. 1947. The differentiation of neural crest cells into visceral cartilage

and odontoblasts in Amblystoma and a re-examination of the germ-layer theory. *Proc. Roy. Soc., Ser. B*134:377–98.

Beynon, A. D. 1967. Oxytalan fibers in the developing mouse molar. *J. Dent. Res.* 46:1272–73.

Chibon, P. 1967. Etude expérimentale par ablations, greffes et autoradiographie, de l'origine des dents chez l'amphibien urodele pleurodeles waltlii michah. *Arch. Oral. Biol.* 12:745–53.

Fullmer, H. M., and Lillie, R. D. 1958. The oxytalan fiber: A previously unde-scribed connective tissue fiber. *J. Histochem. Cytochem.* 6:425–30.

Glasstone, S. 1967. Morphodifferentiation of teeth in embryonic mandibular seg-ments in tissue culture. *J. Dent. Res.* 46:611–14.

Goggins, J. F. 1966. The distribution of oxytalan connective tissue fibers in perio-dontal ligaments of deciduous teeth. *Periodontics* 4:182–86.

Halley, G. 1955. The placodal relations of the neural crest in the domestic cat. *J. Anat., Lond.* 89:133–52.

Hertig, A. T., and Rock, J. 1945. Two human ova of the pre-villous stage, having an ovulation age of about seven and nine days respectively. *Contrib. Embryol. Carneg. Inst.* 31:65–84.

———. 1951. Implantation and early development of human ovum. *Amer. J. Obst. Gynec.* (suppl.) 61A:8–14.

Hertig, A. T.; Rock, J.; and Adams, E. C. 1956. A description of 34 human ova within the first 17 days of development. *Amer. J. Anat.* 98: 435–93.

Holmgren, N. 1940. Studies on the head in fishes. *Acta Zool. (Stockholm)* 21:51–267.

Horstadius, S., and Sellman, S. 1942. Experimental studies on the determination of the chondrocranium in Amblystoma mexicanum. *Arch. Zool.* 33A (no. 13); 1–8.

Kollar, E. J. 1966. An in vitro study of hair and vibrissae development in embryonic mouse skin. *J. Invest. Derm.* 46:254–62.

———. 1968. The inhibition of vibrissae development in vitro by beta-2-thienyl-alanine. *J. Invest. Derm.* 50:319–22.

Kollar, E. J., and Baird, G. R. 1968. Effect of beta-2-thienylalanine on developing mouse tooth germs in vitro. *J. Dent. Res.* 47:433–43.

Kvam, T. 1950. The development of mesodermal enamel on piscine teeth. *Kgl. Norske Videnskab. Selskabs Forh.* 23:1–115.

MacIntyre, I. 1967. Calcitonin: A general review. *Calc. Tiss. Res.* 1:173–82.

Mcloughlin, C. B. 1961a. The importance of mesenchymal factors in the differentia-tion of chick epidermis. I. The differentiation in culture of the isolated epidermis of the embryonic chick and its response to excess vitamin A. *J. Embryol. Exp. Morph.* 9:370–84.

———. 1961b. The importance of mesenchymal factors in the differentiation of chick epidermis. II. Modification of epidermal differentiation by contact with different types of mesenchyme. *J. Embryol. Exp. Morph.* 9:385–409.

Moss, M. L. 1968. Bone, dentin, and enamel and the evolution of vertebrates. In *Biology of the mouth,* publ. no. 89, Amer. Ass. Adv. Sci., pp. 37–65.

Newth, D. R. 1951. Experiments on the neural crest of the lamprey embryo. *J. Exp. Biol.* 28:247–60.

Ørvig, T. 1966. Phylogeny of tooth tissue: Evolution of some calcified tissue in early vertebrates. In *Structural and chemical organization of teeth,* ed. E. A. W. Miles, 1:45–110. New York: Academic Press.

Pourtois, M. 1964. Comportement en culture in vitro des ébauches dentaires de rongeurs prelevées aux stades de prédifférentiation. *J. Embryol. Exp. Morph.* 12:391–405.

Raisz, L. G., and Hiemann, I. 1967. Early effects of parathyroid hormone and thyrocalcitonin on bone in organ culture. *Nature* 214:486–87.

Sellman, S. 1946. Some experiments on the determination of the larval teeth in Amblystoma mexicanum. *Odont. Tidskr.* 54:1–128.

Shulman, L. B. 1964. Transplantation antigenicity of tooth homografts. *Oral Surg.* 17:389–94.

Tonge, C. H. 1963. The development and arrangement of the dental follicle. *Trans. Eur. Orth. Soc.* 39:1–9.

———. 1967. Identification of cell patterns in human tooth differentiation. *J. Dent. Res.* 46:876–78.

Waddington, C. H. 1956. *Principles of embryology.* London: Allen and Unwin.

5   Relative Rates of Weight Gain in Human Deciduous Teeth

M. V. Stack   *Medical Research Council, Dental Unit, Dental School, University of Bristol, England*

Simple mathematical relationships between ages of developing deciduous teeth and their dimensions and weights have been described (Stack 1967). It has been shown empirically that the correlation coefficient is greatest when ages are compared with square roots of mineralized tissue weights (Stack 1964). In this case significant curvilinear regression was not demonstrable, and a set of linear equations could therefore be derived in order to define rates of gain in weight of all types of deciduous teeth during the period of optimum growth. Such equations suggest threshold ages at which tooth weight first becomes significant, as well as allowing a comparison of growth rates and their variances. The deciduous second molar and permanent first molar have already been compared in these respects (Stack 1968).

The same procedure has now been applied to all dissected teeth from thirty selected deciduous dentitions (fetal age range 28–42 wk). These formed a group characterized by failure to survive birth because of some acute condition of short duration. No dentition was included if the cause of death suggested that growth might have been retarded.

A relative growth relationship between W, the weight of a tooth pair, and $(T - T_o)$, the dental age (chronological age less threshold age), may be expressed in the form

$$dw/W = 2dT/(T - T_o), \text{ accepting that } \sqrt{W} = K(T - T_o).$$

An estimate of tooth weight at a given age thus depends not only upon an estimate of the slope of the regression line but also upon an estimate of $(T - T_o)$. Maximum-likelihood estimates, assuming a log-normal distribution, may then

59

be obtained (Angleton and Pettus, 1966) by trials of a sequence of values for T_o in order to arrive at a minimum value for the sum of squares of

$$ln \sqrt{W} - ln\ K - ln\ (T - T_o),$$

where $\sqrt{W}$ and T here represent each pair of values of the variables.

Values for K, T_o, and the sum of squares are most conveniently obtained by electronic computation in which one of the program statements provides for the incorporation of the weight data in the square root form. A statistical program in Fortran II for performing such estimates with an IBM 1620 computer has been developed by Angleton and Pettus (1966) and tested by them on the problem of defining the dependence of total egg mass on body length in frogs. This program appeared suitable for the present problem since it included a means of estimating threshold age for initiation of mineralization with reference to chronological age.

Dry mineralized tissue weights (in milligrams) of all teeth were listed for the thirty dentitions, arranged approximately in order of fetal age, as derived from expected dates of birth at a fetal age of 280 days according to the clinical records. The data were distributed equitably among three groups (mean ages 33–35 wk). This grouping allowed estimates of the standard error of K, the growth rate constant, for each type of tooth, and suggested whether the various rates were significantly different. It was observed that the values for K were 30 times their standard errors. The standard deviation of the square root of the summed variance ($= 20$) per unit slope (K) for the thirty sets of values for $\sqrt{W}$ was as low as 1, one-half of the variance of this variance in relation to slope being contributed by the upper lateral incisor.

A typical equation representing a mean growth rate and mean intercept is $\sqrt{W} = 0.45T - 10$. For $T = 40$ wk (full-term birth), the weight of such a tooth pair is thus $(18 - 10)^2 = 64$ mg. Values for the growth rate constants varied between 0.35 and 0.56 (Table 1). Most of the calculated threshold ages fell within the sixth month of fetal life. For the ten types of deciduous teeth only three growth rates were found to be significantly different. Growth rates of canines and lower incisors were less rapid than those of upper incisors and second molars; the most rapid growth was evident in first molars. Statistically, growth of lower lateral incisors could be said to be significantly faster than the rates for lower central incisors and for upper and lower canines only if these three types were considered together as a group.

Growth rates of upper incisors were one-third faster than those of the corresponding lower incisors, but growth rates of the upper teeth of the remaining types were not significantly different from those of the corresponding teeth in the lower jaw.

Angleton and Pettus (1966) pointed out the disadvantage of having to test their growth model on a system where the variance was rather large. The present application allows tests on ten related sets of data having considerably smaller variance. The corresponding standard deviations fell within a narrow range when related to growth rates. More confidence may be placed in these two types of estimates than in the estimates of threshold ages, where the calculations imply a process to which the growth rate constant applies at the threshold age. However, the initial growth rate is more nearly represented by $1/\sqrt{2}$ times the overall rate, since mineralization begins first in the dentin, and increases in weight of dentin and enamel are seen to run parallel (Kraus 1959) in the weight range 5–25 mg.

In order to attribute meaning to the calculated threshold ages, those for molars were compared with chronologies for initial mineralization of these teeth, as given by Kraus and Jordan (1965). There was a mean difference of 1 wk between the calculated ages and the mean ages at which the second and third cusps first showed mineralization (Table 2). Threshold ages thus appear to be representative of age ranges during which mineralization begins in the several cusps. Threshold ages for central incisors may be compared with plots of mesiodistal diameters against age (fig. 3 of Kraus 1959). The calculated threshold age of 19 wk for these teeth matches the age at which the mesiodistal width is no longer increasing rapidly.

TABLE 1

GROWTH RATES AND THRESHOLD AGES OF FETAL DECIDUOUS TEETH

Estimate[a]		Central Incisor	Lateral Incisor	Canine	First Molar	Second Molar
Maxilla	$K (\times 100)$	50	49	35	56	49
	T_0 (wk)	19	23	25	22	24
	$\sqrt{V}/Kn (\times 100)$	67	60	68	69	68
Mandible	$K (\times 100)$	36	38	35	56	51
	T_0 (wk)	19	23	25	24	25
	$\sqrt{V}/Kn (\times 100)$	66	65	66	66	67

[a] From $\sqrt{W} = K(T - T_0)$. The value $\sqrt{V}/Kn$ gives the mean square root of the difference between the sum of tooth weights and the mean square of the sum of square roots of tooth weights, divided by the growth rate.

ACKNOWLEDGMENTS

The author thanks Dr. George Angleton, associate professor at the University of Colorado, for providing the Fortran II program, and Miss Christine Faithfull, University of Bristol Computer Unit, for processing the data through the IBM 1620 computer.

TABLE 2

CALCULATED THRESHOLD AGES FOR MOLARS IN RELATION TO OBSERVED
MEAN AGES FOR INITIAL MINERALIZATION OF SECOND AND THIRD CUSPS

Tooth		Mean Fetal Ages (wk)			
		Calculated[a]		Observed[b]	
		From $K, T, \sqrt{W}$	Kraus and Jordan (1965)	Nomata (1964)	Turner (1963)
		N = 30	N = 314	N = 117	N = 35
First	Upper	22	20½	21½	20½
molar	Lower	24	23½	20½	21
Second	Upper	24	25½	24	24
Molar	Lower	25	24½	23	22

[a] As table 1.
[b] Table 5, Kraus and Jordan 1965.

REFERENCES

Angleton, G. M., and Pettus, D. 1966. Relative growth law with a threshold. *Perspect. Biol. Med.* 9:421–24.

Kraus, B. S. 1959. Differential calcification rates in the human primary dentition. *Arch. Oral Biol.* 1:133–44.

Kraus, B. S., and Jordan, R. E. 1965. *The human dentition before birth.* London: Kimpton.

Stack, M. V. 1964. A gravimetric study of crown growth rate of the human deciduous dentition. *Biol. Neonat.* 6:197–224.

———. 1967. Vertical growth rates of the deciduous teeth. *J. Dent. Res.* 46:879–82.

———. 1968. Relative growth of the deciduous second molar and permanent first molar. *J. Dent. Res.* 47:1013–14.

Part II

Phylogeny

6 An Introduction to the Phylogeny of Calcified Tissues

D. F. G. Poole   *Medical Research Council Dental Unit,*
Dental School, University of Bristol, England

Because of their importance in medicine, general biology, and paleonotology, calcified tissues have excited the interest of research workers to such an extent that it is now a formidable task to summarize the present state of knowledge in this field. However, as is shown by recent reviews (Ørvig 1967; Moss 1968), there exists a whole range of problems concerning the structure of bones and teeth. If this introduction does no more than draw attention to some of the more important issues, it will perhaps have served a useful purpose.

In considering the phylogeny of calcified tissues, bearing in mind the various disciplines involved, a difficulty arises at the very beginning over the question of definitions. Thus, the dental tissues of mammals, especially those of man, about which most is known, are relatively discrete and easy to define. But as we go back in time to consider tissues in older vertebrates, distinctions often become blurred and definitions less appropriate.

In mammals the tooth crown is covered by *enamel,* which is a highly calcified tissue, protective in function and produced by an epithelial dental organ. It is different in composition, structure, and origin from the next three tissues and will be considered in detail later. The root of a tooth, as well as the internal mass of the crown, consists of *dentin,* which is a calcified collagen of meso-dermal origin. Running from the outer contour of the dentin inward toward the single pulp cavity are parallel dentinal tubules, each housing the process of an odontoblast cell. Odontoblasts lay down dentin but their cell bodies are never enclosed in the calcified tissue. The root of the tooth is covered by another calcified collagen which is cell free, is associated with the suspension of the

65

tooth in its alveolus, and is known as primary *cementum*.[1] Suspensory fibers run from the cementum into the alveolar *bone*, yet another calcified collagen containing vascular channels around which are concentric layers of hard tissue. Osteoblasts, which produce bone, are finally enclosed in the tissue as osteocytes. Bone dentin and cementum are similar in chemical composition and, when a tooth with its surrounding bone is decalcified, all three tissues stain similarly. Thus we have three tissues easily distinguished histologically but fundamentally similar in composition.

In the dermal armor of early vertebrates the presence of bone is readily established because of the existence of osteons (Haversian systems). This bone (fig. 1), like recent bone, shows in polarized light a well-marked pattern of dark crosses superimposed on the transverse sections of the osteons, reflecting the concentric arrangement of structural elements within the laminae surrounding the vascular channels. Figure 2 shows the principal tissues of the tooth of a fossil elasmobranch and of the dermal armor of an osteostracan, also in polarized light. The similarity to bone is immediately apparent and, in fact, the arrangement of submicroscopic elements is essentially the same. Yet in the last two examples, the tissue illustrated is dentin, and because of its superficial resemblance to bone it has long been referred to as *osteodentin* and the vascular channels with associated laminae are now known as denteons (Ørvig 1967). The distinction between osteodentin and bone still rests on the one diagnostic feature referred to above, that bone contains whole cells enclosed within it, dentin enclosed cell processes only.

This brief description of bone and dentin is sufficient to suggest a close phylogenetic relationship between the two, and several questions come to mind: for example, Did one of these two tissues precede the other? and What is the nature of the earliest type of calcified tissue?

What is believed to be the most primitive form of dentin occurs in the dermal armor of Upper Silurian Osteostraci such as *Tremataspis* and *Dartmuthia* (fig. 3). Here we can identify a central tissue with osteocyte-like cavities, which may confidently be described as bone, and an outer tissue which is different. According to Ørvig (1967), from whose detailed work these illustrations are taken, the cell spaces in the outer tissue differ from odontoblast processes in having a number of canaliculi-like projections as well as a main elongated process. At the same time, they cannot be regarded as typical osteocytes. Therefore, it is proposed that we are concerned with a cell intermediate between the osteoblast and the odontoblast and that this primitive dentin should be called

[1] Secondary cementum, which forms around the tooth root during function, contains cells and bears a stronger resemblance to bone. Neither this tissue nor coronal cementum, which occurs in rodents and ungulates, is considered here.

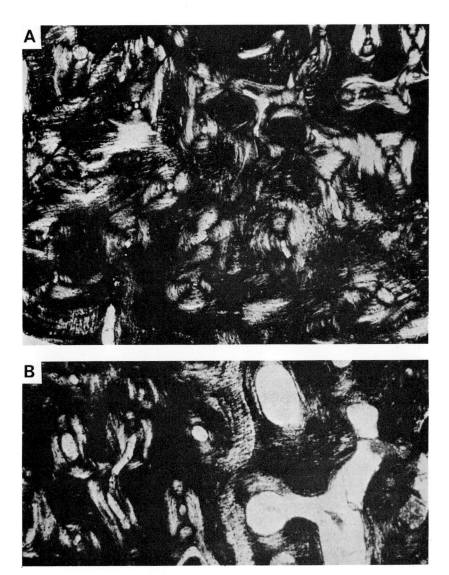

Fig. 1. (*a*) Section of bone with Haversian systems (osteons). The dark crosses are due to the circular arrangement of structural elements (collagen fibres and mineral crystallites in living bone) in the laminae surrounding the vascular channels. Polarizing microscope, × 65.

(*b*) Similar section showing osteons on the left and trabecular tissue without osteons on the right. Polarizing microscope, × 65.

Both preparations are from the dermal skeleton of a coccosteomorph arthrodire (*Plourdosteus*). From Ørvig 1967.

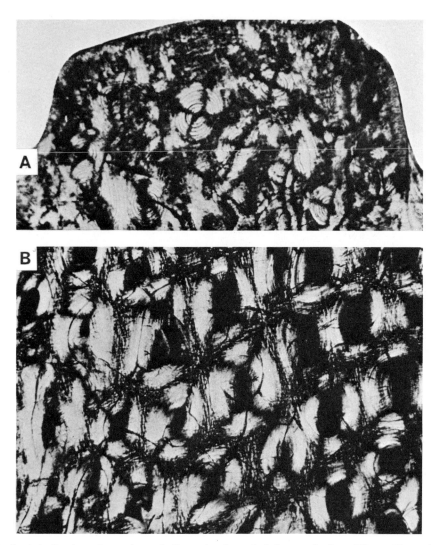

Fig. 2. (*a*) Section of an odontode from the dermal skeleton of a late (Upper Devonian) osteostracan (*Alaspis*). Polarizing microscope, × 200.

(*b*) Section of osteodentin from the tooth of a Tertiary ray. Polarizing microscope, × 65.

The appearance between crossed polars of these two examples of dentin demonstrates the similarity between denteons and the osteons of bone. From Ørvig 1967.

mesodentin. Ørvig (1967) further suggests that the term scleroblast should be used for a basic type of connective tissue cell related to the fibroblast which became hard tissue producing and gave rise, phylogenetically, to both the osteoblast and the odontoblast.

In later Osteostraci a tendency is seen in the dermal armor toward a reduc-

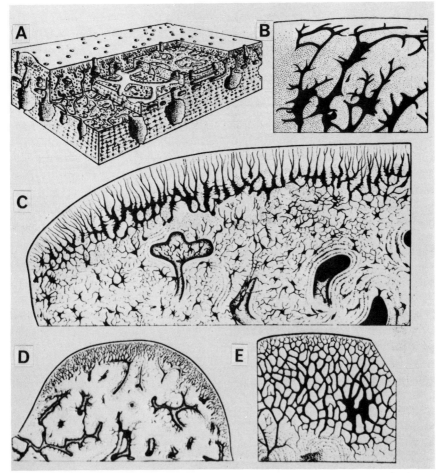

Fig. 3. Mesodentin in the Osteostraci: (*a*) Dermal armor of a Silurian form *Tremataspis* (redrawn from Denison 1947).

(*b*) Mesodentin from an odontode of *Tremataspis* (modified from Denison 1947). × 200.

(*c*) Section of an odontode from another Silurian form, *Dartmuthia*, consisting of an outer pallial mesodentin and an inner bone tissue. × 320.

(*d*) Section of an odontode from an Upper Devonian form, *Alaspis*, consisting of outer pallial mesodentin and inner osteomesodentin. × 150.

(*e*) Detail of the pallial mesodentin of *Alaspis*. × 450. From Ørvig 1967.

tion in the number of enclosed cell spaces, and in some cases the tissue is essentially cell free. Apparently the same tendency is seen in other lines, for example, some acanthodian fishes (*Climatius* and its allies), Jurassic ray-finned fishes and in some modern teleosts (Ørvig 1967; see also Moss 1968). Moreover, in members of the Gadidae, the teeth are composed of a kind of dentin lacking tubules (*vasodentin*, see below). Evidence such as this has led Ørvig to conclude that mesodentin is the most primitive type of dental tissue and is probably derived from primitive bone. In bone and dentin, cell-containing or cell-process-containing tissue is often succeeded phylogenetically by acellular tissue, and the earliest form of calcified tissue is most likely to have been of a cellular nature.

Various authors in the past have taken a different view and have suggested that the basic type of calcified tissue was acellular (Tarlo 1964). Perhaps it is true that the simplest conceivable situation is a bundle of calcified collagen fibers lacking cells, and even in mammals collagen frequently calcifies with age as, for example, in rat tail tendon. In thinking of cell-free, calcified collagens, attention turns again to the primary cementum covering the roots of mammalian, and at least some reptilian, teeth. In fact in modern vertebrates generally teeth are attached to jaws by collagen fibers which are usually, but not always, calcified, suggesting that when support is required the mesoderm has the capacity to produce a cell-free, cementum-like substance to serve this function. Is it possible that this potential of the connective tissue is the same one that gave rise to the basic type of calcified tissue? In this same context, the calcified tissue known as aspidin, which occurs in the Heterostraci, has been the center of its own controversy. Aspidin, like bone, possesses vascular channels surrounded by concentric laminae but, unlike bone, it lacks osteocyte spaces. It is therefore (Ørvig 1967) regarded as a cell-free tissue derived from bone. However, aspidin does possess randomly arranged, spindle-shaped structures regarded by some (e.g. Gross 1935) as spaces originally occupied by thick collagen bundles rather like the Sharpey's fibers in the cementum of higher vertebrates. Tarlo (1964) points out that Sharpey's fibers are associated with the anchoring mechanism of tooth to bone, which is not the case in aspidin. Tarlo prefers to believe that the elongated spaces are the sites of cells (aspidinoblasts) which originally produced the aspidin and that they should be called aspidinocytes. It is also suggested that aspidin is a primitive type of bone or at least a precursor of that tissue, a view which is disputed by Ørvig (1967).

In the dermal armor of the later, arthrodiran fishes, another type of dentinous tissue occurs, containing cells more like odontoblasts but still completely enclosed (fig. 4). Ørvig (1967) uses the term *semidentin* for this tissue and suggests that, phylogenetically, mesodentin was succeeded by semidentin; in turn semidentin was succeeded by true dentin (*metadentin*). Structurally, the relationship between these types of dentin supports this hypothesis, although the evidence that this sequence did in fact occur is not complete. Furthermore, it has been proposed that metadentin possibly exists even in the dermal armor of some of the oldest known vertebrates (Ørvig 1951; Denison 1963). There must, therefore, be some doubt whether, at the moment, the various forms of dentinous tissues can be arranged in any true phylogenetic sequence or whether,

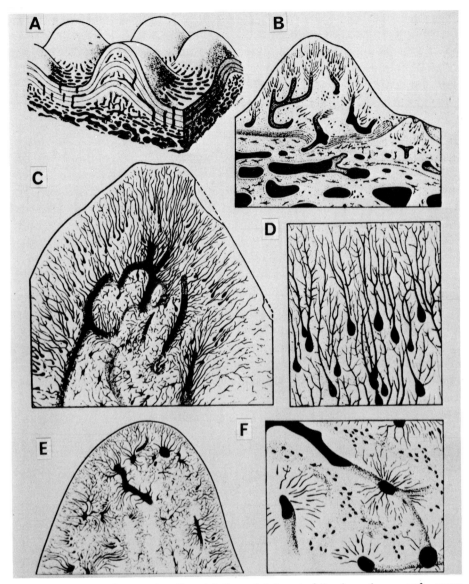

Fig. 4. Semidentin of the Arthrodira: (*a*) Superficial part of the dermal armor of a coccosteomorph, *Plourdosteus,* showing three generations of vestigially developed semidentin
odontodes.

    (*b*) Section of an odontode from the Lower Devonian *Phlyctaenaspis.* × 50.
    (*c*) Section of a tooth from a dermal jaw element of *Phlyctaenaspis.* × 100.
    (*d*) Detail of cell spaces in semidentin of *Phlyctaenaspis.* × 400.
    (*e*) Section of a jaw element of a Middle Devonian form, *Coccosteus.* × 50.
    (*f*) Osteosemidentin from a dermal jaw element of the coccosteomorph *Plourdosteus*
showing osteocyte spaces in the interstitial bone tissue between semidenteons. × 100. From
Ørvig 1967.

because calcified tissues have a polyphyletic history, we are seeing only parts of a spectrum of histological structure, the elements of which are not necessarily related sequentially. To add to the difficulties, various kinds of calcified cartilage are to be found in early vertebrates and the relationships between these and bone and dentin are far from clear.

By the time dermal armor became reduced to denticles and placoid teeth had emerged on jaws, metadentin, with two structural varieties, osteodentin and *orthodentin,* was the established tissue. Both of these varieties are found in the teeth of modern elasmobranchs and teleosts, whereas only orthodentin occurs in the teeth of amphibians, reptiles, and mammals. In some teleosts the calcified tissue of the teeth may contain vascular tubes but enclose no cell processes (*vasodentin*), and in some labyrinthodonts, some reptiles (e.g., *Varanus*) and some mammals (e.g., *Orycteropus*), the dental papilla may infold secondarily to give a complex orthodentin (*plicidentin*) superficially resembling osteodentine. A review of dentin in recent vertebrates is given by Bradford (1967).

Turning now to the question of the history of enamel, it is simplest to start with a consideration of this tissue in mammals. Mammalian enamel contains by weight 95% crystalline calcium phosphate (hydroxyapatite) and 5% organic material and water. It is in the form of a thick covering over the crown of the tooth and is composed of histologically identifiable units, the enamel prisms or rods, which are about 5μ in diameter and run throughout the thickness of the enamel. Incremental markings perpendicular to the axes of the prisms are present and the prisms are often arranged in layers, those of one layer running in a different direction from those of adjacent layers, producing a banded appearance in certain section planes (fig. 5). Features of prism shape in different orders of mammals and the relationship between prism characters and the arrangement of submicroscopic crystallites in enamel have been described by Boyde (1965).

In contrast, reptilian enamel is usually thin and shows a relatively homogeneous structure. The only regularly occurring characteristic is the appearance of approximately parallel, incremental lines with a spacing of the same order as the cross striations of mammalian prisms. It is thus possible to distinguish between typically reptilian and typically mammalian enamels. Because of this difference, interesting questions arise concerning the point in history when prismatic enamel arose and the possibility of using enamel structure as an aid in taxonomy.

It is known that the structure of mammalian enamel is preserved in fossil material and, with this in mind, it is significant that the enamel of a number of early reptiles (cotylosaur and pelycosaur) and Therapsida (gorgonopsid and cynodont) is typically reptilian in structure (Poole 1956, 1957). In all of these,

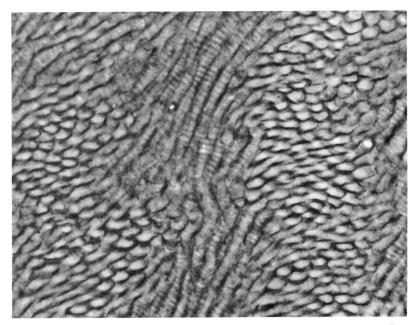

Fig. 5. Part of a longitudinal section through a human tooth showing an appearance in the enamel known as Hunter-Schreger bands. The appearance is due to the arrangement of structural units, the enamel prisms or rods, in layers, the prisms of one layer running in a different direction from those in adjacent layers. Phase contrast microscope, × 600.

as well as the ictidosaurian *Oligokyphus,* incremental marking of the enamel is the only obvious histological feature, although certain sites are darkly stained with mineral inclusions. In the enamel of recent reptiles corresponding areas are often imperfectly mineralized. To date, the enamel of nontherian mammals also appears to be reptilian in character, but in one dryolestid (figs. 6 & 7) evidence of prismatic structure has been obtained (Poole 1967). Probably as concluded by Moss (1968), after examining the teeth of a wide range of early mammalian genera, prismatic enamel only became generally established in therian mammals. Whether this tissue had a single or multiple origin remains to be discovered, but there is some hope that the histological structure of tooth enamel may be useful in the future as a taxonomic criterion.

Below the level of reptiles the understanding of the nature of the hard tissue covering the tooth becomes much more problematical. Teeth in most fishes and some amphibians do possess a highly calcified enamellike tissue, but the variation in the histological and physical character is so great that considerably different interpretations of its nature have been made. This is reflected in the variety of names accorded to the tissue (see Poole 1966), of which the term enameloid will be used here. There is one outstanding ontogenetic difference

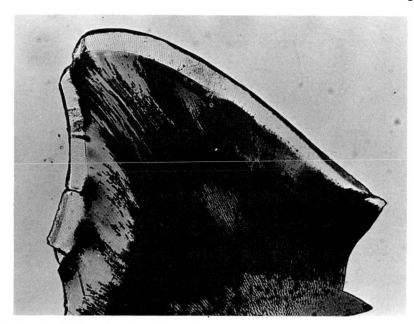

Fig. 6. Longitudinal section through a molar cusp of an early (dryolestid) mammal. The enamel possesses prisms running out from the amelodentinal junction to the surface of the tooth. Bright field microscope, × 60.

between the true enamel of mammals and reptiles and the enameloid of fishes. Enamel formation is carried out by ectodermal, epithelial cells (ameloblasts) of the enamel organ and it is preceded by dentin formation. Enameloid differentiates and begins to calcify before dentin formation begins and it appears to be the first-formed tissue of the mesodermal dental papilla. Structurally there are also differences; true enamel results from the mineralization of a nonstructured organic matrix which consists of a number of relatively low molecular weight protein moieties (amelogenins, Eastoe 1966), whereas enameloid is formed by the mineralization of a collagenous matrix and often possesses dentinal tubules in its mature condition (Schmidt and Keil 1958). Because of the seemingly discrete differences between enamel and enameloid it was at one time believed that at some point in the phylogeny an abrupt change occurred in the origin and nature of the outer layer of the tooth.

However, in this field a number of problems have always existed. For example, although no certain function could be ascribed to them, the epithelial cells covering the developing tooth in fishes undergo changes during the period of enameloid formation similar to changes occurring in ameloblasts as true enamel develops. Further, although the evidence for the presence of collagen fibers in the developing enameloid is strong, fibers are not present in the mature tissue, and the problem is to understand the mechanism whereby they disappear. Solutions to such problems are by no means complete, but a better understanding of them is slowly being achieved.

It is now known that in some fish and amphibians a tooth, even though it possesses enameloid, may be invested with a membrane which is probably derived from the epithelial cells covering the tooth germ (Schmidt and Keil 1958; Kerr 1960). Electron microscopy has shown that, in adult amphibians at least, a thin layer of true enamel exists (Meredith Smith 1967), and autoradiographic studies reveal that the epithelial cells secrete labeled amino acids into the surface of the tooth (Smith and Miles 1969). Other electron microscope studies have shown that collagen fibers are present in immature enameloid of dogfishes (figs. 8, 9, 10), but they disappear as mineralization occurs (Poole 1969). An earlier amino-acid analysis of developing shark enameloid proteins indicated the presence of collagen, and the suggestion was made that such collagen is ecto-dermal in origin (Moss, Jones, and Piez 1964; Moss 1968). Finally, and more interesting, a recent amino-acid analysis of mature shark enameloid proteins showed a composition similar to the proteins of mature mammalian enamel (Levine, Glimcher, and Seyer 1966).

Thus, with many parts of this phylogenetic story still to be investigated it is already clear that that the relationship between enameloid and enamel is much closer than has previously been supposed. Taking into consideration all available evidence, it would appear possible that, primitively, the combined secretory activity of the epithelial sheet and the adjacent, inner odontoblast layer gives rise to an enameloid tissue which initially possesses collagen fibers and rapidly begins to mineralize. As mineralization occurs collagen fibers revert to a labile form and become extruded as crystal growth takes place, the epithelial cells perhaps assisting in its final removal. Otherwise the odontoblasts continue with the production of dentin within the enameloid. Phylogenetically, the main change would have been that, after the first layer of the tooth has been formed, the epithelial cells did not cease secreting but either continued to produce a mineralizing matrix or continued to mineralize the proteins being extruded from between the first-formed crystals. In this way true enamel formation would necessarily lag behind the formation of the first differentiated tissue, the so-called von Korff's layer (Schmidt and Keil 1958).

Whatever the true relationship between enameloid and enamel may eventually prove to be, it is clear that the change occurred before the emergence of reptiles, most likely in the fishes. And finally, although it is necessary to consider living species in order to follow developmental processes, it must be remem-

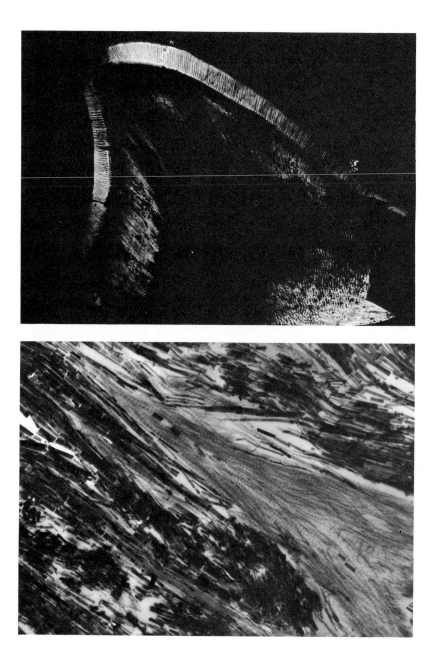

Fig. 7. The same section as fig. 6 viewed between crossed polars. The alternating white and black stripes in the enamel are related to prism structure and are due to the fact that, as in human enamel, the submicroscopic apatite crystallites gradually change direction across each prism. Polarizing microscope, × 60.

Fig. 8. Apatite crystallites and a bundle of fibers in developing enameloid of a dogfish, *Scyliorhinus*. Electron microscope, phosphotungstic-acid stained, × 17,000.

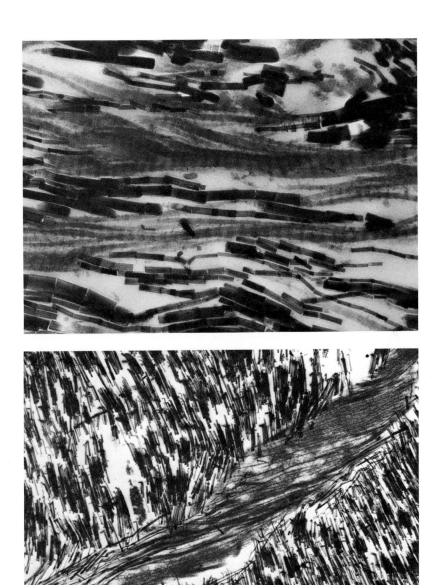

Fig. 9. Fibers in developing enameloid of a dogfish, *Scyliorhinus,* showing the cross-banding of collagen. Electron microscope, phosphotungstic-acid stained, × 57,000.

Fig. 10. An area in the developing enameloid of a dogfish, *Scyliorhinus,* in which new, very fine crystallites are emerging from an amorphous background of organic material derived from collagen. Electron microscope, phosphotungstic-acid stained, × 17,850.

bered that, like all other calcified tissues, enameloid is very old and has been identified in the tubercles (odontodes) of the dermal armor of the ancient Heterostraci (Ørvig 1967).

ACKNOWLEDGMENTS

The author is indebted to Academic Press for permission to reproduce figures 1–4, to the *British Dental Journal* for figure 5, and to the publishers of the *Portuguese Journal of Mining* for figures 6–7.

REFERENCES

Boyde, A. 1965. The structure of developing mamalian dental enamel. In *Tooth enamel: Its composition, properties, and fundamental structure,* ed. M. V. Stack and R. W. Fearnhead, pp. 163–67, 192–94. Bristol: Wright.

Bradford, E. W. 1967. Microanatomy and histochemistry of dentine. In *Structural and chemical organization of teeth,* ed. A. E. W. Miles, 2:3–32. New York: Academic Press.

Denison, R. H. 1947. The exoskeleton of *Tremataspis. Amer. J. Sci.* 245:337–65.

Denison, R. H. 1963. The early history of the vertebrate calcified skeleton. *Clin. Orthop.* 31:141–52.

Eastoe, J. E. 1966. The changing nature of developing dental enamel. *Brit. Dent. J.* 121:451–54.

Gross, W. 1935. Histologische Studien am Aussenskelet fossiler Agnathen Fische. *Palaeontolographica,* A83:1–60.

Kerr, T. 1960. Development and structure of some actinopterygian teeth. *Proc. Zool. Soc. Lond.* 133:401–22.

Levine, P. T.; Glimcher, M. J.; Seyer, J. M.; Huddleston, J. I.; and Hein, J. W. 1966. Noncollagenous nature of the proteins in shark enamel. *Science* 154:1192–94.

Meredith Smith, M. 1967. Studies on the structure and development of urodele teeth. Ph.D. thesis, London.

Moss, M. L. 1968. Bone, dentin and enamel and the evolution of vertebrates. In *Biology of the mouth,* ed. P. Person, pp. 37–66. Proceedings A.A.A.S. Symposium, Washington, 1966.

Moss, M. L.; Jones, S. J.; and Piez, K. A. 1964. Calcified ectodermal collagens of shark-tooth enamel and teleost scale. *Science* 145:940–42.

Ørvig, T. 1951. Histologic studies of placoderms and fossil elasmobranchs. I. The endoskeleton, with remarks on the hard tissues of lower vertebrates in general. *Ark. Zool.* 2:321–454.

————. 1967. The phylogeny of tooth tissues: Evolution of some calcified tissues in early vertebrates. In *Structural and chemical organization of teeth,* ed. A. E. W. Miles, 1:45–105. New York: Academic Press.

Poole, D. F. G. 1956. The structure of the teeth of some mammal-like reptiles. *Quart. J. Micr. Sci.* 97:303–12.

————. 1957. The formation and properties of the organic matrix of reptilian enamel. *Quart. J. Micr. Sci.* 98:349–67.

————. 1967*a*. Enamel structure in primitive mammals. *J. Dent. Res.* 44:1175–76.

————. 1967*b*. The phylogeny of tooth tissues: Enameloid and enamel in recent vertebrates. In *Structure and chemical organization of teeth,* ed. A. E. W. Miles, 1:111–47. New York: Academic Press.

————. 1969. Collagen in dogfish enameloid. *J. Dent. Res.* 48:1119.

Schmidt, W. J., and Keil, A. 1958. *Die gesunden und die erkrankten Zahngewebe des Menschen und der Wirbeltiere im Polarisationsmikroskop.* Munich: Carl Hanser.

Smith, M. M., and Miles, A. E. W. 1969. An autoradiographic investigation with the light microscope of proline-H[3] incorporation during tooth development in the crested newt (*Triturus cristatus*). *Arch. Oral Biol.* 14:479–90.

Tarlo, L. B. H. 1964. The origin of bone. In *Bone and tooth,* ed. H. J. J. Blackwood, pp. 3–17. Oxford: Pergamon Press.

7 Comparative Histology of Mammalian Teeth

A. Boyde

Department of Anatomy and Embryology,
University College, London

Introduction

A large part of the information used to classify fossil vertebrates is derived from the teeth. This is so because the teeth, as the most mineralized portions of the skeleton, are usually the best preserved skeletal remains. The best preserved portion of the teeth is again that which is most highly mineralized, the enamel. It has been known for a long time that certain features of the histological organization of enamel are sufficiently characteristic of a taxonomic group to be used for identification. However, little attention has been given to this problem in recent years, and with the new methods of microscopic examination available it now seems appropriate to summarize the present state of our knowledge and to indicate where further study might be profitable. It is probable that intensive study will follow only where a particular taxonomic problem has arisen that cannot be tackled in another way. Nevertheless, it is important for workers in this field to have some idea of the potential usefulness of dental histology and, in particular, of enamel histology.

Enamel

Enamel Tubules. The first feature of the organization of enamel to receive intensive investigation from the taxonomic viewpoint was the occurrence of enamel tubules (Tomes 1849). They are characteristically abundant in the marsupial mammals with the exception of the wombats, in which they are absent. Enamel tubules are also found in certain members of the orders Rodentia (e.g., the jerbca), Insectivora (e.g., hedgehog, mole, shrew), Lemuroidea, and Chiroptera.

Electron microscopic examination of fractures (figs. 1, 2) across the enamel-dentin junction show that the enamel tubules are far more common than was previously realized in other mammals, but they are of a size which normally precludes study by light microscopy (Boyde and Lester 1967).

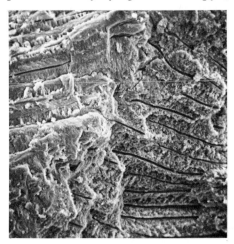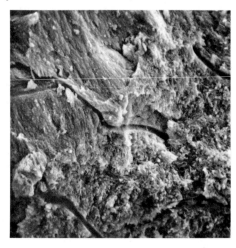

Figs. 1, 2. *Macropus* molar. Scanning electron micrographs of fracture through enamel- (*left*) dentin (*right*) junction. Dentin tubules (complete with peritubular zones) are continuous with tubules in the enamel. Fig. 1, × 930; fig. 2, × 930.

Enamel tubules are continuous with the dentine tubules across the enamel-dentin junction. Lester (1969) has recently shown that enamel tubules are formed in similar manner to that of the dentin tubules, in that the ameloblast leaves behind a fine cytoplasmic process: this is often juxtaposed to an odontoblast process at the enamel-dentin junction.

Decussation of Enamel Prisms. Enamel prisms are the basic, light-microscopically visible units of this tissue. They are demarcated by boundaries commonly called prism sheaths. The prisms extend from a zone a very few microns removed from the enamel-dentin junction to usually some 10 or more μ short of the surface of the tissue. In the Cetacea, Sirenia, Chiroptera, and Insectivora, the prisms proceed in a uniform direction, often almost in straight parallel lines. They usually have a simple cross-sectional shape. In the majority of mammals, however, the prisms deviate in their course from the enamel-dentin junction outward, the deviation being generally in the side-to-side direction of the tooth. This gives rise to an often characteristic distribution of *zones* of prisms that are cut in different planes in a microscopical section. The exact details of whether, as implied in the term decussation, adjacent prisms actually cross over their neighbors do not concern us here (see Boyde 1969). Many features of the various possible arrangements can be and have been measured.

Korvenkontio's (1934–35) detailed study of the rodents and lagomorphs probably provides sufficient information to enable the familial identification of even small fragments of "rodent" teeth (fig. 3). Kawai (1955) measured the average width of zones of prisms proceeding in different directions, as well as the angle at which the zones meet the enamel-dentin junction, for several mammalian groups. This work could certainly be extended to include the apparent decussation angle and to bring it nearer to the degree of completeness reached by Korvenkontio's (1934) study of the rodents.

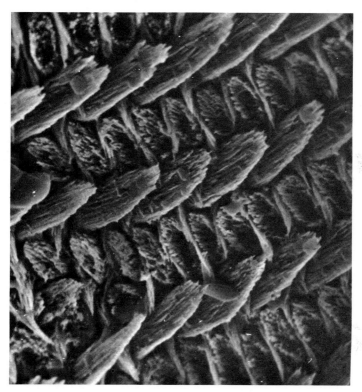

Fig. 3. Figures 3, 4, 5, and 6 are scanning electron micrographs of enamel surfaces prepared by etching polished ground sections cut transverse to the prism direction: Rat incisor inner-enamel. The decussation pattern shown is typical of those of the myomorph group of rodents (× 4,600).

Cross-sectional Shape of Enamel Prisms. The cross-sectional form of enamel prisms can be studied in sections cut transverse to the mean prism direction, or in etched surfaces ground and polished perpendicular to the mean prism direction. The latter type of preparation is particularly suited to examination by replica techniques for transmission electron microscopy or directly in the scanning electron microscope. The latter instrument also enables small fragments of fractured enamel to be used to obtain this type of information, since it is generally possible to discover a region in which some of the prisms have been fractured transversely.

The first comprehensive comparative study of the cross-sectional shape of enamel prisms was that of Shobusawa (1952). The conclusions of this work were confirmed by Boyde (1964, 1965), and could be further substantiated by many illustrations in the literature. Briefly, three characteristic prism-packing patterns can be described. In pattern 1 (fig. 4; Boyde 1964, 1965) the prisms

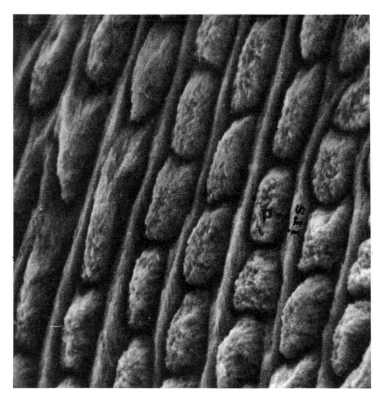

Fig. 4. Pig deciduous molar. Pattern 2. The enamel prisms (*P*) are arranged in longitudinal rows separated by interrow sheets (*IRS*). This arrangement is found in the Artiodactyla, Equidae, and Marsupialia. × 5,000.

are hexagonally packed, with complete cylindrical boundaries, and are often nearly straight in their course; this pattern is found in the Chiroptera, Insectivora, Cetacea, Sirenia (e.g., fig. 5), Tapiridae, and some, if not all, Lemuroidea. In pattern 2 (fig. 4) the prisms are organized as longitudinal rows separated by interrow sheets of interprismatic "substance." The prism boundaries have a horseshoe-shaped cross section, with the open side of one horseshoe

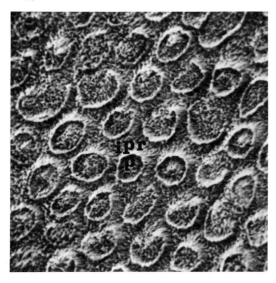

Fig. 5. Manatee molar. Pattern 1. The enamel prisms usually have complete cylindrical prism sheaths which enable one to distinguish prisms (*P*) from the interprismatic regions (*IPR*). They are usually found in the Cetacea, Sirenia, Insectivora, Chiroptera, and Tapiridae. × 1,550.

fitting closely to the closed (cuspal) side of its neighbor. This arrangement is found in the Marsupialia, Artiodactyla, and Equidae. In pattern 3 (fig. 6) it is conventional to refer *all* the enamel to the prisms. They are described as having winged processes or "tail" regions, whereas the topographically equivalent regions of pattern 1 enamels are called "interprismatic regions" and in the pattern 2 enamels, "interrow sheets" (Boyde 1964, 1965). Pattern 3 enamels are found in the Primates (fig. 6), Proboscidea, Pinnipedia, and Carnivora.

The marked decussation of the prisms that is found in the inner enamel of rodent incisor teeth gives rise to a further set of variations in the shape of the prisms (fig. 3) (Tomes 1850; Korvenkontio 1934–35).

It has recently been found (Boyde 1969) that the cross-sectional shape of the enamel prisms may also be correlated with the area of the secretory territories of the enamel-forming cells. This finding suggests that it might be useful to measure prism sizes as well as shapes in any pilot study directed at determining taxonomic affinities. In the mature tooth, one may use the cross-sectional area of the enamel prisms in a plane parallel with the incremental lines as the area of the secretory territories.

It is important to realize that the distinction between the various prism patterns is by no means absolute. Intermediate forms are common, and examples of all of the basic arrangements mentioned above will usually be found in any mammalian enamel sample. Nevertheless, the great majority of fully differenti-

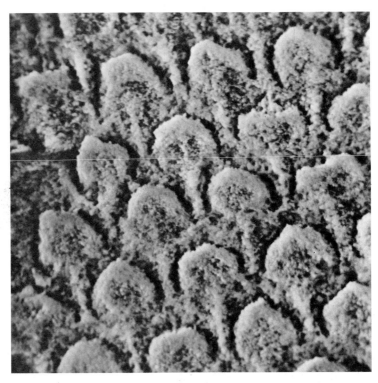

Fig. 6. Human enamel. Pattern 3, "keyhole" shape. The largest enamel prisms, found in the orders Primates, Proboscidea, Carnivora, and Pinnipedia most commonly show this packing arrangement. × 3,600.

ated prisms will more nearly fit one of the arrangements described. Thus, for example, local regions of pattern 2 prisms will be found in human (pattern 3) enamel, but the distinctive lamellar arrangement imposed by the extensive interrow sheets found in ungulate enamels is not encountered. Pattern 1, hexagonal prisms, are often found in dog and cat enamel, but the large majority are pattern 3 (for details see Boyde 1969).

Surface Zone Enamel. The formation of the most superficial layer of mammalian enamels is associated with a reduction in the secretory potential of the respective ameloblasts. The loss of their Tomes's processes allows a prism-free surface zone to be formed: all the crystallites stand parallel and perpendicular to the surface. So far, the distribution of this true surface-zone enamel has not been studied closely from a comparative viewpoint.

Perikymata are circumferential deficiencies in the thickness of the (outer) enamel layer representing the outcrop of the incremental lines, or brown striae of Retzius. They indicate the premature cessation of enamel formation and show the pits which were occupied the enamel-forming cells. Perikymata are, therefore, presumed to reflect variations in the environment experienced by the individual animal during the development of enamel. These may, however, be of sufficiently regular character in any one species or group to be of some practical value.

Dentin

Minor variations in the arrangement of microscopically visible structural features of dentin have not, so far, been used in any direct way to indicate taxonomic affinities. However, such comparative anatomical surveys as have already been made do indicate a promising potential in this respect.

The packing density and dimensions of the dentin tubules were considered in detail as early as 1837 in the work of Retzius, which was translated into English by Nasmyth in 1839. The degree of side-branching of the dentin tubules (fig. 7) and the frequency with which these side-branches anastomose are very

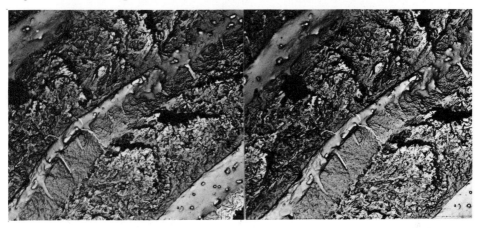

Fig. 7. Calf dentin. Transmission electron micrograph stereo-pair of carbon replica of fractured dentin showing the remarkable number of small side-branches of the dentin tubules which penetrate the peritubular dentin. × 5,000.

variable among different mammalian orders, and it is probable that after some further study one could at least confine the origin of a particular piece of dentin to a small group of mammalian orders on this basis alone.

Most mammalian dentins possess a layer of densely mineralized material lining the dentinal canals. Although it has been widely considered that in human teeth this peritubular dentin forms as a result of an aging process or as a response to an altered environment, this view cannot be accepted if we examine a variety of mammals. Peritubular dentin may form in advance of the mineralizing front in the intertubular dentin in the elephant molar, and this should be sufficiently distinctive a character to permit identification. Peritubular dentin forms synchronously with the mineralizing front of the intertubular dentin in the dog and cat (Carnivora) and in the cow, sheep, and pig (Artiodactyla). In the latter group, peritubular dentin forms predominantly on one side of the tubules (figs. 7, 8). In many other mammals, including man, the peritubular

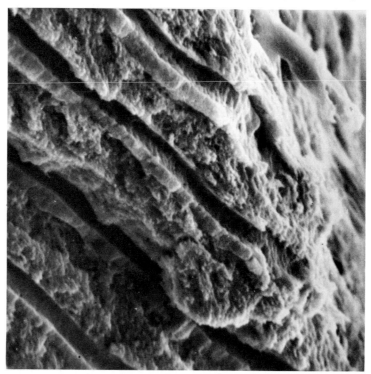

Fig. 8. Calf dentin. Scanning electron micrograph of fractured, anorganic developing dentin showing the eccentric formation of the peritubular dentin at the level of the mineralizing front in the intertubular dentin. × 4,500.

dentin forms at some distance from the mineralizing front in the intertubular dentin. A close analysis of these variations seems to offer particular promise.

The mantle, or Von Korff, layer of dentin is also variable in its development in the different mammals (Lester and Boyde 1968). We have encountered the greatest development of the Von Korff fibers in the Odontoceti (see also Schmidt and Keil, 1958). The examination of fractured dentin surfaces in the scanning electron microscope should suffice to determine whether a piece of dentin has derived from this group. At the other extreme, the mantle dentin layer is missing altogether in the marsupials, with the one exception of the wombat. There is, therefore, a correlation between the extension of the dentin into the enamel and the absence of Von Korff fibers (Boyde and Lester 1967).

In mammals other than marsupials, enamel tubules may develop where there is a localized absence of the Von Korff fiber layer at the enamel-dentin junction. An exact categorization of the other mammalian orders between these two extremes would be valuable.

The incidence of secondary dentin and pulpal calcification is again, like that of the peritubular dentin, widely supposed to be related to the functional experience of a particular tooth, and this would suggest that the variability between individuals of the same species may be too great for the histology of these secondary repair tissues to be of practical taxonomic value. However, there are many species, particularly among the Cetacea, in which the formation of secondary dentin and pulpal calcification is the normal event in unworn teeth.

Certain variations in dentin structure can be seen on naked eye examination. These may generally be ascribed to two particular sources. In the first, variations in the degree of mineralization affect the translucency of the tissues. Thus incremental lines of more and less transparent dentin are formed (fig. 9). Strongly marked incremental variations in dentin mineralization are found in the Odontoceti and Pinnipedia, though by no means in every member of these groups. They are also found in the elephants.

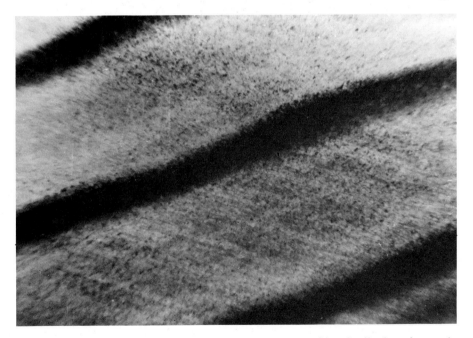

Fig. 9. *Hyperoodon ampullatus* (bottlenosed whale). Part of longitudinal section to show prominent, dark incremental lines of poorly mineralized dentin. Light micrograph, × 100 approx.

A second type of naked eye feature of the dentin is related to the course of the dentinal tubules. Where all the tubules show the same change in direction, light will be reflected differently and a "Schreger line of the dentine" may be formed. Bradford (1967) states that such lines are a common feature of walrus dentine, and Schmidt and Keil (1958) describe them in the *Babyrousa babyrussa* and hippopotamus. The checkerboard pattern of more and less translucent areas seen in sections cut transverse to the long axis of the tusks and molar roots of recent elephants and mammoths (together with some of their more immediate fossil forebears) has a somewhat similar origin. For descriptive purposes we may consider these teeth as divided into longitudinal wedge-shaped segments. In any one such segment the tubules show the same pattern of curves: a primary curvature with a wave length of the order of a few microns and a secondary curvature with a wave length between 1 and 3 mm. The secondary waves are 90° out of phase in alternative wedge segments. Variations in translucency or reflectance are related to the angle of incidence of the light on the cut tubules.

Longitudinal wedge segmentation of the dentin is a marked feature in the narwhal tusk. This segmentation is brought about by poorly mineralized radial planes related to concavities between ridges in the developing dentin surface (fig. 10).

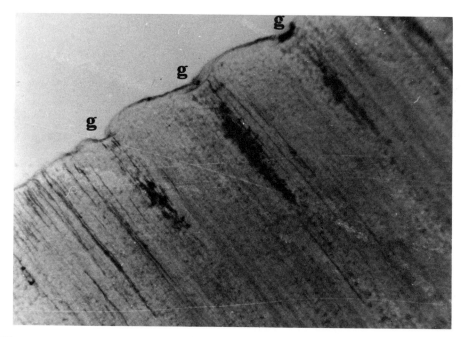

Fig. 10. *Monodon monoceros* (narwhal). Part of transverse section of tusk at internal, developing surface. Poorly mineralized dark radial planes are related to (longitudinal) grooves (*G*) at pulpal surface. Light micrograph, × 100 approx.

Vasodentin. Dentins containing tubular spaces of a size which might reasonably be taken to indicate that they may once have been occupied by capillary blood vessels have been reported in several mammalian orders (for list, see Arsuffi 1938). In most of these cases the original observations have not been substantiated by further reports. However, there seems to be no doubt of its occurrence in the Edentata (in *Bradypus tridactylus, Dasypus,* and *Megatherium* [extinct]) and in the *Mesoplodon* species of the ziphioid odontocetes (personal observation). Several other instances will, no doubt, be confirmed and others discovered. I have been unable to confirm Tomes's (1876) observation of vasodentin in the manatee (order Sirenia).

Cementum

Acellular Cement. The acellular (attachment) cement which covers the surface of the roots of the teeth of a great many mammals probably does not possess sufficiently distinctive variations to enable examination of a small piece of this tissue alone to lead to an identification.

Cellular Cementum. Cellular cementum is found covering both the crowns and the roots of teeth in many members of the orders Odontoceti, Artiodactyla, Perissodactyla, Proboscidea, and Rodentia. This tissue occurs in sufficient bulk to permit generalizations about its structure. Variable features include the

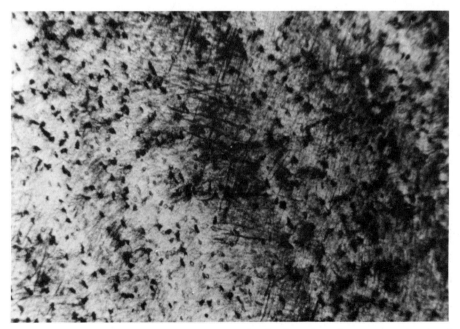

Fig. 11. *Physeter catodon* (sperm whale). Longitudinal section of cementum showing decussation of Sharpey fibers. Light micrograph, × 100 approx.

cellular (lacunar) packing density, the prominence of incremental lines due to the variations in the degree of mineralization, and the proportion of the tissue occupied by the Sharpey fibers. Decussation of the Sharpey fibers can be found in some instances, for example, in the sperm whale (fig. 11) and elephant.

The external coronal cementum of the hypsodont molars of herbivores may have to serve the same attachment function and shows the same structure as normal root cementum—these teeth may begin to be used before they have "anatomical roots." The "internal" coronal cementum can have no attachment function, but presumably serves only to cement together the high ridges (cusps) or plates of grinding lophodont molar teeth. Oriented Sharpey fiber bundles are usually absent in this situation. "Internal" coronal cementum may be extremely cellular.

Vasocementum. Both coronal and root cellular cementum may at some stage in their development possess a vascular supply (fig. 12). The capillary blood vessel canals may remain patent (e.g., *Mesoplodon layardi* root cementum and horse coronal cementum).

The degree of vascularity of the first-formed layer of cementum in the root region of the *Mesoplodon* species is much the greatest we have encountered. This cementum is also unusual in that it contains neither cell spaces nor Sharpey fibers and therefore presumably serves only as a packing material.

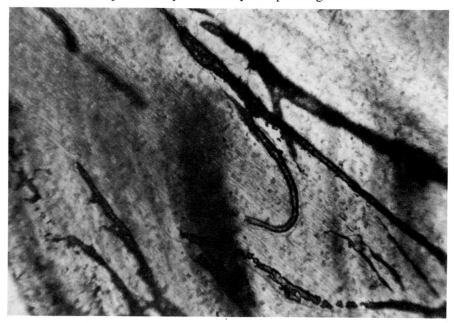

Fig. 12. *Ziphius cavirostris* (Cuviers beaked whale). L.S. cementum showing what are presumed to be capillary blood vessel spaces. Light micrograph, × 100 approx.

A vascularized cementum apparently containing both Sharpey fibers and cells has been described by Owen (1842) in the extinct giant sloth *Mylodon* (*Megatherium*). A less well vascularized tissue is found in Cuviers beaked whale (*Ziphius cavirostris*) (fig. 12).

The new techniques of electron microscopy have made it possible to designate and define taxonomic groups more precisely with descriptions of mineralized tissues.

REFERENCES

Arsuffi, E. 1938. Beiträge zur Kenntniss das Vasodentins. *Z. Anat. Entwicklungesch.* 108:749–60.

Boyde, A. 1964. The structure and development of mammalian enamel. Ph.D. diss., University of London.

———. 1965. The structure of developing mammalian dental enamel. In *Tooth enamel,* ed. M. V. Stack and R. W. Fearnhead. Bristol: Wright.

———. 1969. Correlation of ameloblast size with enamel prism pattern: Use of scanning electron miscroscope to make surface area measurements. *Z. Zellforsch.* 93:583–93.

———. 1969. Electron microscopic observations relating to the nature and development of prism decussation in mammalian dental enamel. *Bull. Group Int. Rech. Sci. Stomatol.* 12:151–208.

Boyde, A., and Lester, K. S. 1967. An electron microscope study of fractured dentinal surfaces. *Calc. Tiss. Res.* 1:122–36.

———. 1967. The structure and development of marsupial enamel tubules. *Z. Zellforsch.* 82:558–76.

Bradford, E. W. 1967. Microanatomy and histochemistry of dentine. In *Structural and chemical organization of teeth,* ed. A. E. W. Miles, 2:3–32. New York: Academic Press.

Kawai, N. 1955. Comparative anatomy of the bands of Schreger. *Okajimas Folia Anat. Jap.* 27:115–31.

Korvenkontio, V. A. 1934–35. Mikroskopische Untersuchungen an Nagerincisiven unter Hinweis auf die Schmelzstruktur der Backenzähne: Histologisch-Phyletische Studie. *Annal. Zool. Soc. Zool-Bot. Fenn. Vanamo (Helsinki)* 2:1–274.

Lester, K. S. 1969. On the nature of "fibrils" and tubules in the developing enamel of the opossum, *Didelphius marsupialis. J. Ultrastruct. Res.* In press.

Lester, K. S., and Boyde, A. 1968. The question of Von Korff fibres in mammalian dentines. *Calc. Tiss. Res.* 1:273–87.

Owen, R. 1842. Description of the skeleton of an extinct gigantic sloth *Mylodon robustus.* London: John van Voorst. (*Odontography.* London: Ballière, 1845).

Shobusawa, M. 1952. Vergleichende Untersuchungen über die Form der Schmelzprismen der Säugetiere. *Okajimas Folia Anat. Jap.* 24:371–92.

Schmidt, W. J., and Keil, A. 1958. *Die gesunden und die erkrankten Zahngewebe des Menschen und der Wirbeltiere im Polarisationsmikroskop.* Munich: Carl Hanser.

Tomes, C. S. 1876. *Dental anatomy*. London: Churchill.

Tomes, J. 1849. On the structure of the dental tissues of marsupial animals and more especially of the enamel. *Phil. Trans.* 139:402–12.

———. 1850. On the structure of the dental tissues of the order Rodentia. *Phil. Trans.* 140:529–67.

8 Basic Crown Patterns and Cusp Homologies of Mammalian Teeth

Philip Hershkovitz *Field Museum of Natural History, Chicago, Illinois*

Introduction

This account, which stems from a study of dental variation and evolution in platyrrhine monkeys, attempts to establish a scientific basis for tracing dental elements in living marsupials and placentals to their inception in earliest mammals.

The much criticized but widely used Osbornian terminology for dental elements was first devised to serve precisely such aims. Unfortunately, the terms, as has been repeatedly shown, are equivocally based and their definitions obscure, when they do not distort or flatly contradict the messages they were designed to convey. One result has been the proliferation of makeshift terminologies, all cast in the Osbornian mold but with some modifications or additions to fit special problems. Another dire consequence has been the corruption of dental evolutionary thought through use of similar terms for nonhomologous upper and lower dental elements, and dissimilar terms for the homologous elements.

A radical departure from the traditional school is the system of dental terminology proposed in 1961 by Vandebroek. The scheme is founded on the primitive pattern of crests and cusps common to all postincisor teeth of eutherian (marsupial and placental) grade, and to most teeth of subeutherian grade, specifically Triconodonta, Docodonta, Symmetrodonta and Pantotheria.

Reaction to the Vandebroek thesis has been for the most part reserved and sometimes hostile. General acceptance of his important contributions to knowledge of mammalian dental evolution was probably hindered by minor flaws in arguments, some controversial statements, use of strange terms for familiar dental elements, and, perhaps more than anything else, by his assaults on cherished dogmas. Notwithstanding, my independent investigations of dental evolution and homologies based on large series of teeth of living species, mostly primates, insectivores, and marsupials, led to conclusions reached by Vandebroek. There appears to be no choice, therefore, but to adopt names proposed by this authority for dental elements not previously described in formal terms, and as replacements for those Osbornian terms which more perniciously than others deprive dental descriptions of evolutionary significance. Concepts or interpretations of dental homologies and evolution presented here and not anticipated by Vandebroek, or by Cope, Osborn, Gregory, Simpson, Butler, Remane, Patterson, and others cited in text, are derived as much from data and discussions presented by these authorities as from the specimens I studied.

The Tridentate Tooth and Primary Evolutionary Processes

The primitive mammalian tooth, or its reptilian prototype, is single- or double-rooted, sagittate in outline, subovate in cross section, with main cusp, the eocone (-id, or paracone-protoconid) rising to a conical peak; a small tubercle, the mesiostyle (-id), is usually present at the anterior base of the cusp, and another, the distostyle (-id), is present at the posterior base of the cusp. The crest of the eocone (-id) from tubercle to tubercle, is the eocrista (-id). The axis of the eocrista from end to end of the three cusps is the primary or eocone (-id) axis. Either or both tubercles or styles (-ids), may become specialized, usually by hypertrophy, or either element, most often the mesiostyle (-id), may disappear altogether. The ledge at the base of the crown which supports each style (-id) may disappear with it, or it may spread horizontally as a narrow band, the *cingulum* (-id), along the buccal or the lingual, or on both sides to engirdle the base of the crown. This primitive, tricuspidate tooth, dominated by the comparatively enormous eocone (-id), is often called tritubercular, and sometimes triconodont. The equivalent term *tridentate* (fig. 1A, B), proposed here for the primitive mammalian tooth, avoids confusion with the homonomous term tritubercular, and avoids the taxonomic connotation of the term triconodont.

Specialization of the tridentate tooth is achieved through the evolutionary processes of (*a*) *caninization*, (*b*) *molarization* or complication, and (*c*) *degeneration* or secondary simplification through reduction and elimination of dental elements.

Fig. 1. (A) Primitive mammalian tridentate tooth, buccal and occlusal views of left upper or right lower; (B) tridentate lower incisors in pygmy marmoset, *Cebuella pygmaea* (Primates, Callithricidae); (C) caninized lower right incisor in the extinct *Phenacolemur pagei* (Primates, Phenacolemuridae, U. Paleocene), redrawn from Simpson (1955, pl. 32); absence of terminal stylids (*a, b*) and cingulum is a degenerative character; (D) nu-

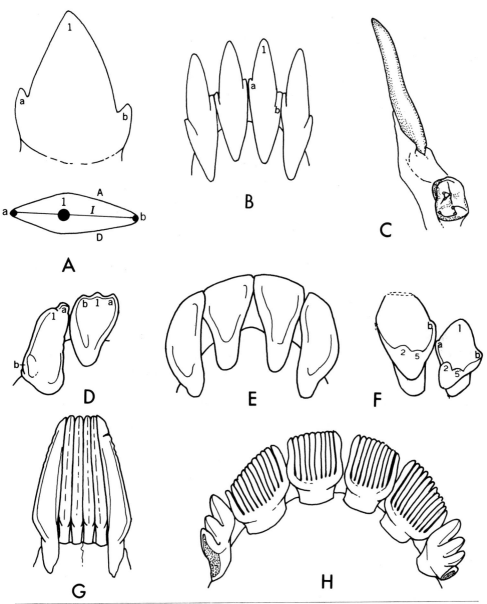

tricial lower left incisors in cotton-top tamarin, *Saguinus oedipus* (Primates, Callithricidae) —compare with following; (E) adult lower incisors in cotton-top tamarin, *Saguinus oedipus*, example of caninization by expansion of main cusp and fusion with terminal stylids; (F) left upper tritubercular incisors of *Callicebus torquatus*, example of molarization; (G) comblike lower incisors and canines in the ringtail lemur (*Lemur catta*), an example of caninization with secondary simplification or degeneration; (H) comblike lower incisors (and canines?) in the colugo, *Cynocephalus volans*, an example of pectinization through complication or molarization, with each process (or crenule) of the morphogenetic field of the main cusp developing into an independent cuspulid. See page 136 and figure 17 for complete list of symbols and their respective conventional names.

Caninization

Caninization is specialization, usually through hypertrophy, of the main cusp and of either or both primary cuspules of the tridentate tooth. Caninization may act on any primitive tooth, but it never transgresses the tridentate stage in dental complication.

The true canine, for all its exaggeration in many mammals, often as a sexual character of adult males, departs least from the tridentate model. The primitive canine, like primitive incisors and premolars, is a simple tridentate tooth. Specialization by hypertrophy and curvature or hooking of the main cone and cuspules are results of caninization. Formation of the lingual bulge, or torus, and vertical grooves, and addition of cusps or talon (-id), are manifestations of molarization. Obsolescence or loss of cingulum and primitive mesial and distal tubercles are consequences of degeneration.

The primitive or caninized anterior premolar is, in effect, a second and smaller canine. It still retains the form and function of a secondary canine in the maxillary arcade of prosimians, notably in *Galago elegantulus* and lorisoids, most marmosets, as well as most primitive mammals. Some expansion or caninization of the main cusp of the second premolar (pm^3) is also common among species with three premolars. In primates, extreme enlargement occurs in pm_4 of some early Tertiary prosimians (e.g., Carpolestidae). Departures from the caninized or tridentate model are products of molarization.

Incisors, like the lower central of *Cebuella*, may remain tridentate or primitively caniniform (fig. 1B). In many prosimians, especially early Tertiary Omomyidae and Paramomyidae, the lower incisors are caninized into thick elongate procumbent tusks (fig. 1C). A more common and more successful form of incisor caninization results in expansion or spatulation of the main cusp, including fusion with one or both tubercles. In marmosets, and indeed in most higher mammals, the mesial tubercle, or mesiostylid, loses its identity first, as in i_{1-2} of *Callithrix,* then mesial and distal tubercles disappear from all incisors as in *Saguinus* (fig. 1E). In most higher primates, however, the distal tubercle, or distostylid, persists on the lateral incisor.

Lower incisors of living lemuroids are narrow, subcylindrical, elongate, and rake- or comblike (fig. 1G). The hypertrophy may well be the result of caninization, but loss of tubercles is degenerative. The upper lemuroid incisors degenerated into peglike structures, perhaps directly from the primitive tridentate stage.

The trifid cutting edge of the spatulate upper central incisor of *Cebuella*, and many other primates, appears to be an indication of the lingual vertical grooves and torus between, noted in the upper canines.

Incisivization, as conceived by Butler (1939a, p. 3), refers to differentiation of the incisor field. Incisors per se, however, are highly diversified. They may be primitively tridentate or simplified tusks, premolarlike, or peculiarly structured. Whatever their forms, the evolutionary processes leading to them are *caninization, molarization* including nutricialization (fig. 1D and p. 115) and pectinization or formation of comblike complications as in Dermoptera (fig. 1H), and, finally, *degeneration*.

Degeneration

Degeneration is the process of simplification through *reduction, obsolescence,* and *loss* of a tooth or its parts. Reduction often results in distortions of the original proportions and relationships of parts. As a rule, parts diminish and disappear inversely to the order in which they appeared in phylogeny. Some exceptions to the rule, however, may be more apparent than real. Older dental elements such as the paraconid may have disappeared or were in process of disappearing before later elements arose in the same tooth. Small size as a characteristic can be the primitive size and not the result of secondary reduction. Many styles and crenulations are plastic and often transient. Their absence in an individual or a population may be followed by full or partial reappearance in another individual or the population of a succeeding generation.

Molarization

Molarization is the evolutionary process of complication of the primitive tridentate crown (fig. 2A) by addition of secondary cusps, crests, cingula, or shelves, and other dental elements. Molarization usually progresses from canine to incisors, and from canine to molars. In other words, the more distant from the canine, the more molarized or cuspidate the tooth. In some eutherians, the gradient of increasing complexity is from incisors to molars. Attendant modifications in size, form, and functional relations of teeth and their components are also phenomena of molarization. The end product of molarization is the true molar with a multiple root system and the persistent eocone (-id) forming part of a complex crown pattern. The crown of the mammalian lower molar, a trigonid with or without talonid, conforms to the single basic type described below (p. 108). All therian upper molar crowns conform to one of three basic enamel patterns defined as follows.

BASIC UPPER CORONAL PATTERNS

1. *Zalambdomorphic* (fig. 2B; fig. 3C-D). A single cone, the eocone (paracone), present; true metacone absent; eocrista V- to nearly U-shaped relative

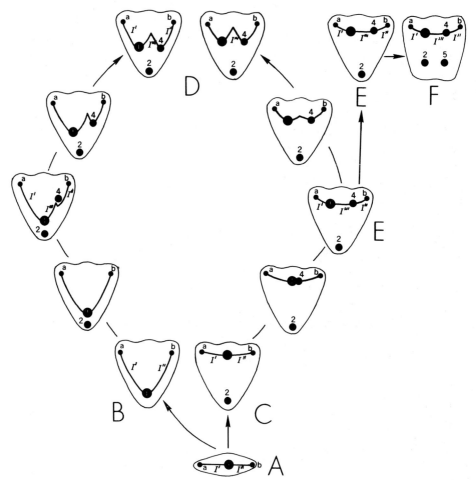

Fig. 2. Evolution of dilambdomorphic upper molar crown pattern (*D*) from primitive tridentate (*A*) through zalambdomorphic (*B*), and euthemorphic (*C*). The euthemorphic line may progress from tritubercular (*E–E*) to quadritubercular (*F*) grades. The same applies to the dilambdomorphic lines. Note mechanics of differentiation of metacone (*4*) from eocone (*1*), in each lineage. Cingula and crests of cones 2 and 5 not shown.

to buccal edge of crown; buccal cingulum expanded laterally into a broad shelf supporting mesiostyle, distostyle, and two to five or more ectostyles; lingual shelf, protocone or hypocone or both undifferentiated, rudimentary, or not more than moderately developed.

2. *Euthemorphic* (fig. 2E, F). Two cones, the eocone and true metacone, the last always present and often as well developed as the first; eocrista roughly parallel to buccal edge of crown, the portion between eocone and metacone more or less straight or folded into a weak angle; mesiostyle and distostyle present, ectostyles, if present, variable in size and number but usually not ex-

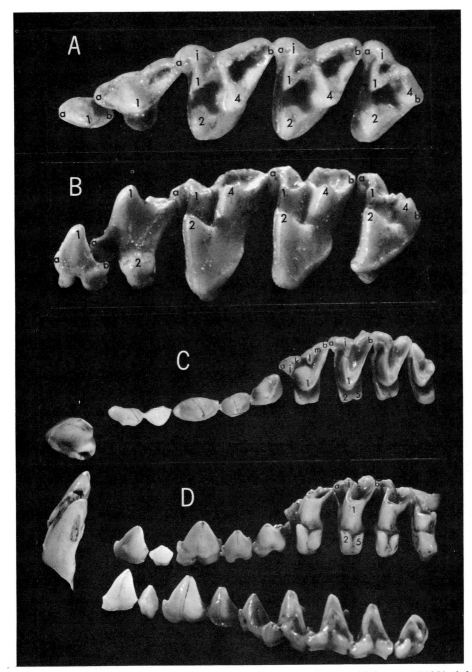

Fig. 3. (A, B) *Nesophontes edithae* (American Museum of Natural History, 17109), left pm$^{3-4}$, m$^{1-3}$, occlusal, and lingual aspects. Compare m^1 with fig. 5M. (C, D) *Solenodon paradoxus* (FMNH 18505), left I^1–m^3, occlusal, and left and right oblique views. Compare m^1 with fig. 5J.

ceeding six; lingual cingulum expanded into a prominent shelf, triangular to nearly square in outline and supporting a protocone or hypocone, or both, and frequently one or more entostyles.

3. *Dilambdomorphic* (fig. 2D, fig. 3A, B). Metacone always present, often larger than eocone; eocrista W-shaped relative to buccal edge; buccal cingulum always expanded into a broad shelf subdivided by a distinctive notch or fold into parastylar and metastylar areas with one to three or four ectostyles; lingual shelf produced into a triangular base supporting a distinct protocone; one or more minute lingual styles, or entostyles, sometimes present.

Remarks. The euthemorphic (fig. 2E, F, fig. 4C) molar could have evolved directly from the primitive tridentate tooth by differentiation of metacone from eocrista, and formation of buccal and lingual cingula, or shelves, with their respective complement of styles, conules, and cones. This molar type characterizes most orders of mammals including primates, rodents, ungulates, and carnivores. It is the tritubercular molar of Butler's arrangement (1939, p. 8). Retention of the more or less straight eocrista and persistence of high domed or conical cusps are the most primitive characteristic of euthemorphic molars.

The zalambdomorphic or V-shaped molar (fig. 2B) is a tridentate tooth with an extensive buccal stylar shelf. A high conical eocone on a low crown appears to have been retained by the Pantotheria and Symmetrodonta. In living zalambdodont insectivores, such as most tenrecoids and *Chrysochloris*, the buccal aspect of the eocone is triangular in outline, tilted about 45° to nearly horizontal, and serves as the main occlusal surface.

Advanced complications of the zalambdomorphic tooth include rise of the plesioconule and eoconule on the eocrista, expansion of anterior and posterior cingular shelves and their union into a lingual shelf, differentiation of protocone, hypocone, and frequently, a second generation lingual cingulum (e.g., m^2 in *Tenrec*, figs. 4A-B, 5K). The first sign of indentation or infolding of the distal enamel border of the eocone marks the appearance of a true metacone and transition from a zalambdomorphic to a dilambdomorphic pattern (fig. 2D).

The dilambdomorphic or W-shaped molar crown can be derived from both a primitive euthemorphic molar and from an advanced zalambdomorphic molar. In the first instance (fig. 2), the W-shaped crown in the E–D series results from a mediad tilting of the buccal aspect of the eocone and metacone accompanied by a flexure of the portion of eocrista (the centrocrista, I'') between eocone and metacone. In the second instance (fig. 1B–D series), a V-shaped metacone is differentiated through flexure of the distal border of the V-shaped eocone. The product in either case is the double V-, or W-shaped dilambdomorphic crown. For example, in the first molar of *Potamogale* (fig. 5L, fig. 7)

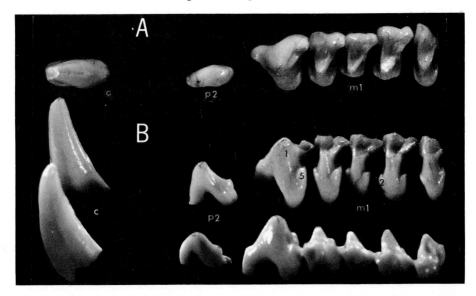

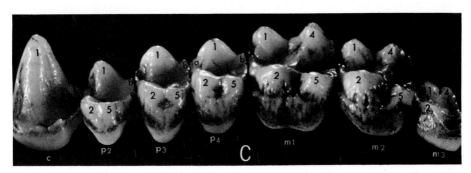

Fig. 4. (A, B) *Tenrec ecaudatus* (FMNH 85515), left c–m³ occlusal, and left and right oblique views. Compare p⁴ with fig. 5K. (C) *Callicebus torquatus* (FMNH 70700), left c–m³, oblique view from lingual aspect. Compare m¹ with fig. 5W.

the first indication of the metacone is a wedgelike indentation of the distal enamel border of the triangular eocone. The deeper and broader the wedge the larger the metacone, and the more evenly subdivided or W-shaped the molar crown. The metacone continues to increase in size at the expense of the eocone. Ultimately, as in *Nesophontes* (fig. 5M, fig. 3A, B), it may become the larger of the two cones in all molars except the last.

So nearly complete is convergence of the two independently evolved W-shaped molars, the one from the euthemorphic molar, the other from the zalambdomorphic molar, that only a dilambdomorphic molar is recognized without distinction of origin (fig. 2).

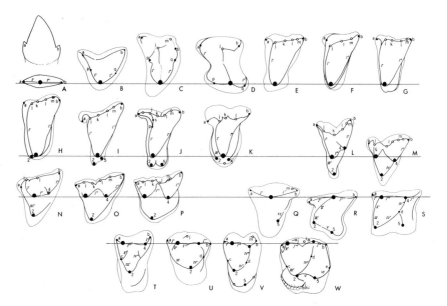

Fig. 5. Basic crown types and patterns of upper cheek teeth. Models are arranged in independent and increasingly complex morphological series. Identical symbols are used for homologous upper and lower dental elements. Red line passing through eocones separates buccal (*upper*) from lingual (*lower*) portions of crowns. Medium-sized black dots are secondary main cones, small black dots are terminal styles (*a*, *b*) and conules, open dots are ectostyles and entostyles, not always labeled. See figs. 13 and 17, and page 136 for complete list of symbols and their respective conventional terms.

Ancestral Mammalian
(A) Primitive tridentate tooth pattern, buccal and occlusal views.

Simple Zalambdomorphic; Crown Buccal or Archaic
(B) *Peralestes* (Symmetrodonta, Spalacotheriidae, U. Jurassic); molar from Butler (1939*b*; p. 342).
(C) *Melanodon oweni* Simpson (Pantotheria, Dryolestidae, U. Jurassic); m² from Simpson (1929, p. 76); see also Patterson (1956, p. 37); dotted lines added on basis of *Melanodon goodrichi* Simpson, Yale Peabody Museum 13748 (cf. Simpson 1929, p. 77).
(D) *Docodon* (Docodonta; Docodontidae, U. Jurassic); molar composite from Butler (1939*b*, p. 331), and Vandebroek (1961, pls. 1, 6, 7, 9); see also Patterson (1956, p. 69) and Jenkins (1969, p. 6).

Complex Zalambdomorphic; Crown dominantly Buccal, Lingual Shelf Present
(E) *Nesogale talazaci* (Insectivora [Zalambdodonta], Tenrecidae, Madagascar); m¹, FMNH 99800.
(F) *Echinops telfairi* (Insectivora [Zalambdodonta], Tenrecidae, Madagascar); pm⁴, FMNH 33948.
(G) *Setifer setosus* (Insectivora [Zalambdodonta], Tenrecidae, Madagascar); m¹, FMNH 85513.

Complex Zalambdomorphic with Lingual Cusps and Styles
(H) *Echinops telfairi* (Insectivora [Zalambdodonta], Tenrecidae, Madagascar); m¹, FMNH 33948.
(I) *Oryzoryctes hova* (Insectivora [Zalambdodonta], Tenrecidae, Madagascar), m¹, FMNH 5641.
(J) *Solenodon paradoxus* (Insectivora [Zalambdodonta], Solenodontidae, Dominican Republic, Hispaniola); m¹, FMNH 18505 (lingual style present in m², as in K. Compare with McDowell (1958, p. 150, fig. 13).
(K) *Tenrec* (= *Centetes*) *ecaudatus* (Insectivora [Zalambdodonta], Tenrecidae, Madagascar); pm⁴, FMNH 85514.

According to Butler (1941, p. 437) the zalambdodont molar, as typified by *Potamogale* and *Tenrec*, could give rise to the dilambdodont molar, as typified by *Didelphis* and *Tupaia*. The tritubercular (i.e., euthemorphic), he believed, could evolve from the dilambdodont. Transition from zalambdodont, or zalambdomorphic to dilambdomorphic can indeed be demonstrated in some cases, notably through the several species of *Potamogale* (cf. fig. 7). On the other hand, the possibility that the dilambdomorphic molar pattern of *Didelphis* and *Tupaia* derives from the euthemorphic as typified by the Forestburg molars (fig. 5N), may be entertained. In this event, at least insofar as marsupials are concerned, it would be necessary to demonstrate that the zalambdomorphic molars of the South American Miocene *Necrolestes*, and those of the extant Australian *Notoryctes*, are secondarily simplified, or degenerate, or that the animals themselves are not marsupials. As for Butler's tritubercular (i.e., euthemorphic) molar, it is certain that the generalized form of the tooth could give rise to, but cannot be derived from, a dilambdomorphic pattern (fig. 2).

CORONAL TYPES AND BUCCAL AND LINGUAL HOMOLOGIES

All elements of the eoconal axis of the tridentate tooth, namely, eocone (-id), mesiostyle (-id), distostyle (-id), plesioconule (-id), eoconule (-id), metacone

---

Zalambdomorphic-Dilambdomorphic; Crown Buccolingual
(L) *Potamogale velox* (Insectivora [Zalambdodonta], Tenrecidae [Potamogalidae], Congo); m¹, FMNH 25973.
(M) *Nesophontes edithae* (Insectivora [Zalambdodonta (dilambdomorphic)], Solenodontidae, Pleistocene, Porto Rico); m¹, American Museum of Natural History 17109. Compare with McDowell (1958, p. 150, fig. 13).

Euthemorphic-Dilambdomorphic; Crown Buccolingual
(N) Therian molar (Subclass Eutheria; E. Cretaceous); molars PM-FMNH nos. 884 and 999 from Patterson (1956, p. 17), the figure reversed, specimens also examined. For discussion and analysis of structure, see Turnbull (this volume).
(O) *Marmosa cinerea* (Marsupialia, Didelphidae, Ecuador); m², FMNH 53351.
(P) *Tupaia glis* (Insectivora, Tupaiidae); m¹, FMNH 76826. Molars of other tupaiids (cf. *Tupaia palawanensis*, *Ptilocercus*), are quadritubercular. The dilambdomorphic molars excludes tupaiids from Primates whose molars are characteristically euthemorphic.

Simple Euthemorphic; Crown Dominantly Lingual
(Q) *Tenrec ecaudatus* (Insectivora [Zalambdodonta], Tenrecidae, Madagascar); pm³, FMNH 85514.
(R) *Podogymnura truei* (Insectivora, Erinaceidae, Philippines); pm⁴, FMNH 74852.
(S) *Podogymnura truei* (Insectivora, Erinaceidae, Philippines); m¹, 74852.

Progressive Euthemorphic; Crown Dominantly Lingual
(T) *Purgatorius* (Primates [?], Middle Paleocene); m², from Van Valen and Sloan (1965, p. 744), the figure reversed.
(U) *Cebuella* (Primates, Callithricidae, Peru); m¹, FMNH 88998.
(V) *Callimico* (Primates, Callimiconidae, Colombia); m¹, Instituto de Ciencias Naturales, Bogotá, 084.
(W) *Callicebus torquatus* (Primates, Cebidae, Colombia); m¹, FMNH 70700. Note the densely crenulated secondary or neolingual cingulum (*D'*) and compare with fig. 1H, where each such process becomes a distinct cuspulid.

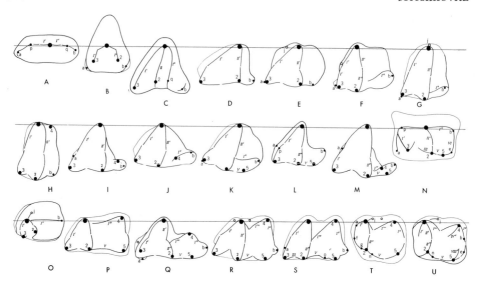

Fig. 6. Basic crown types and patterns of lower cheek teeth. Models are arranged in independent and increasingly complex morphological series. Identical symbols are used for homologous upper and lower dental elements. Red line passing through eoconids separates buccal (*upper*) from lingual (*lower*) portions of crowns. Medium-sized black dots are secondary main conids, small black dots are terminal stylids (*a, b*) and conulids, open dots are ectostylids and entostylids, not always labeled. See fig. 17, and page 00 for complete list of symbols and their respective conventional terms.

Primitive Mammalian
(A) *Triconodon* (Triconodonta; Triconodontidae, U. Jurassic); molar from Butler (1939*b*, p. 352).

Crown Buccolingual
(B) *Spalacotherium* (Symmetrodonta, Spalacotheriidae, U. Jurassic); molar, from Butler (1939*b*, p. 352).

Crown Dominantly Lingual, Primitive Talonid Rudimentary
(C) *Laolestes* (Pantotheria, Dryolestidae, U. Jurassic); molar from Vandebroek (1961, p. 260).
(D) *Nesogale talazaci* (Insectivora [Zalambdodonta], Tenrecidae, Madagascar); m_1, FMNH 99800.
(E) *Tenrec ecaudatus* (Insectivora [Zalambdodonta], Tenrecidae, Madagascar); m_1, FMNH 85514.
(F) *Potamogale velox* (Insectivora [Zalambdodonta], Tenrecidae [Potamogalidae], Congo); m_2, FMNH 25973.
(G) *Echinops telfairi* (Insectivora [Zalambdodonta], Tenrecidae, Madagascar); m_1, FMNH 33948.

Crown Dominantly Lingual, Primitive Talonid Simple to Complex
(H) *Setifer setosus* (Insectivora [Zalambdodonta], Tenrecidae, Madagascar); m_1, FMNH 85513.
(I) *Oryzoryctes hova* (Insectivora [Zalambdodonta], Tenrecidae, Madagascar); m_1, FMNH 5461.
(J) *Nesogale talazaci* (Insectivora [Zalambdodonta], Tenrecidae, Madagascar); m_3, FMNH 99800.

(hypoconid) and connecting eocrista (-id), are strictly homologous wherever they occur in upper and lower teeth whether incisors, canines, premolars, or molars. Elements resulting from molarization of either buccal or lingual sides of the eoconal axis are also homologous with corresponding elements of the same respective sides of other teeth, upper or lower. Conversely, no element of the buccal side of the eoconal axis is homologous with any element of the lingual side of the axis (figs. 5, 6, 8). The coronal types described below serve to keep the morphological distinctions in focus, whatever the coronal patterns derived from them.

1. *Buccal or Archaic Upper Crown.* The essentially buccal crown is characterized by expansion of the buccal cingulum into a stylar shelf supporting two or more cuspules or styles, frequently with one, sometimes two, comparable to the eocone in size. The buccal crown is the primary "trigon" of Gregory (1922, pp. 105–6) and the earliest known form of the molarized tridentate tooth. It is virtually the entire molar crown of Triconodonta, Symmetrodonta, and Panto-

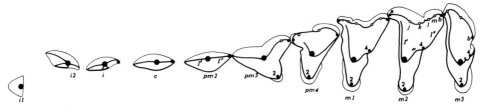

Fig. 7. *Potamogale velox*, occlusal view of upper left tooth row; dental elements labeled in m2, also compare with figure 5J. See page 136 and figure 17 for list of symbols and their respective conventional names.

(K) *Solenodon paradoxus* (Insectivora [Zalambdodonta], Solenodontidae, Dominican Republic, Hispaniola), m_1, FMNH 18505.
(L) *Oryzoryctes hova* (Insectivora [Zalambdodonta], Tenrecidae, Madagascar); pm_4, FMNH 5641.
(M) *Oryzoryctes hova* (Insectivora [Zalambdodonta], Tenrecidae, Madagascar); m_3, FMNH 5641.
(N) *Docodon* (Docodonta, Docodontidae, U. Jurassic); molar after Butler 1939*b*, p. 352), and Vandebroek (1960, pl 8); see also Jenkins (1969, p. 6).

Crown Dominantly Lingual, Progressive Talonid Simple
(O) *Echinosorex gymnurus* (Insectivora, Erinaceidae, Sarawak); pm_4, FMNH 88323.

Crown Dominantly Lingual, Progressive Talonid Simple to Complex
(P) *Echinosorex gymnurus* (Insectivora, Erinaceidae, Sarawak); m_1, FMNH 88323.
(Q) Therian (Subclass Eutheria); molar PM-FMNH 965, diagram based on Patterson (1956, p. 22) only, but specimens also examined. For discussion and complete analysis of structure, see Turnbull (this volume).
(R) *Marmosa cinerea* (Marsupialia, Didelphidae, Ecuador); m_1, FMNH 53351.
(S) *Tupaia glas* (Insectivora, Tupaiidae); m_1, FMNH 76825, 76826.
(T) *Cebuella pygmaea* (Primates, Callithricidae, Peru); m_1, FMNH 88998–99.
(U) *Callicebus torquatus* (Primates, Cebidae, Colombia); m_1, FMNH 70700 (also *C. torquatus*, 70694, Colombia, and *moloch*, 87810, Colombia).

theria, and nearly the whole of most zalambdomorphic or tenrecoid molar crowns (figs. 5, 8A, B).

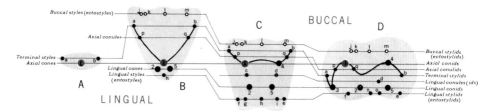

Fig. 8. Cusp homologies: (A) primitive tridentate crown; (B) dominantly buccal zalambdomorphic crown; (C) dominantly lingual euthemorphic crown; (D) common lower crown. Red line passing through red eocones and eoconid separates buccal (*upper*) from lingual (*lower*) portions of crowns; main crest or eocrista (eocristid) shown by heavy line; fine lines connect cusps of similar grade including homologues.

2. *Buccal Lower Crown.* The buccal side of the eoconal axis is unmodified, or marked by a complete or interrupted cingulum bearing one or a few small styles. At best, the buccal crown of lower teeth remains relatively uncomplicated (figs. 6, 8).

3. *Lingual or Tritubercular Upper Crown.* The predominantly lingual upper crown is distinguished by usually well defined axial elements, that is, eocone, mesiostyle, distostyle, and eocrista, with the addition of the protocone, which rises from the anterolingual shelf, and either hypocone, which originates on the posterolingual shelf, or metacone, derived from the distal slope of the eocone. The three cones, whichever the combination, are the tritubercular elements of the lingual crown of the euthemorphic tooth. When all four cones are present, the quadritubercular stage of molarization is achieved, but the coronal type remains tritubercular (figs. 5, 8C).

4. *Lingual Lower Crown.* Molarization of the lower teeth with its proliferations and hypertrophy of secondary cusps, cingula, and crests, occurs nearly or quite entirely on the lingual side of the eoconid axis. This basic or lingual lower molar crown, characterized by a metaconid, is primitive and universal and occludes with all upper molar types (figs. 6, 8D). It is not the homologue of the archaic or primary trigon of Gregory (1922, p. 105) as asserted by that authority.

The conservative nature of the lower molar crown is determined partly by the narrowly limited transverse dimensions of the alveolar space, but mainly by mandibular mobility which permits a set of generalized lower teeth to function effectively against a variety of specialized sets of upper teeth. Upper molar crown evolution is more likely geared to mandibular movements than to possible modifications per se in lower molar form. In some mammalian lines, including all higher primates, the one most important modification in the lower molars, after attainment of their highest grade of complexity, has been the obsolescence and disappearance of the paraconid.

5. *Buccolingual Upper Crown*

A. *Dominantly Archaic.* Most of crown buccal, stylar shelf elaborate; lingual shelf with anterior or posterior cingula or both, rudimentary protocone or hypocone or both; metacone absent (fig. 8B).

B. *Dominantly Tritubercular.* Approximately half of crown buccal, stylar shelf complex; lingual shelf with protocone the dominant if not sole cusp; metacone present but derivation from eocrista identifies it as a cusp of eoconal axis (fig. 8C).

6. *Buccolingual Lower Crown.* Dominantly lingual, the extensive buccal shelf uncomplicated (fig. 8D).

Remarks. Failure to understand or recognize the several coronal types described here and their applicability to *all* teeth, not molars alone, has resulted in confusion of buccal crown elements with analogous lingual crown elements, particularly in comparing upper and lower teeth. The Cope-Osbornian system of dental terminology, discussed later, reflects this confusion.

MOLARIZATION STAGES

Evolution from the tridentate to the zalambdomorphic, euthemorphic, and dilambdomorphic tooth is summarized herewith in terms of stages, each significantly more complex than the preceding. The stages cut across phylogenetic lines and morphogenetic fields. The examples are individual teeth. The taxa they represent range from Mesozoic subeutherians to modern primates. Dental elements are identified by the conventional terms adopted here, and by their respective symbols (cf. p. 136 and fig. 17).

Upper Teeth (fig. 9)

A. *Unicuspid or Tridentate Stage (Eocone and Axial Conules).* Eocone (1) generally large; mesiostyle (*a*), distostyle (*b*), and cingulum usually present; bulge or torus (crista *II*) usually occurs on slope of eocone in system leading to the euthemorphic (tritubercular-quadritubercular) pattern.

Examples: Incisors and canines of most mammals, including many primates, one or more anterior premolars of many eutherians including *Didelphis,* most tenrecoids and all teeth of *Nesogale* except m^3 and variables of m^{1-2} with rudimentary protocone. Most, if not all teeth of Symmetrodonta, Pantotheria, and perhaps Triconodonta belong here.

B. *Biscupid Stage (Eocone and either Protocone [type 1], Hypocone [type 2], or Metacone [type 3])*

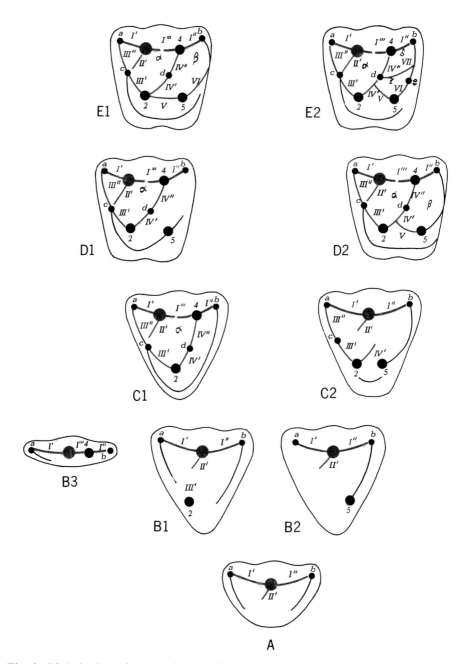

Fig. 9. Molarization of upper cheek teeth; eocone and cristas in red. (A) unicuspid or tridentate stage; (B) (1–3), three types of bicuspid stage; (C) two types or tritubercular stage; (D) two types of quadritubercular stage; (E1) quadritubercular talon stage, (E2) quinquetubercular talon stage.

Type 1. Protocone *(2)* appears on lingual shelf; anterolingual angle of primitive cingulum hypertrophies at this stage or next (Stage C), into crista *III* (protoloph) connecting protocone and mesiostyle *(a)*; protoconule *(c)* present or absent.

Examples: Incisors and canines of many placental mammals including many primates; one or more premolars in all primates; one or more molars in some Insectivora (cf. *Microgale, Echinops, Nesogale, Setifer, Chrysochloris*[1].

Type 2. Hypocone *(5)* appears on lingual end of posterior cingulum; protocone, metacone absent.

Example: Tenrec (penultimate premolar, fig. 4B). The phylogenetic significance of the difference between types 1 and 2 are evident.

Type 3. Metacone *(4)* defined by enamel fold on distal slope of eocone; protocone, hypocone absent.

Examples: Macroscelididae (the canine in all species, and one or two premolars in many species (fig. 10).

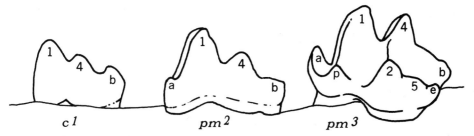

Fig. 10. *Nasilio brachyrhynchus* (Insectivora, Macroscelididae, Kenya), upper canine and anterior premolars; absence of protocone *(2)* in bicuspid c[1] and pm[2] is regarded as a secondary loss. Note differentiation of metacone *(4)* from eocone *(1)*.

The eocone-metacone biscuspid of macroscelidids is not a primary combination. Extensive palatal fenestration has led to degeneration with transverse contraction and apparent loss of lingual shelf including protocone in the canine and premolars of many species. Degeneration of the lingual shelf can be traced through the various described forms of *Elephantulus.*

C. *Tritubercular or Trigon Stage (Eocone, Protocone, and either Metacone [type 1], or Hypocone [type 2])*

Type 1. Metacone *(4)* differentiates from distal slope of eocone *(1)*; crista *IV* (metaloph) extends from protocone to metacone enclosing trigon basin *(a)*; hypocone absent.

Examples: Last deciduous premolar of most living primates; molars of

[1] Van Valen (1967) includes tenrecoids and chrysochlorids in his Deltatheridia, a new order which, as he points out (1966, p. 109 n) should have been called Zalambdodonta Gill, as redefined by Vandebroek (1961, p. 308).

tritubercular primates (notably marmosets), insectivores, marsupials, bats; the tritubercular and dilambdodont molar of authors.

Type 2. Hypocone (5) rises from posterolingual border of posterior cingulum; eocone and protocone present, metacone absent.

Examples: Incisors (variable) and premolars of *Callicebus* (fig. *1*F), premolars of *Alouatta* (variable). In Tupaiidae, last premolar of *Ptilocercus;* in tenrecoids, last premolars and molars of *Solenodon* and *Oryzoryctes;* first molar of *Tenrec* (variable).

D. *Quadritubercular Stage (Eocone, Protocone, and either Metacone Followed Chronologically by Hypocone [type 1], or Hypocone Followed Chronologically by Metacone [type 2])*

Type 1. Eocone, protocone, and metacone present, as in stage C, type 1; hypocone differentiates from posterior lingual angle of posterior cingulum; mesial crista of hypocone may fuse with anterior crista of protocone, or with metaloph.

Examples: Molars of most higher mammals including nearly all primates.

Type 2. Eocone, protocone, and hypocone present as in stage C, type 2; metacone appears fully differentiated.

Examples: Molars of Echinosoricinae and Erinaceinae among Insectivora; possibly *Callicebus* among platyrrhine Primates, and others of the C 2 premolar stage.

E. *Talon Stage (With Four or Five Permanent Molar Cones)*

1. Quadritubercular. Modification of posterior cingulum into broad shelf often with posterior margin modified into crista (*VI*) enclosing shallow talon basin (β).

Examples: Quadritubercular molars of many mammals including those of many primates.

2. Quinquetubercular. Appearance or hypertrophy of postentoconule (*e*); crista *VI* well defined; oblique crista (*VII*) between metaconule and distostyle often present and bisecting talon basin (β) into sub-basins (γ) and (δ).

Examples: Molars of *Saimiri* and *Callicebus* (with individual exceptions).

Lower Teeth (fig. 11)

A. *Unicuspid or Tridentate Stage (Eoconid and Axial Stylids).* Eoconid (1) dominant, mesiostylid (*a*) usually, and distostylid (*b*) always present; pronounced bulge or torus, often with sharp crest (II), frequently present on lingual slope of eoconid.

Examples: Molars of Triconodonta, canines and anterior premolars of most other mammals.

B. *Bicuspid Stage (Eoconid, Metaconid).* In euthemorphic dental systems with paraconid obsolete or absent; metaconid (2) rises from lingual cingulum to coalesce with epicristid (II) on lingual slope of eoconid.

Examples: Bicuspid carnassials; premolars, usually pm_2, often pm_3, rarely pm_4, of higher mammals; molars of many Megachiroptera (e.g., *Acerodon*).

Note: The bicuspid stage, as described here, is a degenerate stage. Phylogenetically, it would follow stage C, D, or E, with loss of paraconid.

   C. *Trigonid Stage (Eoconid and Metaconid with Well Developed Paraconid [type 1], or with Paraconid Obsolete or Absent [type 2].*

Type 1. Paraconid (3) originates on eocrista of anterior slope of eoconid of premolar, moves linguad on molars, enlarging meanwhile; metaconid arises nearly simultaneously from lingual cingulum; resultant trigonid encloses basin (α); distostylid usually well developed, small low talonid basin (β) sometimes indicated.

Examples: Molars of Symmetrodonta, Pantotheria, posterior premolars of zalambdomorphic systems.

Type 2. Like type 1, but with paraconid obsolete or absent, trigonid basin open anteriorly, or more or less enclosed by raised anterior cingulum.

Examples: Posterior premolars of most mammals with euthemorphic dental system.

   D. *Early Talonid Stage (Trigonid, Plus the Talonid Distostylid and either Entoconid or Hypoconid).* Trigonid cones and basin elevated and well defined; talonid with low distostylid and either weak hypoconid (4) rising from eocristid or small entoconid (5) originating on lingual cingulid; short shallow talonid basin (β) usually defined.

Examples: Molars of zalambdomorphic dental system, such as those of *Solenodon* and *Potamogale* (distostylid and entoconid in m_1), *Nesogale* (distostylid and hypoconid in m_3), *Echinops* (distostylid and hypoconid in m_1).

   E. *Advanced Talonid Stage (Trigonid as in C, Plus the Talonid Distostylid, Hypoconid, and Entoconid).* Trigonid elevated above talonid, distostylid as in D, hypoconid completely differentiated by upward thrust and infolding of eocristid; conulids and stylids often present on talonid rim; transverse extension of inner torus of entoconid or hypoconid or both sometimes differentiated as cristid; plagioconulid (d) present or absent.

Examples: Molars of early euthemorphic and dilambdomorphic dental systems. The Trinity Sands therian lower molar (Patterson 1956, fig. 7 [FMNH no. 965]) belongs here.

   F. *Specialized Talonid Stage (Trigonid and Talonid as in E but with Paraconid Reduced, Obsolete, or Absent)*

Examples: Molars of advanced euthemorphic systems such as those of platyrrhines and catarrhines, rodents, most ungulates.

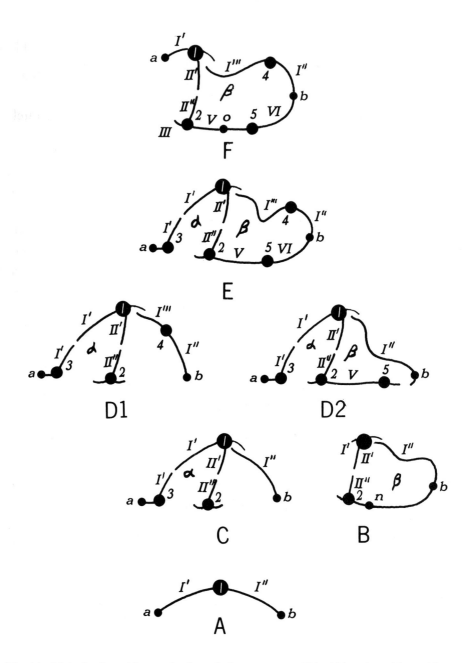

Fig. 11. Molarization of lower cheek teeth (see text page 00); (A) unicuspid or tridentate stage; (B) bicuspid stage; (C) trigonid stage; (D1) early talonid stage, with hypoconid; (D2) early talonid stage with entoconid; (E) advanced talonid stage; (F) specialized talonid stage. See page 136 and fig. 17 for list of symbols and their respective conventional names.

NUTRICIALIZATION

Nutricialization is the adaptation of the newborn's milk incisors, usually the lower, for teat gripping and ingestion of premasticated food. Nutricialization usually involves the splaying of procumbent deciduous tridentate incisors into volar-shaped feeding implements. During expansion, eoconid usually fuses with mesiostylid and, often, the distostylid as well. The shallow spoon-shaped depression, formed at least on the superior portion of the lingual aspect of each incisor, is probably homologous with the trigonid basin of cheek teeth. The lower milk canine also appears to be somewhat nutricialized in some species and may perform a subsidiary or peripheral nutricial function. Milk incisors erode rapidly as solid food becomes a regular part of the juvenal diet.

Nutricial incisors are present in some species of newborn marmosets (fig. 1D). They are also common among cebids (e.g., *Saimiri,* atelines) and Old World monkeys (e.g., colobines). Only those of marmosets have been studied in detail or from an evolutionary point of view.

The least-specialized nutricial incisors among marmosets are the deciduous lateral pair in *Cebuella.* The single worn tooth at hand appears to be caninized as much as nutricialized, but the impression is probably heightened by the fact that the canine is partly nutricialized. The lateral incisor in *Callithrix* is similar, with eoconid remaining dominant, the mesiostylid fused with it, with the distostylid, metaconid, and trigonid basin distinct. Culmination of nutricialization is attained in the splayed lower lateral incisor of *Saguinus oedipus* with main cusp, the two primary tubercles, and the metaconid subequal and surrounding the "trigonid" depression. The more symmetrical central incisor of *oedipus* is expanded distally, the cutting edge trifid as in the spatulate permanent central incisors.

Striking similarities in form, and perhaps secondarily in function, are noted between marmoset nutricial incisors and the simplified upper molariform teeth of Megachiroptera and such fruit-eating phyllostomid bats as *Vampyrops.* Mention might also be made of the first upper and lower molars of the Paleocene picrodontids, as illustrated and described by Szalay (1968: pp. 49, 53, fig. 21). In the living forms, at least of those mentioned, mushy foods, particularly the soft fruits, are dietary mainstays.

Cusp Homologies and the Tritubercular Theory of Molar Evolution

Cope-Osborn Tritubercular Theory of Molar Evolution

Recognition of a common plan in dental morphology based on homologous cusps dates from the discovery by Cope (1883, pp. 407–8) of a basic tritubercular pattern in the crowns of upper molars in Eocene mammals. The theory of molar evolution predicated on this primitive pattern was developed in later works by Cope (cf. 1887, p. 359; 1896, pp. 135, 331), and more extensively and independently by Osborn (1888*a, b,* 1897, 1907). The theory was critically reviewed by numerous authors including Woodward (1896), Osborn (1897, 1907), Gidley (1906), Gregory (1916, 1922, 1934), Simpson (1936), Butler (1941), Patterson (1956), Vandebroek (1961), and Romer (1966). Several rival theories of dental evolution and systems of molar cusp terminology were also proposed and have been reviewed by many authorities, including those cited above. These proposals have had little acceptance and need not be considered here. On the other hand, concepts of cusp homologies derived from the generally adopted Cope-Osborn tritubercular theory must be reexamined in the light of the foregoing discussions of dental evolutionary processes, crown patterns, and types.

In his definitive work on trituberculy, Osborn (1907, pp. 2–7) presented the main tenets of the Cope-Osborn theory of molar evolution in the form of four principles from which I quote or abstract the essence.

I. *First Principle. The Primitive Tritubercular Type.*
   The tritubercular type was ancestral to many if not all of the higher types of molar teeth.

II. *Second Principle. The Origin of the Tritubercular Type from the Single Reptilian Cone.*
   The tritubercular type sprang from a single conical type by the addition of lateral denticles.

III. *Third Principle: Cusp Addition or Differentiation.*
   New dentules, cuspules or smaller cones on the sides of the original reptilian cone [are added by] budding or outgrowth [not by concrescence of discrete elements].

IV. *Fourth Principle. Reversed Upper and Lower Triangles.*
   In the lower molars the reptilian cone is external and the two denticles internal, while in the upper molars the reverse is the case, namely, the reptilian cone is internal and the denticles are external. This principle, if a true one, enables us to establish a kind of [reversed] serial homology between the main primary cone and secondary denticles or cusps of the upper and lower teeth respectively. Osborn expressed such a homology in a system of nomenclature (protocone, paracone, metacone, etc.).

In the same work, Osborn (p. 9) admonished that the

> four great principles of molar evolution *do not stand or fall together.*
> The first or *primitive trituberculy* principle is now almost undeniable
> for the majority of mammals; entirely apart from the disputed ques-
> tion of the original homology of the cusps of the upper and lower
> teeth, there is no question whatsoever as to the beautiful and almost
> incredible homologies between the cusps of the molar teeth in the
> most diverse orders of mammals.

The first principle is indeed generally accepted, but it is ambiguous. Only
the trigon of euthemorphic upper molars is tritubercular, that is, defined by
three main cusps, here the eocone, metacone, and protocone. Upper molars of
zalambdodonts, and the subeutherian pantotheres, symmetrodonts, triconodonts, and multituberculates, are not tritubercular. The trigonid, on the other
hand, is nearly universally tritubercular, although only two of the three cusps
are homologues of trigon cusps.

Simpson (1936, p. 5) suggested that the first principle "alone and without
prejudice to the other three principles," be called the Cope-Osborn theory. At
the same time he coined (1936, p. 8) the single term *tribosphenic* for replacing
the somewhat awkward Cope-Osbornian "tritubercular" and "tuberculo-sectorial," used respectively for the essentially euthemorphic upper and lower
molars.

The second principle of tritubercular origin, as shown by Gidley (1906),
Simpson (1936, p. 16), and others, lacks firm support. The cheek teeth of
earliest known mammals and their probable ancestors among mammal-like
reptiles are not haplodont, and the eutherian tritubercular cheek tooth need not
be derived from a triconodont (s.s.) tooth. Even the apparently haplodont or
conical canines and incisors, present in many eutherians, are secondary simpli-
fications of tridentate teeth.

The third principle, to the effect that new crown elements originate by budding or outgrowth, is basically correct, as is demonstrated by embryological
studies. It fails to allow, however, for proliferation of elements by infolding or
subdivision, or by crenulation (cf. fig. 1H, fig. 5W, fig. 14C, fig. 15C). Nevertheless, the principle as enunciated is an essential part, if not the only valid
part, of the restricted Cope-Osborn theory, and contradicts the next or fourth
principle.

The fourth principle of reversed upper and lower triangles is equivocal and
gave rise to controversies regarding interpretations of cusp homologies, and
cusp terminologies based on such interpretations. Osborn (1907, p. 227)

recognized but failed to resolve serious conflicts between his ideas regarding origin and position of cones forming the trigon (-id), and competing, often conflicting ideas based on evidence from paleontology, embryology, and serial homology.

The hypothesis of cusp rotation, migration, or circumduction, as an explanation for seemingly reversed upper and lower triangles, is usually attributed to Cope (1884, p. 239). This authority, however, only suggested that "shifting of the two subordinate cusps to the inner sides of the principal one will give a tritubercular [lower] molar." Osborn (1888c, p. 1073) concurred but noted that "it has been *assumed* [italics mine] by Cope and the writer [Osborn 1888a, p. 243] that the para- and metaconid were first formed upon the anterior and posterior slopes of the protoconid and then rotated inwards, *but it is also possible that they were originally formed upon the inner slopes* [italics mine]." Unfortunately, Osborn did not elect the alternative. In his diagram (1895, fig. 8; 1907, fig. 4) illustrating origin and evolution of primitive molars, the rotation of supposed homologous upper and lower cusps to occupy vertices of upper and lower reversed triangles, respectively, is explicit. Osborn's diagram is reproduced here with addition of my symbols for cusp identifications to show the true homologies (fig. 12). Evidently, the primary reptilian cusp (eocone) was homologized with the mammalian protocone (*2*), and the mesiostyle (*a*) and distostyle (*b*) of the primary reptilian-mammalian tooth, with the mammalian paracone or eocone (*1*) and metacone (*4*), respectively. In the lower teeth, the mesiostylid (*a*) and distostylid (*b*), were confused with the mammalian paraconid (*3*) and metaconid (*2*). Although the archaic styles (-ids) may shift position with each flexure of the eocrista (-id), the shifting and rotation of cusps described by Osborn are only the shifting and rotation of names applied to inversely analogous upper and lower dental elements.

Evidence for Cusp Homologies

PALEONTOLOGICAL EVIDENCE

Paleontological evidence, as deduced by Winge (1882), Scott (1893), Wortman (1902, p. 41; 1903, p. 365; 1921, p. 178), Gregory (1922, p. 103), Simpson (1928, p. 172), Butler (1937; 1939a) and others show that the main cusp of all upper and lower cheek teeth is the *anteroexternal* (mesiobuccal) cone, the paracone and protoconid, respectively, of the Cope-Osborn terminology, and the eocone (-id) of this paper, following Vandebroek (1961). The same evidence also reveals that all so-called primary cones originating on the lingual and buccal cingula evolved independently, and that rotation of such cusps from buccal to lingual or from lingual to buccal positions relative to the main cone or axis never occurred.

Support by Crompton and Jenkins (1968) of the Cope-Osborn concept of rotating cusps and reversed triangles is based on new material and old explanations but with emphasis on the role of occlusion in molar evolution. The authors (1968, pp. 447, 453) speak of a trigon in the upper molars of Triconodonta, Docodonta, Symmetrodonta, and Pantotheria where the eocone is the only cusp of the eutherian trigon. Likewise, their trigonid in Triconodonta consists of only the eoconid. Paraconid and metaconid, however, are present and complete the trigonid in molars of the remaining subeutherians. These conids are derived from the lingual cingulum and ought not to be misconstrued as errant homologues of cusps which originated on the buccal cingulum of the upper molars. External flexure of the eocone axis with its subsidiary cusps, and internal flexure of the eoconid with homologous subsidiary cusps have also been construed by Crompton and Jenkins as rotation in the sense of a continuous migration of the subsidiary cusps from buccal to lingual zone, or vice versa. The flexures, however, began on a primitively longitudinal axis and curved away from each other in opposite directions, buccally in the upper molars, lingually in the lower. The position of the pivotal eocone (-id) remains fixed. In molars of Triconodonta, with comparatively narrow external and internal shelves and a nearly longitudinal axis, the eocone (-id) is central relative to the entire crown surface. As the external shelf enlarged, the locus of the main cone became more lingual relative to the total occlusal surface. With expansion of the lingual shelf and contraction of the buccal, the pole became more buccal. Changes in relative size and importance of occluding buccal and lingual shelves involve no migration of the eocone (-id), no rotation of cusps, and no inversion of triangles.

It was also suggested (Crompton and Jenkins, 1968, p. 451) that acquisition of transverse movements of the lower jaw during mastication was coupled with cusp rotation. It seems to me, rather, that the transverse jaw movement is correlated with hypertrophy of the internal shelf and differentiation of metacone and lingual protocone in the upper molars, and lingual metaconid and paraconid in the lower.

SERIAL ARRANGEMENT

Serial arrangement from the primitive or tridentate tooth to the complex molar of higher mammals involves a progressive accumulation of homologous elements. This is reflected in the gradient of increasing complexity beginning in most eutherians with the canine and advancing forward to incisors and backward to molars. In other eutherians the gradient is from incisors to molars. The

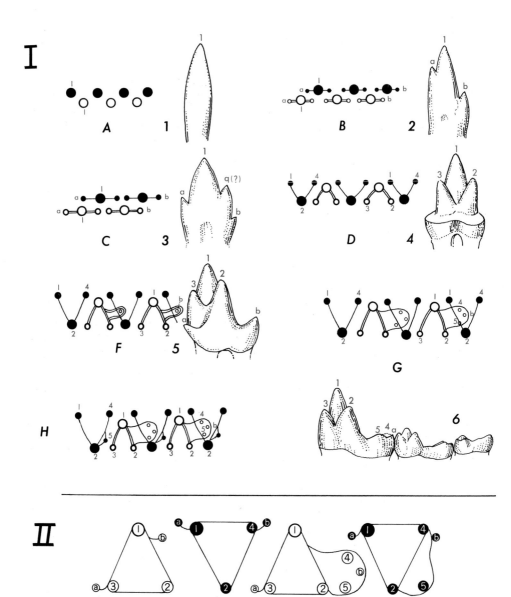

Fig. 12. 1. Reproduction of a combination of essential parts of the original figure 38 (lower teeth) and 41 (diagrams), after Osborn (1907), with the original captions (quoted below), explaining his theory of cusp addition and rotation, or circumduction. Osborn labeled the dental cusps in figure 38, but not the corresponding parts of the diagrams in figure 41. My identification of the cusps and corresponding dots of the diagrams are shown in red, and my comments in square brackets, are interpolated in Osborn's captions for the figures, as follows.

"Figure 41. Mechanics of Cusp Addition (diagrammatic). Compare with shaded drawings [*of lower teeth*] in Figure 38 [p. 50].

resulting molar pattern is well defined and permits the identification of each part of a tooth in any part of the dental system (fig. 16).

The serial arrangement of similar parts is a clear expression of serial homology. It is not a recapitulation of molar evolution. Rather, it presents a morphological gradient from which phylogeny may be inferred. Serial homology is the basis for the so-called *premolar analogy theory* developed by Scott (1893) and Wortman (1902, p. 41; 1903, p. 365; 1921, p. 178), and strongly supported by Gregory (1922, p. 103), Simpson (1933, pp. 265, 269–70), Butler (1937, 1941), Van Valen (1966, p. 2), and others. In the light of present interpretations, it may be more appropriate to refer to the premolar analogy theory as the Scott-Wortman theory of serial homology.

ONTOGENY

Ontogeny reflects phylogeny with respect to the place and sequence of molar cusp origins, and verifies homologies inferred from the serial arrangement of cusps in the tooth row. The first cone of the euthemorphic system to develop and calcify in ontogeny is invariably the eocone (*1*) in the upper teeth and the eoconid (*1*) in the lower. The second cone to develop in the upper teeth, usually the cheek teeth, is the protocone (*2*), doubtfully the metacone (*4*), which

---

"A, the conical stage* (No. 1 [*the conical, reptilian fang shown*].) *Note that the upper teeth (black) bite outside the lower teeth.

"B, C, the triconodont stages (Nos. 2, 3 ['2. *Dromatherium*, 3. *Microconodon*']).

[*Comment: Dromatherium and Microconodon are reptiles, according to Simpson* (1929, p. 2), *the cusp pattern of each tooth, however, is tridentate, the terminal cusps are the terminal stylids* **a** *and* **b**, *not paraconid* (**3**) *and metaconid* (**2**), *as labeled by Osborn in the original figure 38. My labels (red) for cusps of the triangles in diagrams A, B, C, accord with those of the sample lower teeth labeled* **a, b.**]

"D, the first triangular stage† (no. 4 ['*Spalacotherium*']). "† Note that the protocones bite inside of and between the lower teeth.

[*Comment: The lingual cusps of Spalacotherium are paraconid* (**3**) *and metaconid* (**2**). *The lingual cusps of the triangles in diagram D, are meant to represent the same cusps. These cusps are also indistinguishable from those in diagrams B, C. The latter, however, are mesiostylid* (**a**) *and distostylid* (**b**). *Evidently, Osborn overlooked stylids* **a** *and* **b**, *present but not shown in Spalacotherium (cf. fig. 6B) and therefore, confused conids* **2** *and* **3** *with them. This, and other errors of identification, resulted in Osborn's hypothesis of cusp rotation and system of false homologies between upper and lower dental elements.*]

"E, F, G, the triangular upper molar, the lower molars, with triangle and heel (Nos. 5, 6, 7, 9 [5. *Amphitherium*, 6. *Miacis*, 7. *Anaptomorphus*]).

[*Comment: Osborn's no. 7 is an occlusal view, not essential to the present demonstration. The same applies to an occlusal view of 6. Nothing is labeled no. 9 in Osborn's figure 38, but separate occlusal and buccal views of a Homo molar are labeled 8. The primitive stylid* **a** *(in red) is not labeled in the original drawing of no. 5; stylid* **b** *(in red) is labeled hypoconulid in the orignal nos. 6, 7 and in the two original views of 8.*]

"H [*I, omitted*], upper and lower molars with triangle and heel."

II. Diagram showing relationship between homologous cusps of upper and lower molars. There is no rotation or shifting of cones (-ids), only the terminal styles, -ids (a, b) shift as new cones arise between them and the eocone, -id (1). See page 136 and figure 17 for a complete list of symbols and their respective cusp names.

is usually third; the hypocone (5) is usually fourth in the quadritubercular tooth, but it is sometimes third in the tritubercular premolar and molar. Lower cones of the euthemorphic molar system usually develop in the same sequence and in the same position as the uppers relative to each other. Thus, the protoconid (1) is followed by the metaconid (2) or the paraconid (3), if present; the entoconid (5) is followed, sometimes preceded by, the hypoconid (4) in the increasingly complex tooth. The hypoconule (1b) and hypoconulid (1b) are emergent cones and are last to develop in the more highly complex upper and lower molars, respectively. Judged by adult dentition, the order of cone development in zalambdomorphic and dilambdomorphic systems deviates from the euthemorphic in several respects (cf. figs. 5, 6). In the multicuspidate upper teeth of *Tenrec,* for example, the eocone and hypocone are often the only principal cones present.

The ontogenetic sequence of cusp development and calcification outlined above has been demonstrated in man (Röse 1892*a*; Kraus 1963; Kraus and Jordan 1965; Butler 1956; and others), rhesus monkey, *Macaca mulatta* (Swindler and McCoy 1964, 1965), opossum, *Didelphis marsupialia* (Röse 1892*a, b*), insectivores, *Erinaceus, Gymnura, Sorex, Centetes* (= *Tenrec*), *Ericulus* (= *Setifer*), *Talpa* (Woodward 1896), dog, *Canis familiaris* (Tims 1896), cat, *Felis catus* (Gaunt 1959), mink, *Mustela vison* (Aulerich and Swindler 1968), ungulates *Equus, Sus, Hyemoschus, Cervus, Capreolus, Capra, Bos* (Taeker, in Röse 1892*a*; and Osborn 1893), rodents, including *Rattus rattus* (Glasstone 1967), mouse, *Mus musculus,* golden hamster, *Mesocricetus auratus* (Gaunt 1955, 1961).

Summary of Cope-Osbornian Cusp Homologies

Evidence from phylogeny, ontogeny, and the serial arrangement of cusps establishes the homologies between upper and lower dental elements. Cristas (ridges and lophs) and cristids connecting serially homologous cusps are likewise homologous. Minor conules (-ids) and styles (-ids) appearing regularly in similar positions are also homologous. Where the chronological sequence of appearance in either archaic (buccal) or tritubercular (lingual) crown appears to deviate, place of origin and position relative to other cusps, particularly the eocone (-id) are crucial for determination of cusp homologies.

In the following list, the same number is used for homologous upper and lower cusps. The number in parentheses refers to the usual order of appearance of each cusp in ontogeny and in most, if not all cases, phylogeny. Cusp names are from Osborn (1888*b*, p. 927), the synonyms in brackets are from Vandebroek (1961).

	Upper Cusps		*Lower Cusps*
1 (1*a*)	Paracone [eocone]	1 (1*a*)	Protoconid [eoconid]
2 (2)	Protocone [epicone] (see note 3, p. 125)	2 (2)	Metaconid [epiconid]
3	—	3 (3)	Paraconid [mesioconid] (see note 4, p. 126)
4 (4)	Metacone [distocone] (rarely precedes protocone) (see note 5, p. 127)	4 (5)	Hypoconid [teleconid] (see note 6, p. 128)
5 (5)	Hypocone [endocone] (usually precedes metacone in a few forms including *Callicebus* pm³⁻⁴, *Solenodon* pm–m (see note 7, p. 128)	5 (4)	Entoconid [endoconid]
6 (1*b*)	Hypoconule [distostyle] (see note 8, p. 130)	6 (1*b*)	Hypoconulid [distostylid]

Notes on Dental Elements

1. STYLAR SHELVES AND STYLAR CUSPS

Buccal and lingual stylar shelves are expansions of the buccal and lingual cingula, respectively. They are described in a preceding section. In zalambdo-morphic teeth, buccal styles are differentiated from thickened anterior and posterior areas of the buccal cingulum. In the euthemorphic cheek teeth, buccal styles rise from anterior, median, and posterior swellings of the buccal cingulum. Stylar cusps *B, C,* and *D,* of Simpson (1929, p. 119), or ectostyles -*j* (and -*k*), -*l*, and -*m*, respectively, of this paper, represents the three stylar areas. The principal division, or *ectoflexus,* of the stylar shelf lies between ectostyle -*j* (and -*k*) and ectostyle -*l*. Ectostyle -*j* (stylocone of authors) is often enlarged. Ectostyle -*l* or -*m*, however, is sometimes as large or larger (fig. 13).

Any one or more of the primary buccal styles may divide into two or three stylules. The most frequent and significant stylule is *k* derived from *j*. Other stylules are unlabeled and their homologues must be determined separately. Figure 13 shows the primary styles and possible stylules. Stylar cusps labeled *A* and *E* in Simpson's system, are mesiostyle (*a*) and distostyle (*b*), respectively, in the present terminology. For complete synonymies, see below.

The primary lingual stylar shelf is formed by extension of the posterior cingular shelf to the lingual border of the tooth, or by fusion, lingually, of posterior and anterior cingula. The protocone rises from the anterolingual portion of the shelf, the hypocone from the posterolingual portion. A secondary

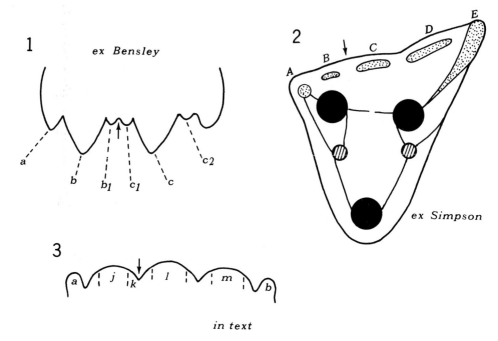

in text

Fig. 13. Stylar cusps, ectostyles, and terminal styles. The arrow has been added to repro-ductions 1 and 2 for showing position of main enamel fold (ectoflexus).

1. Buccal view, from Bensley (1906, p. 6); anterior terminal cusp (a), and three stylar fields ($b + b_1$, $c + c_1$, $c_2 +$ unlabeled cusp), posterior terminal style absent.

2. Occlusal view, from Simpson (1929, p. 119), showing terminal styles (A, E) and three main stylar fields (B [= stylocone], C, D).

3. Occlusal view of system and symbols used in text showing terminal styles (a, b) and three main stylar cusps (j [= stylocone], l, m) with potential subsidiary cuspules indicated by broken lines (k, shown, is most frequently differentiated and helps define position of ectoflexus).

cingulum may then form linguad to but not as high as, the primary lingual cingulum. The secondary lingual cingulum usually supports one to several styles, or may be crenulated. Protocone and stylocone are respective lingual and buccal analogues on the same tooth. The buccal analogue of the lingual hypocone may be either style l or style m.

2. EOCRISTA, PREPARACRISTA, AND STYLOCRISTA

The eocrista extends from mesiostyle through eocone to distostyle. The plesio-conule between eocone and mesiostyle and the eoconule between eocone and distostyle rise from the eocrista. The portion of the eocrista between eocone and mesiostyle, the *preparacrista* (I') is frequently complicated, particularly in zalambdomorphic and dilambdomorphic cheek teeth. The preparacrista may course directly from eocone to mesiostyle (I'_z) through the plesioconule, if present. It may also be diverted (I'_x) to an enlarged stylocone, then continue to the mesiostyle by paralleling the buccal cingulum. This stretch of the preparacrista is labeled I'_v. Finally, the preparacrista may send a branch to the stylocone while the main trunk (I'_y) proceeds to the mesiostyle (fig. 17A).

The stylocrista (IX) from eocone to stylocone may be present, absent or vestigial. It may parallel the preparacrista, and it may become fused or confused with it when the latter passes through the stylocone. One, sometimes, two conules, or *styloconules*, may rise from the stylocrista, or straddle stylocrista and preparacrista should the two run together (fig. 17A).

An analogous case of crista diversion and capture resulting in new alignments can be demonstrated in the transition from the triangular platyrrhine molar pattern to the bilophodont catarrhine pattern as it appears in cercopithecines (fig. 14). Butler (1956, pp. 51–54) discusses the formation and instability of cristas in general with a hypothesis based on ontogenetic processes to account for variation.

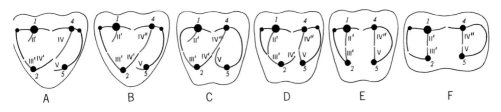

Fig. 14. Mechanics of crista capture and conversion of platyrrhine triangular molar crown pattern to catarrhine bilophodont pattern. (A-E) diagrams showing diversion of crista *III'* and capture of crista *II'* (D-E) connecting cones *1* and *2*, and diversion of crista *V* to capture crista *IV'* connecting cones *4* and *5*. Diagram (A) based on molars of *Callicebus* (with unerupted m³); (B) *Lagothrix;* (C-D) *Cebus;* (E-F) *Macaca.* Stages between B and E are demonstrable in *Cebus* alone. A similar but hypothetical plan for ceropithecoid bilophodonty was devised by Kälin (1962, p. 35).

3. PROTOCONE VERSUS PARACONE IN BUCCAL AND LINGUAL TYPE CROWNS

The main cusp of the buccal or archaic subeutherian crown labeled *protocone* by authors, is not homologous with the protocone of the eutherian (includes Marsupialia) lingual or tritubercular crown (cf. p. 108). The lingual cusp in the buccal crown type molar of the subeutherian *Melanodon* (Pantotheria), identified as protocone by Simpson (1929, p. 7, fig. *e*), is the paracone (= eocone) according to Butler (1939*b*, p. 336). In turn, the lingual cusp of the subeutherian *Docodon,* determined as protocone by Butler (1939*b*, p. 331), shows a crest running buccally to the cusp he labels "paracone." In the primitive lingual or tritubercular crown, a crest of the protocone extends to the mesiostyle, another to the true metacone, but none to the paracone, i.e., eocone. Possibly, the *Docodon* molar belongs to the buccal type and its "protocone" is therefore, like that of pantotheres and symmetrodonts, an eocone. The larger cusp in midcrown labeled "paracone" must then be, as in other subeutherians, a hypertrophied stylar cusp, most likely the stylocone. Patterson (1956, p. 67) doubts that any cusp of the lingual or tritubercular crown save paracone and protoconid (= eocone and eoconid) can be considered homologous with any in triconodont, docodont, and multitubercular teeth.

4. PARACONID AND STYLID-F (PSEUDOPARACONID)

The paraconid in primitive eutherian teeth is nearly as well developed as the metaconid and appears almost simultaneously with it in the molarization progression from anterior premolar to molars. A maxillary homologue of the

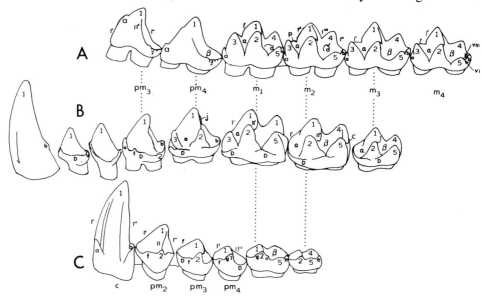

Fig. 15. The paraconid-eoconid, and pseudoparaconid-metaconid relationships. The paraconid (3) originates on the eocristid (*I'*, paracristid), the pseudoparaconid (*f*) rises from the lingual cingulum (*D*) in the metaconid field. (A) pm₃ — m₄ of *Didelphis marsupialis;* plesioconulid (*p*) often present in molariform dpm₄; plagioconulid (*d*), with indications of plagiocristid (*IV'*), often present in one or more unworn molars; cristids *VI* and *VIII* enclose basin γ (not labeled); (**B**) c — m₃ of *Echinosorex gymnurus;* paraconid rudimentary in pm₄, well developed in m₁, absent in remaining cheek teeth; large stylocone (*j*) frequently evident from lingual aspect, as shown. **C.** c — m₂ of *Saguinus oedipus,* stylar process *f* (pseudoparaconid) and *g* are individually variable; additional stylids may be present; eocrista (*I'*) meets lingual cingulum (*D*) in all cheek teeth without indication of paraconid or other cuspids. All parts of each tooth not labeled to avoid clutter; do not confuse label for trigonid basin (*a*) with label for mesiostylid (*a*). See fig. 17 and p. 136 for complete list of symbols and conventional terms.

paraconid is not demonstrable. The "anterior accessory cusp," regarded by Butler (1939*b*, pp. 324, 351, fig. 7*aac*) as the homologue of the paraconid, is probably the plesioconule, an outgrowth of the eocrista. The mandibular homologue of the plesioconule is the plesioconulid, an element sometimes seen on the eocristid between eoconid and paraconid (figs. 6, 15).

The paraconid disappears in most primates (and other mammals) pari passu with advance and increasing specialization of the quadritubercular molar. A reduced or vestigial paraconid may persist in living platyrrhines and catarrhines, but mainly as a rare individual variable, usually in posterior premolars and more frequently in the deciduous than in the permanent series. It appears to be a consistent feature, however, in pm_{3-4} of the Miocene cebid, *Stirtonia tatacoensis* (Hershkovitz 1969). Butler (1939*a*, p. 31) notes a paraconid in dpm_4 of *Brachyteles* and dpm_3 of other genera of Cebidae. He adds that in catarrhines ("platyrrhines" by mistake) the element is present only in dpm_3. I fail to find this cusp in a random sampling of one or two juvenals of most species.

Stylid-*f*, of sporadic occurrence in platyrrhines (and other mammals), rises from the lingual portion of the anterior cingulum anteriad to the metaconid. It is best developed and occurs most frequently in dpm_{3-4}. It may also appear in either or both of the last two permanent premolars, and in the first, and sometimes also the second, molars. The stylid resembles a reduced paraconid and probably functions as such, notably in callithricids which lack the hypocone. Because of the similarities, stylid-*f* is termed pseudoparaconid (fig. 15).

5. METACONE (-ID) VERSUS EOCONULE (-ID) IN BUCCAL AND LINGUAL TYPE CROWNS

The cusp of the subeutherian archaic or buccal type molar crown, labeled metacone by authors including Butler (1939*b*), Patterson (1956), Kermack, Kermack, and Mussett (1968), and as distocone by Vandebroek (1961), cannot be homologous with the same-named cusp of the eutherian tritubercular, or lingual type, crown. This cusp, the eoconule (-id) of my system (cusp *c* of Patterson, 1956, p. 69, and Jenkins, 1969, p. 5), rises as a protrusion or excrescence of the eocrista between eocone (-id) and true metacone (hypoconid) of the tritubercular crown. An analogous cusp, the plesioconule (cusp *a* of Patterson, 1959, p. 69), rises from the mesial slope of the eocrista in the archaic crown, and is sometimes present, usually vestigial, in the tritubercular crown. In contrast with the eoconule (and plesioconule), the true tritubercular metacone differentiates as the result of an *invagination*, or enamel infolding, of the eocrista or distal slope of the eocone. Furthermore, the true metacone appears late in eutherian dental evolution and in molars with lingual portion of the crown well developed. The cusp originates independently in euthemorphic dental systems, and in most advanced eutherian zalambdomorphic systems (cf. *Potamogale*). As a rule, the metacone follows the protocone, sometimes the hypocone, in phylogenetic and ontogenetic sequence of origin and development. The true metacone, like lingual protocone and hypocone, may have its analogue, but evidently no homologue in the archaic or buccal type molar crown of subeutherians.

The eoconule of the buccal type molar crown of late Triassic (Rhaetic) *Kuehneotherium* was correctly identified by McKenna (1969, fig. 2, and p. 219) as a "metacone-like cusp" which together with paracone (eocone) and stylocone (or plesioconule ?) formed a triangle. However, McKenna (1969, p. 224) is ambiguous in his insinuation that this "metacone-like cusp," ostensibly the analogue and not the anlage of the metacone of later mammals, became the homologue of the metacone in such Cretaceous eutherians (includes metatherians) as *Holoclemensia* and *Pappotherium*. His footnote (McKenna 1969, no. 14, p. 225) states that the "metacone-like cusp" tended to disappear in dryolestids but in later protocone bearing zalambdodonts, it is the metacone which "was finally lost as paracone height increased and the protocone decreased." McKenna fails to show a lineal relationship between the subeutherian "metacone-like cusp" and the eutherian metacone, and his detailed sequence of molarization is quite the reverse of what appears to have actually occurred in eutherians.

6. HYPOCONID

The hypoconid, like the metacone, differentiates on the distal slope of the eocristid between eoconid (or eoconulid, if present) and distoconulid. The two cusps, hypoconid and metacone, therefore, are regarded as serially homologous. The hypoconid, however, appears even later in phylogeny and ontogeny than the metacone, and out of phase with it. It is interesting that Butler (1941, p. 446) finds no maxillary homologue (i.e., metacone) for the hypoconid in noneutherian teeth. Thus, of the three cusps of the archaic crown, identified by Butler (1930b; 1941, p. 446) as paracone, "metacone," and "anterior accessory cusp," only the paracone, the acknowledged *main* cusp or eocone, is strictly homologous with the like-named cusp of the lingual or tritubercular upper crown. As I have already suggested above, Butler's "metacone" is the eoconule, his "anterior accessory cusp," the pleisoconule of the lingual crown.

7. HYPOCONE AND PSEUDOHYPOCONE

The hypocone (5) rises from the lingual portion of the primitive posterior cingulum and usually incorporates it. This is often followed by the production of a new cingular shelf on the crown at the base of the hypocone. The anterior crest of the hypocone, or entocrista (V), may connect with the protocone. More commonly, the entocrista curves toward the midline of the tooth and contacts the medial portion of the plagiocrista (IV'), which courses from the buccal slope of the protocone. The relationship between cristas V and IV' is usual in quadritubercular euthemorphic molars like those of cebids and anthropoids. In cercopithecoids, crista V is transverse and meets the buccal or metaconal portion of the plagiocrista (IV'') (fig. 14).

The order of appearance of the hypocone relative to protocone and metacone differs in a number of hierarchies. In a few lineages, the hypocone precedes both protocone and metacone, a phenomenon most apparent in premolars. More frequently, the hypocone follows the protocone and either precedes the metacone, or, most commonly, follows the metacone, thus being the last of the major cones to arise (cf. figs. 4, 5, 9).

Variation in the form and relative sequence of appearance of the hypocone complex and the relationship of the entocrista to other cusps has not been well understood. Gregory (1922, pp. 130, 220) believed that in the presence of a distinct lingual cingulum (actually a neolingual cingulum) a connection between hypocone and protocone, as in notharctids, adapids, and others, indicated differentiation by "budding" of the first cone from the posterior border of the second. The presumed new cusp was named "pseudohypocone," to distinguish it from the hypocone which originates on the cingulum. Some authors accepted the connection between hypocone and protocone as primary, but Hürzeler (1948, p. 19) in comparing the Eocene tarsioids *Necrolemur* and *Nannopithex*, showed that the connection was secondary. Simpson (1955, p. 435n), rejected the discrimination of pseudohypocone from hypocone as a "distinction without a difference." Butler (1956, p. 49), in his discussion of the hypocone, concluded that the "variety of conformations which are observed on the completed teeth may largely be attributed to variations in the time of appearance of the lingual cusps during ontogeny."[2]

In conclusion, the hypocone is the hypertrophied lingual portion of the primitive posterior cingulum. It evolved independently of the protocone, which rises from the lingual portion of the primitive anterior cingulum. Connection of hypocone with protocone by means of the entocrista (V) is secondary and its connection ($V + IV''$) with the metacone is tertiary. Variation in the relationship of the hypocone complex to other cusps is largely determined by the phylogenetic order of appearance of the hypocone relative to those cusps. Ontogenetic variation in the relative sequence of development of the hypocone

[2] In his figure of the *Caenomeryx* m[1], the cusp Butler (1956, p. 48, fig. 9D), labeled "pr[otocone]," is most likely an entostyle on a neolingual cingulum. The protocone, then, is the unlabeled anterolingual cusp, and the hypocone is the posteromedian cusp, as in figures A-C, but with protoconule and metaconule absent.

reflects to some extent phylogenetic variation but also engenders new forms of variation.

The hypocone and entocrista originate and evolve independently in platyrrhines and catarrhines. The hypocone complex increases in size and importance with increasing herbivority. The ultimate expression of the complex appears in the bilophodont or laminate molars of browsing and grazing animals.

Theories regarding the nature of the hypocone and evolution of bilophodonty in catarrhine monkeys were reviewed by Voruz (1970). His conclusions are summarized as follows. (1) The posterointernal cusp of the quadritubercular upper molar is a true hypocone. (2) Bilophodonty in lower molars began with fusion of hypoconulid (*b*) and entoconid (5), an assumption with which I do not agree. (3) Evolution of bilophodonty in upper molars has not yet been satisfactorily explained (but see text above and my figure 14 with explanations). (4) Evolution of the cercopithecoid bilophodont pattern was not completed by the beginning of the Pliocene.

8. HYPOCONULE

The hypoconule (-id) is certainly identical with the Osbornian metastyle (hypoconulid). Historically, the cusp is coeval with the mammalian main cone and so indicated (1*b*). In the tritubercular crown, however, the cusp may appear late in ontogeny, if not wholly suppressed in phylogeny, especially where crowded by an adjacent tooth.

Dental Homologies: Criteria and Generalizations

Most of the foregoing discussion on dental evolution and bases for the determination of cusp homologies can be summarized as follows:

1. All teeth of mammalian dental systems are serially homologous. Deciduous and permanent dental systems evolve independently. Permanent molars are persistent milk molars without successors.

2. Each upper tooth is grossly homologous with the corresponding lower tooth. For example, the first upper molar is homologous with the first lower molar even if all elements of one tooth are not precisely homologous with all elements of the other.

3. Serially homologous (or equivalent) cusps usually originate, develop, and calcify in approximately the same sequence and the same relative positions in upper and lower teeth.

4. Eocone (paracone) and eoconid (protoconid) are the primary, or reptilian cones, respectively, of all mammalian upper and lower teeth. As such, they are strictly homologous and the common base of reference for all cusp homologies. The same cones are also referred to as main cusps or main cones.

5. Serially homologous cusps of upper or lower tooth rows are aligned in a gradient of increasing complexity from canine to incisors, and canine to molars, or incisors to molars, with main cone always conspicuous, if not always largest, and most persistent throughout.

6. Each upper cusp is, as a rule, serially homologous with the lower cusp of same general form and same position relative to other cusps, but particularly the main one (fig. 16).

7. Cingula (-ids) and cristas (-ids) connecting homologous cusps (cuspids) are homologous; conversely, cusps arising in the same position in the same sequence on homologous cingula and cristas are serially homologous. The same applies to mandibular elements. Primitive crest patterns, however, may be disrupted through capture of parts by new crests differentiating from late evolving and rapidly expanding peripheral cones, particularly stylocone and hypocone.

8. The eocone (-id) axis, i.e., the principal axis, is the structural basis of all mammalian teeth. The axial elements, *eocone* (-id), *mesiostyle* (-id) (parastyle [-id]), *distostyle* (-id) (metastyle [hypoconulid]), *plesioconule* (-id), *eoconule* (-id), and connecting *eocrista* (-id), are strictly homologous wherever they occur in upper and lower teeth, whether incisors, canines, premolars, or molars, deciduous or permanent. The teeth of Triconodonta are composed of axial elements only.

9. Buccal side or lingual side, *relative to the primary axis* of each upper tooth is homologous with respective buccal side or lingual side of the corresponding lower tooth (fig. 16), never the reverse, as suggested by Butler (1937, p. 130).

10. The *archaic or buccal crown* (primary trigon of Gregory [1922, pp. 105–6]) evolved by expansion of *buccal* side of eocone axis, usually with addition and complication of buccal cingulum or shelf. The buccal or archaic crown is the only type present in upper teeth of Symmetrodonta and Pantotheria. The upper crown overhangs the lower.

11. The *lingual or tritubercular* crown evolved by expansion of the lingual side of the eocone axis and includes the neomorphic metacone derived from eocone, and protocone derived from lingual shelf.

12. Except for the primitive eocone axial elements common to both types, no cusp of the lingual or tritubercular portion of the crown is homologous with any cusps of the buccal or archaic portion of the crown.

13. The primitive trigonid consists of primary protoconid, that is, eoconid, on the buccal side, and secondary paraconid and metaconid on the lingual

side. The two lingual cusps originated in situ; neither is homologous with the Osbornian like-named cusps of the trigon.

14. Trigon cusps of either archaic or tritubercular crown types are not inverted in position with respect to homologous trigonid cusps; only the Osbornian cusp names are transposed.

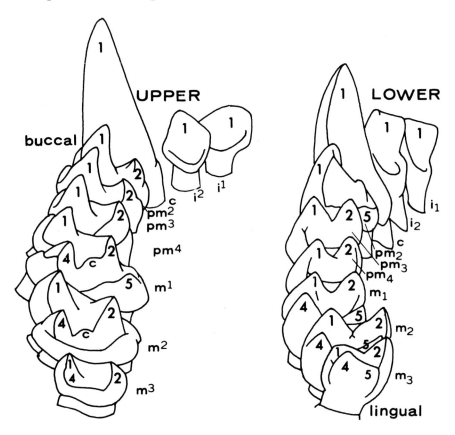

Fig. 16. Right upper and left lower tooth rows of *Callimico goeldii*. Buccal and lingual upper cusps are homologous with respective buccal and lingual lower cusps.

15. Osbornian named homologous cusps of the trigon-trigonid are paracone-protoconid (= eocone-eoconid), protocone-metaconid, parastyle-parastylid (= mesiostyle-mesiostylid), mestastyle-hypoconulid (= distostyle-distostylid). Paraconid without homologue in trigon shears with protocone or occludes with hypocone, by which it ultimately may be replaced as a functional unit. Metacone, with allochronic hypoconid as homologue, shears with protoconid.

16. Talon and talonid are specializations of the distal region of the trituber-cular crown. They extend into or across the embrasure between adjacent teeth and overlap in occlusion with adjacent opposing teeth. The talonid evolved in an early stage tritubercular lower molar (cf. Pantotheria) to permit limited grinding; the talon appears later in the quadritubercular upper molar of special-ized herbivores.

Dental Symbols and Terminologies

The Dual System

The equivocal homologies implicit in the Osbornian terminology were recog-nized early by critics of the tritubercular theory. Nevertheless, the terms have become established and students of dental evolution continue to use them. Others avoid, evade, or change them. In dentistry, purely locational terms for cusps are generally used. Butler (1937, p. 116), in one of a series of papers on dental evolutionary theory, avoided embarrassment by using Osbornian terms for the lower molars only. Vandebroek (1961), guided by true ho-mologies, rejected compromise and proposed an entirely new terminology based on strict homology but patterned on Osborn's system. Those who counter-acted by defending the classical system rejected Vandebroek's nomencla-ture as well as his valid bases for it. Paradoxically, some went on to coin new terms for elements already named by Vandebroek and other workers, including Osborn.

A dual system of symbols and Osbornian type names is employed here. The symbols are used in illustrations and the names in text, but sometimes with their symbols shown in brackets.

In the symbol system, Arabic numerals are used for *cones* (= principal cusps), small letters for *conules* and *styles* (minor cusps), Roman numerals for *cristas* (ridges, lophs), capital letters for *cingula* (peripheral bands or shelves), and Greek letters for *basins* (fossae).

The same symbol is used for serially homologous or equivalent coronal elements of upper and lower teeth. Where confusion might arise, symbols for elements of upper teeth may be underlined, those for mandibular teeth overlined.

The adopted Osbornian terminology is based on a system of prefixes and suf-fixes which signify type, position, and relationships of the dental elements. The suffix *-cone* or *-conid* is employed for the established or principal cusps of trigon (*-id*) and talon (*-id*); *-conule* (*-id*) is used for diminutive cusps or cuspules rising from cristas (*-ids*); *-style* (*-id*) identifies tubercles or "pillars" rising from the cingula or cingulids; -loph (-id) refers to any ridge or crest but the modern term -crista (-id) is preferred. In Osborn's terminology, such prefixes as *proto-*, *para-*, *meta-*, *meso-*, *hypo-*, *ecto-*, and *ento-* referred to the supposed primitive position or order of development of the dental element. Like *proto-* in proto-cone, however, Osborn's prefixes are not consistently valid indicators of phylo-genetic or ontogenetic sequences, or of positions. Nevertheless, many do serve as topographic guides, and the more solidly entrenched Osbornian terms are retained here. The Osbornian terms *trigon* (-id), *talon* (-id), and the suffix -*id*, for distinguishing mandibular elements, are universally recognized.

The Osbornian system of prefixes and suffixes was also intended to imply evolutionary processes and tendencies. In practice, however, the system is typological. It makes no allowance for change in evolutionary grade of a dental element, and as new terms are introduced, the system becomes more confused and contradictory. The Osbornian hypocone for example, is typed as a *cone* despite the fact that it begins as a tiny excrescence in primitive forms. The hypoconid cannot have evolved from a hypoconulid because that name is used for something entirely different which also began as a stylid. Even such Osborn-ian terms as paracone and paraconid, used for supposedly homologous upper and lower dental elements, actually refer to unrelated structures. Revised nomenclatures such as Van Valen's (1966) and the totally new one of Vande-broek (1961) are more precise, but are no less typological. The open-ended symbol system introduced here has the flexibility others lack but does not solve all problems. It provides one sign for each dental element and its homologue, from anlage to the highest evolutionary grade it attains in the mammalian tooth. As new elements appear or previously unused earlier ones need recognition, new letters, numbers, and superscripts can be assigned to them.

A list of explanations of the symbols appears below. It is followed by a cross index which registers all dental terms used here, and others selected from recent literature. Each such term is identified by the name and symbol em-ployed in the text and illustrations.

Names and Symbols for Homologous Dental Crown Elements (fig. 17)

In the following list, the letter or number used as a symbol for each dental crown element is followed by the name or names used in the text. The same symbol is used for homologous upper and lower features in all teeth in all toothed mam-mals. Sources for the nominal terminology are included in the alphabetical list of dental crown elements given below. It is suggested that if symbols are used exclusively for dental crown elements, those for the upper crown may be underlined, and those for the lower crown may be overlined in the conventional manner employed for indicating upper and lower teeth.

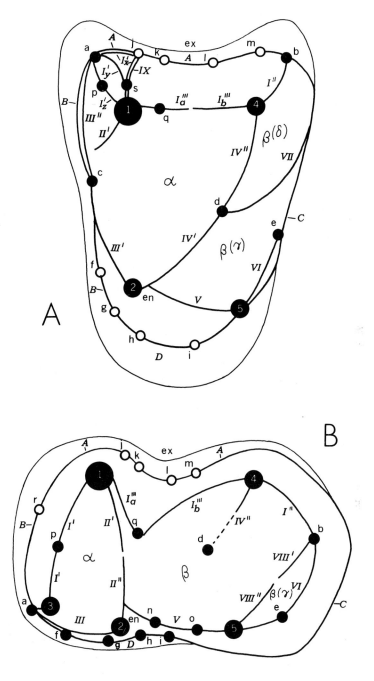

Fig. 17. Master plan of coronal pattern of upper and lower euthemorphic molars. All dental elements present in primitive and early therian mammals are shown: (A) Left upper molar crown; (B) right lower molar crown.

UPPER TEETH	LOWER TEETH
Cones[3]	*Cones*

1	eocone (paracone)	*1*	eoconid (protoconid)
2	protocone	*2*	metaconid
3	—	*3*	paraconid
4	metacone	*4*	hypoconid
5	hypocone	*5*	entoconid

Conules and Styles[4]	*Conulids and Stylids*

a	mesiostyle (parastyle)	*a*	mesiostylid (parastylid)
b	distostyle (metastyle)	*b*	distostylid (hypoconulid)
c	epiconule (protoconule)	*c*	(not identified in specimens examined)
d	plagioconule (metaconule)	*d*	plagioconulid
e	postentoconule	*e*	postentoconulid
f	entostyle-*f*	*f*	entostylid-*f* (pseudoparaconid)
g	entostyle-*g* (pericone, Carabelli's cusp)	*g*	entostylid-*g*
h	entostyle-*h* (pericone)	*h*	entostylid-*h*
i	entostyle-*i*	*i*	entostylid-*i*
j	ectostyle-*j* (stylocone)	*j*	ectostylid-*j* (styloconid)
k	ectostyle-*k*	*k*	ectostylid-*k*
l	ectostyle-*l* (mesostyle)	*l*	ectostylid-*l*
m	ectostyle-m	*m*	ectostylid-*m*
n	—	*n*	postmetaconulid
o	—	*o*	entoconulid
p	plesioconule	*p*	plesioconulid
q	eoconule	*q*	eoconulid
r	—	*r*	stylid-r
s	styloconule	*s*	(not identified in specimens examined)

[3] Most cones are numbered in the order of their origin and development.

[4] Most conules and styles are listed in the order of their position from buccal to lingual and anterior to posterior. Rarer or more variable elements of the tritubercular trigon are listed opportunistically toward the end. Supernumeraries or gemini of established cusps are not distinguished.

Cristas[5]	*Cristids*
[Connecting cusps shown in brackets]	[Connecting cuspids shown in brackets]
I eocrista [*a*–(*j*)–*p*–*1*–*q*–*4*–(*b*)]	*I* eocristid [*a*–*3*–*p*–*1*–*q*–*4*–(*b*)]
I′ paracrista [*a*–*1*]	*I*′ paracristid [*a*–*3*–*p*–*1*]
alternate routes	
I′*x* [*a*–*j*–*1*]	
I′*y* [*a*–(*s*)–*1*]	
I′*z* [*a*–*p*–*1*]	
I″ postmetacrista [*4*–(*b*)]	*I*″ postmetacristid [*4*–*b*]
I‴ centrocrista [*1*–*q*–*4*]	*I*‴ centrocristid *1*–*q*–*4*]
I‴*a* postparacrista	*I*‴*a* postparacristid [*1*–*q*]
I‴*b* premetacrista	*I*‴*b* premetacristid [*q*–*4*]
II epicrista [*1*–*toward 2* or *c*]	*II* epicristid [*1*–*2*]
	II′ [*1*–linguad]
	II″ [*2*–buccad]
III protoloph (protocrista) [*a*–*2*]	*III* protolophid (protocristid)
III′ [*2*–*c*]	[*a*–*2*, anterior (or anterolingual)
III″ [*a*–*c*] crested portion of	portion of cingulum modified as
anterior cingulum.	crest; usually incomplete or
	rudimentary]
IV plagiocrista (metaloph) [*2*–*4*]	*IV* plagiocristid [incomplete or
	obsolete]
IV′ [*2*–*d*]	*IV*′ [absent in present material]
IV″ [*4*–*d*]	*IV*″ [*4*–*d*]
V entocrista [*2*–*5*]	*V* entocristid [*2*–*n*–*o*–*5*]
VI distocrista [*5*–*e*; (*5*–*e*–*b*)]	*VI* distocristid [*5*–*e*–*b*]
VII transcrista [*d*–*b*]	*VII* —
VIII —	*VIII* postentocristid [in two segments;
	5–*b* anteriad to *VI*, but rarely well
	defined]
IX stylocrista [*1*–*j*]	*IX* stylocristid [*1*–*j*; frequently
	obsolete or absent]

Basins or Fossae	*Basins or Fossids*
α trigon basin or fossa	α trigonid basin or fossid
β talon basin or fossa	β talonid basin or fossid
γ post-talon basin or fossa	γ post-talonid basin or fossid
δ pretalon basin or fossa	

[5] Most cristas (-ids) are numbered in the order of their appearance or development in phylogeny, others are numbered opportunistically; all cristas (-ids) except *I*–*I*‴ inclusive, are modified cingula (-ids).

Cingula and Cingulids[6]	*Main Enamel Folds*
A external or buccal	*ex* ectoflexus (between *1–4*)
B anterior or mesial	*en* entoflexus (between *2–5*)
C posterior or distal	
D internal or lingual	

[6] Cingula (-ids) are identified solely on the basis of position relative to the mesiodistal axis of the tooth. The various cingula (-ids) may be continuous between some points and each may be interrupted between any points. Portions of cingula (-ids) may become modified as cristas (-ids), hypertrophied into cusps (e.g., protocone, hypocone), and new cingula may be produced after the old ones, or portion of them, have been incorporated into cusps or modified into crests. Secondary or neocingula (-ids) may be distinguished from the primary ones by adding a prime sign (′) to the positional symbol.

Alphabetical List of Terms for Dental Elements with Synonyms and Symbols

Dental terms used here and by authors listed below are arranged alphabetically; some descriptive and geographic terms are also listed. Each term is followed by a definition, a note, or the equivalent name or symbol used in the text and illustrations of this article. Letters in brackets are abbreviations for the authors of dental terms. Universally understood dental terms and new ones proposed here are listed without reference to source.

[B 37] = Butler 1937
[B 39] = Butler 1939
[Be] = Bensley 1903, 1906
[CJ] = Crompton and Jenkins 1968; Hopson and Crompton 1969
[O] = Osborn 1888, 1907
[P] = Patterson 1956

[R] = Remane 1960
[S] = Simpson 1929
[Sc] = Scott 1893
[Sz] = Szalay 1968, 1969
[Vb] = Vandebroek 1961
[Vv] = Van Valen 1966

amphicone—name sometimes applied to eocone before separation of metacone.

anterior accessory cusp [B 39b] (plesioconule)—**p**

anterior buccal cusp [B 37] (stylocone or ectostyle-*j*)—**j**

anterior buccal cusp [B 39a] (ectostyle-*k*)—**k**

anterior buccal ledge [B 37] (in upper molars, anterior cingulum)—**B**

anterior buccal region [B 39a]—paraconal portion of stylar shelf in dilambdomorph molars.

anterior cingulum—**B**

anterior cingulum cusp [P] (mesiostyle)—**a**

anterior cusp [B 37, 39] (mesiostyle and mesiostylid)—**a**

anterior labial cusp [B 37]—used alternatively for anterior buccal cusp—**k**

anterior ledge [B 39b] (anterior cingulum)—**B**

anterior lingual ledge [B 37] (anterior cingulum)—**B**

anterobuccal cusp [B 37] (mesiostyle)—**a**

anterobuccal ridge [B 37] (paracrista)—**I′x**

antero-internal cingulum cusp [P] (para-conid)—**3**

anticone [Vb] (ectostyle-*j* [stylocone] or ectostyle-*k*)—**j** or **k**

anticonid [Vb]—styloconid in *Docodon* (Docodonta).

anticrista [Vb] (transverse crest of archaic trigon connecting eocone and anticone, but I do not find the combination consistent or the parts always homologous in Vandebroek's samples—see stylocrista and stylocone.

anticristid [Vb]—(anticristid, mandibular homologue of anticrista). See preceding note.

arch—curve of the combined tooth rows in upper jaws or mandible.

äussental [R] (mandibular ectoflexus) —**ex** (mandibular).

äusseres Basalband [R] (external cingulum and cingulid)—**A**

äussere Hypoconulid-Randleiste [R] (distal part of postmetacristid)—**I″** (part).

äussere Talonid-Randleiste [R] (talonid portion of centrocristid, or cristid obliqua)—**I‴b**

Basalband [R]—cingulum or cingulid.

bicuspid—tooth, usually antemolar, with two cones usually eocone and either protocone, hypocone, or metaconid; also human premolar.

buccal—external or cheek side of teeth.

buccal cingulum (external cingulum)— **A**

buccal cusp [B 39*b*] (ectostyle-*j* or stylocone)—**j**

buccal shelf—lateral extension of buccal cingulum.

Carabelli's cusp (entostyle -*g*)—**g**

centrocrista [Vv]—**I‴**

centrocristid—**I‴** (trigonid and talonid parts combined).

cervix—neck of tooth, usually at gum line between crown and root.

cingulum—enamel shelf on one or more sides of upper crown base.

cingulid—mandibular homologue of cingulum (q.v.).

cone—any major upper cusp for which the term may be used as a suffix; the primary cone is the eocone.

conid—any major lower cusp for which the term may be used as a suffix.

conule—primary conules (plesioconule and eoconule) rise as evaginations from primary crista of upper teeth, all other conules evaginate from secondary cristas.

conulid—mandibular homologue of conule (q.v.).

coronal—of or pertaining to crown of tooth.

crenellate—with a series of minute cuspules or beadlike elevations, particularly on cristas or cingula.

crista—crests or ridges of cones and conules, often interconnecting.

crista anterior [R] (epicrista)—**II′**

crista nova [R]—crest from eocone to protocone formed by union of diverted epicrista (**II′**) and lingual portion of protoloph (**III′**)

crista obliqua [R] (metaloph)—**IV**

crista obliqua (see cristid obliqua).

crista posterior [R] (mesiolingual portion of postentocristid)—**VIII** (part).

cristid—mandibular homologue of crista (q.v.).

cristid obliqua [Sz] (talonid part of centrocristid; homologue of premetacrista)—**I‴b**

cusp a [CJ] (eoconid in *Eozostrodon* and relatives)—**1**

cusp a [P] (plesioconule [id] in Triconodonta and Docodonta)—**p** cusp b [CJ] (plesioconulid in *Eozostro-don* and relatives)—**p**

cusp B [CJ] (plesioconule) in *Eozostro-don* and relatives)—**p**

cusp c [CJ] (eoconulid in *Eozostrodon* and relatives)—**q**

cusp C [CJ] (eoconule in *Eozostrodon* and relatives)—**q**

cusp d [CJ] (distostylid or hypoconulid in *Eozostrodon* and relatives)—**b**

cusp D [CJ] (distostyle or metastyle in *Eozostrodon* and relatives)—**b**

cusp e [CJ] (mesiostylid or parastylid in *Eozostrodon* and relatives)—**a**

cusp E [CJ] (mesiostyle or parastyle in *Eozostrodon* and relatives)—**a**

cusp g [CJ] (stylid in *Eozostrodon* and relatives)—figured by Crompton and Jenkins (1968, p. 434) and Hobson and Crompton (1969, p. 22) as the largest of a string of stylids on the lingual shelf. Topographically it compares with the metaconid (2) a cusp joined to the eoconid by the epicristid (II) which is absent in *Eozostrodon* and all Triconodonta. Possibly stylid-*g* evolved into the metaconid of symmetrodonts, pantotheres and eutherians. The same stylid in the very similar molar of *Morganucodon* (= *Eozostrodon, fide* Parrington, 1967, p. 171) was described by Vandebroek as a "cingular denticle."

cusp x [B39a] (entostyle-*g*, or -*h*)— **g** or **h**

cusp y [B39a]—a small supernumerary ectostyle between *k* and *l*

deuterocone [Sc] (protocone or epicone) —**2**

diastema—gap between successive teeth which do not normally touch

dilambdodont—upper molar with main crest (eocrista) W shaped in occlusal view; also the dental system characterized by one or more dilambdomorphic teeth as in many Marsupialia, Insectivora, Chiroptera.

dilambdomorphic—of or pertaining to upper dental crowns with W or dilambdomorphic enamel pattern; used to avoid the taxonomic connotation of Dilambdodonta.

diphyodont—with two sets of teeth, the deciduous or milk teeth and the permanent teeth, including the replacements for the milk teeth.

distal—posterior to or away from line between anteromedian pair of teeth.

distal style (distostyle)—**b**

distoanticone [Vb] (ectostyle-*m*)—**m**

distobuccal cusp [dentistry] (metacone and hypoconid)—**4**

distocone [Vb]—metacone of lingual crown; probably eoconule of buccal crown.

distoconid [Vb] (eoconulid)—**q**

distoconulus [R]—posterior style or styles including postentoconule (*e*) and, possibly, distostylid (*b*) in pongids.

distocrista—**VI**

distocristid—**VI**

distolingual cusp [dentistry] (hypocone and entoconid)—**5**

distostyle [Vb] (distostyle or metastyle) —**b**

distostylid [Vb] (distostylid or hypoconulid)—**b**

Dryopithecus pattern—an inconstant Y-shaped figure formed by union of the main lingual fold (**en**) with the transverse folds or grooves delimiting the hypoconid (**4**) in lower molars of dryopithecines and other hominoids.

ectocingulid [Sz] (external cingulid)—
A

ectocingulum [Vv]—stylar shelf.

ectoflexus [Vv] (ectoflexus, median enamel fold from buccal wall of tooth to eocrista)—**ex**

ectoflexid—**ex**

ectoloph [O] (eocrista)—**I**

ectostyle (any style on external cingulum)
—**j, k, l,** or **m**

ectostylid (any stylid on external cingulid)—**j, k, l,** or **m**

ectostylid [authors] (usually ectostylid-1)
—**l**

endocone [Vb] (hypocone)—**5**

endoconid [Vb] (entoconid)—**5**

endocrista [Vb] (entocrista)—**V**

entoconid [O]—**5**

entoconulid [Vv]—**o**

entocrista—**V**

entocristid [Vv]—**V**

entoflexus—**en**

entoflexid—**en**

entostyle (any style on lingual cingulum)
—**g, h,** or **i**

entostylid [O] (entoconulid)—**o**

eocone [Vb] (eocone or paracone)—**1**

eoconid [Vb] (eoconid or protoconid)—
I

eoconule—**q**

eoconulid—**q**

eocrista [Vb]—**I**

eocristid [Vb]—**I**

epicone [Vb] (epicone or protocone)—
2

epiconid [Vb] (epiconid or metaconid)
—**2**

epiconule [Vb] (epiconule or protoconule)—**c**

epicrista [Vb]—**II**

epicristid [Vb]—**II**

euthemorphic [Vb]—upper molar with main crest (eocrista) more or less

parallel to buccal edge of crown; also, the dental system characterized by one or more euthemorphic teeth.

external cingulum—**A**

fifth cusp [anthropology] (entostyle or Carabelli's cusp)—**g**

fossa externa [Vb] (major fold in lower teeth)—**mf**

fovea anterior [R] (trigonid basin)—α

fovea centralis [R] (talonid basin)—β

fovea externa [R] (deep part or depression of ectoflexid)—**en**

fovea posterior [R] (post-talonid basin)
—γ

Gothic arch—form of dental arch between the V- and U-shaped arches.

haplodont—simple conical tooth with undivided crown.

haplodont primary tooth [Vb]—essentially the tridentate tooth.

Hauptleiste [R]—a principal, or primitive, crest or loph.

heterodont—dental system with teeth of same jaw modified into distinct structural and functional types such as typical incisors, canines, molars.

hintere Entoconid-Randleiste [R] (distolingual part of distocristid)—**VI** (part).

hintere Hauptleiste [R] (mesiolingual part of postentocristid)—**VIII″**

hintere Hypoconid-Randleiste [R] (mesial part of postmetacristid)—**I″** (part).

hintere Metaconid-Randleiste [R] (mesial part of entocristid)—**V** (part).

hintere Protoconid-Randleiste [R] (postparacristid)—**I‴a**

hintere Randleiste [R]—**VI**

hintere Talonid-Randleiste [R] (post-metacristid)—**I″**

hintere Trigonid-Hauptleiste [R] (epicristid)—**II**

homodont—all teeth of the same jaw more or less similar in form and function.

hypocone [O]—**5**

hypoconid [O]—**4**

hypoconule [O] (distostyle)—**b**

hypoconulid [O] (or distostylid)—**b**

hypoflexid [Vv] (entoflexid)—**en**

hypolophid [O] (postmetacristid + distocristid)—**I″ + VI**

hypostyle [O] (postentoconule)—**e**

innere Hypoconulid-Randleiste (distobuccal part of distocristid)—**VI** (part)

inneres Basalband [R] (internal or lingual cingulum)—**D**

interconulid [R] (ectostylid-*l*)—**l**

interconulus [R] (entostyle-*h*)—**h**

internal—lingual aspect of tooth.

internal cingulum—lingual cingulum (-id) formed by union of anterior and posterior cingula (-ides)—**D**

labial—external or lip side of teeth generally, but usually restricted to front teeth in primates.

Leiste [R]—crest.

lingual—inner or tongue side of tooth.

lingual cingulum—internal cingulum (-id) formed by union of anterior and posterior cingula (-ides)—**D**

lingual shelf—medial extension of lingual cingulum.

loph—ridge or crista on occlusal surface of crown.

lophid—mandibular homologue of loph (q.v.).

main cusp (upper)—(eocone or paracone)—**1**

main cusp (lower) (eoconid or protoconid)—**1**

main internal cingulum cusp [P] (eocone and metaconid in upper and lower molars, respectively, of *Docodon*)—**1, 2**

mesial—anterior aspect of tooth relative to long axis of dental arch.

mesial tubercle (mesiostyle [-id])—**a**

mesioanticone [Vb] (ectostyle-j or stylocone)—**j**

mesiobuccal cusp [dentistry] (eocone or paracone and eoconid or protoconid)—**1**

mesiocone [Vb] (plesiocone, cusp of mesial slope of eocone, [Vandebroek] 1967: p. 800]) (plesioconule)—**p**

mesioconid [Vb] (paraconid of trituber-cular trigonid; plesioconulid of non-eutherian trigonid)—**3; p**

mesioendocone [Vb] (plesioconule?)—**p** (?)

mesiolingual cusp [dentistry] (protocone and metaconid)—**2**

mesiostyle [Vb] (or parastyle, often reduced or absent especially if crowded by tooth in front)—**a**

mesiostylid [Vb] (mesiostylid or parastylid)—**a**

mesoconid [Vv] cusp said to be on mid-portion of centrocristid (I‴ **b**); may be the plagioconulid (**d**).

mesoconid—name applied by various authors (cf. Gregory 1916, p. 293, 1922, p. 328) to the hypoconulid or distostylid of *Dryopithecus* molars—**b**

mesostyle [O] (ectostyle-l)—**l**

metacingulum [Vv] (cingular or unmodified stage of distocrista)—**VI**

metaconal area—posterior portion of stylar shelf buccal to metacone.

metacone [O]—**4**

metacone [B]—metacone (**4**) of tritubercular crown; also applied by authors to eoconule (**q**) of archaic crown.

metacone-like cusps (McKenna 1969; 219, fig. 2) (econule)—**q**

metaconid [O] (or epiconid)—**2**

metaconid [Sc] (hypoconid)—**4**

metaconule [O] (plagioconule)—**d**

metaconule wing (Vv)—postmetaconule wing.

metacrista [Vv] (postmetacrista)—**I″**

metacristid [Vv] (protolophid or protocristid)—**III**

metaloph [O] (plagiocrista)—**IV**

metalophid [O] (epicristid)—**II**

metastylar area—portion of stylar shelf distad to the primary fold or ectoflexus.

metastyle [O] (distostyle or metastyle) —**b**

metastylid [O] (postmetaconulid)—**n**

monophyodont—with one set of teeth none of which is replaced during life.

Nannopithex Falte [R; also Hürzeler, 1948, pp. 13–20] (lingual portion of plagiocrista)—**IV′**

Nebenleiste [R] -accessory crest.

nutricial teeth—usually deciduous lower incisors, often reinforced by deciduous canines, specialized for teat grasping and ingestion of premasticated food.

occlusal—crown surface of tooth.

paracingulum [Vv] (anterior cingulum) —**B**

paracingulum [Sz]—area of lingual shelf between **II′** and **III″**, or the anterior cingular or unmodified stage of **III″**

paraconal area (= eoconal area)—anterior portion of buccal shelf buccal to eocone in teeth with metacone present.

paracone [O] (or eocone)—**1**

paracone in *Docodon* [P]—large median ectostyle (or stylocone) in *Docodon*.

paraconid [O]—**3**

paraconule [Vv] (epiconule or protoconule)—**c**

paraconule wing (Vv)—preparaconule wing.

paracrista [Vv] (paracrista)—**I′**$_x$

paracristid [Sz] (paracristid)—**I′**

paralophid [Vv] (paracristid)—**I′**

paramolar cusp (ectostyle-*j*)—**j**

parastylar area—portion of stylar shelf mesiad to the primary fold or ectoflexus.

parastyle [O] (or mesiostyle)—**a**

parastylid (or mesiostylid)—**a**

pericone (any entostyle)—**g, h,** or **i**

plagioconule [Vb] (metaconule)—**d**

plagioconulid—**d**

plagiocrista [Vb] (or metaloph)—**IV**

plagiocristid (plagiocristid)—**IV″**

plagiocristid [Vb] (entocristid)—**V**

plesiocone [Vb] (plesioconule, cusp of mesial slope of eocone present in archaic trigon, usually absent or vestigial in tritubercular trigon)—**p**

plesioconid [Vb] (plesioconulid of archaic trigon)—**p**

plesioconule—**p**

postcingulid [Sz] (posterior cingulid)— **C**

See following note.

postcingulum [Vv] (posterior cingulum) —**C**

Note: *Postcingulum* was proposed earlier by Hershkovitz (1962, p. 74) for the posterior cingulum and the complex of dental elements derived from it, particularly in rodent molars.

postcristid [Sz]—**I″** and **VI** combined.

postentoconule—**e**

postentoconulid—**e**

postentocristid—**VIII**

posterior accessory cusp [B 37, 39] (part, conulid on eocristid between *l* and *b* only)—**q**

posterior buccal cusp [B 37] (ectostyle-l) —**l**

posterior buccal cusp [B 39a] (ectostyle-m)—**m**

posterior buccal ledge [B 39a]—metaconal area of stylar shelf in tritubercular molars.

posterior buccal region [B 39a]—metaconal area of stylar shelf in dilambdomorphic molars.

posterior cingulum—**C**

posterior cingulum cusp [P] (distostyle) —**b**

posterior cusp [B 37] (distostyle [-id]) —**b**

posterior labial cusp [B 37]—used alternatively with posterior buccal cusp —**m**

posterior lingual ledge [B 37]—lingual portion of posterior cingulum—**D** (part).

posterior ridge [B 37] (postentocrista)— **I″**

posterobuccal ledge [B 37] (posterior portion of buccal cingulum)—**A** (part).

postero-external cingulum cusp [P] (mesiostyle)—**a**

postero-internal cingulum [P] (eoconule and entoconid in upper and lower molars, respectively, of *Docodon*)— **q, 5**

postfossid [Vv] (talonid basin)—β

postmetaconule crista [Sz] (transcrista) —**VII**

postmetaconule wing [Vv] (transcrista) —**VII**

postmetaconulid—**n**

postmetacrista [Sz]—**I″**

postmetacristid—**I″**

postparaconule wing [Vv] (epicrista)— **II′**

postparaconule crista [Sz] (epicrista)— **II′**

postparacrista [Sz] (mesial part of centrocrista)—**I‴a**

postparacristid (mesial part of centrocristid)—**I‴a** (mesial part).

postprotocrista [Vv] (metaloph or plagiocrista)—**IV′**

post-talon basin—γ

post-talonid basin—γ

postvallid [Vv]—posterior shearing surfaces of lower teeth.

postvallum [Vv]—posterior shearing surfaces of upper teeth.

precingulid [Sz] (anterior cingulid)—**B**

precingulum [Vv] (anterior cingulum) —**B**[7]

prefossid [Vv] (trigonid basin)—α

premetaconule wing [Vv] (metaloph, part)—**IV″**

premetaconule crista [Sz] (metaloph, part)—**IV″**

premetacrista [Sz] (distal part of centrocrista)—**I‴**

preparacrista [Sz]—**I′**

preparaconule crista [Sz] (portion of anterior cingulum modified as crest)— **III″**

preparaconule wing [Vv] (portion of anterior cingulum modified as crest)— **III″**

preprotocrista [Vv] (protoloph or proto-

---

[7] The term *procingulum* had been proposed by Hershkovitz (1962, p. 74) for the anterior cingulum and the complex of dental elements derived from it, particularly in rodent molars.

crista, part)—**III′**

pretalon basin—δ

prevallid [Vv]—anterior shearing surfaces of lower teeth.

prevallum [Vv]—anterior shearing surfaces of upper teeth.

protocone [O] (or epicone)—**2**

protocone [Sc] (paracone)—**1**

protoconid [O] (or eoconid)—**1**

protoconule [O] (epiconule)—**c**

protoconulus [R] (epiconule)—**c**

protocrista (protoloph)—**III**

protocristid (or protolophid; cingulid C modified as cristid)—**III**

protocristid [Sz] (epicristid)—**II**

protofossa [Vv] (trigon basin)—α

protoloph [O] (or protocrista, primitive anterior cingulum)—**III**

protolophid [O] (or protocristid)—**III**

protolophid [Vv] (epicristid)—**II**

protostyle [O] ("or *tuberculus anomalus.* On the anterior side of the protocone in the upper molars . . . in many of the lower mammals" Osborn 1907, p. 158)—perhaps = entostyle-f

protostylid [Vv] (eoconulid)—**q**

pseudoparaconid [R] (stylid-f or pseudoparaconid)—**f**

quadritubercular molar—upper cheek tooth with eocone, metacone, protocone and hypocone; derived from the tritubercular molar.

Randleiste [R]—marginal crest.

ridge—crista or cristid

seventh cusp [anthropology] (postmetaconulid or tuberculum intermedium) —**n**

shelf—horizontally expanded portion of cingulum (-id)

sixth cusp [anthropology] (postentocon-

ulid or tuberculum sextum)—**e**

style—tubercle rising from cingulum.

style [Vb]—restricted to mesiostyle and distostyle.

style a [B] (mesiostyle)—**a**

style b [B] (ectostyle-j or stylocone)—**j**

style b_1 [B] (ectostyle-k)—**k**

style c_1 [B] (ectostyle-l)—**l**

style c [B] (ectostyle-m geminus)—**m** (part).

style c_2 [B] (ectostyle-m geminus)—**m** (part).

stylar cusp A [S] (mesiostyle)—**a**

stylar cusp B [S] (ectostyle-j or stylocone)—**j**

stylar cusp C [S] (ectostyle-l)—**l**

stylar cusp D [S] (ectostyle-m)—**m**

stylar cusp E (distal portion) [S] (distostyle)—**b**

stylar shelf (expanded buccal cingulum, especially of archaic crown)—**A**

stylid—tubercle rising from cingulid.

stylocone [P] (cusp of stylar shelf usually present in teeth with well developed buccal crown and often joined to eocrista by stylocrista)—**j**

stylocrista—**IX**

talon—heel formed on primitive upper crown by expansion of posterior cingulum, and, usually, by rise of one or more new cusps including hypocone.

talon basin—β

talonid—heel, usually with basin, formed on distal end of primitive lower crown by extension and expansion of distosylid and posterior or lingual cingulum; addition of cristids and new cusps add to the complexity.

talonid basin—β

talonidmulde [R] (talonid basin)—β

talonid notch [Sz]—trough often present in distocristid (**VI**) between hypoconulid and entoconid (or entoconulid).

teleconid [Vb] (hypoconid; "may be considered as developed from the distostylid," Vandebroek 1961, p. 285, footnote 1)—**4**

terminal style (-id)—either mesiostyle (id)—**a,** or distostyle (id)—**b**

tetartocone [Sc] (hypocone)—**5**

transcrista—**VII**

tribosphenic molar [Simpson 1936, 8, fig. 1]—molar type of the basically tritubercular upper and tuberculo-sectorial lower permanent molars of marsupials and placentals.

tridentate tooth—the primitive mammalian upper or lower tooth consisting of a single high cusp, the eocone (-id) and an anterior and posterior tubercle, the mesiostyle (-id) and distostyle (-id) rising from a more or less complete cingulum.

trigon—as currently used, the triangle of the lingual or tritubercular crown formed by eocone (paracone), metacone, and protocone; also applied to the subtriangular buccal or *archaic crown* defined by eocone, mesiostyle, distostyle and stylar shelf.

trigon basin—*a*

trigonid—triangle of the anterior part of the crown formed by eoconid (protoconid), metaconid and paraconid, the latter often absent in systems with advanced quadritubercular upper molars.

trigonid basin—*a*

trigonid notch [Sz]—trough between buccal and lingual portions of epicristid (**II**).

tritocone [Sc] (metacone)—**4**

tritubercular molar—upper cheek tooth with three major cusps (eocone, and any two of metacone, protocone and hypocone); lower with trigonid (eoconid, metaconid, paraconid) but no talonid except, commonly, an unspecialized distostylid.

tubercle—any cusp; usually restricted to a style (-id) or conule (-id), especially mesiostyle (-id) and distostyle (-id).

tubercular-sectorial—see tuberculosectorial.

tuberculosectorial—therian lower cheek tooth characterized by an elevated trigonid and low talonid.

tuberculum intermedium [anthropology] (postentoconulid)—**n**

tuberculum internum accessorius anterius [R] (postmetaconulid)—**n**

tuberculum internum accessorius posterius [R] (entoconulid)—**o**

tuberculum paramolare [R] (ectostyle-*j*; stylocone)—**j**

tuberculum sextum [R] (postentoconulid)—**e**

tuberculus anomalus—see protostyle.

unicuspid—a single-cusped tooth, haplodont; as used in text, a tooth with the main cone only, accessory tubercles present or absent, primitively the tridentate tooth.

vallis externus [R] (ectoflexid)—**ex**

vordere entoconid-Randleiste [R] (distal part of entocristid)—**V** (part)

vorder Hypoconid-Randleiste [R] (distal or talonid part of centrocristid, the cristid obliqua)—**I'''** (talonid part).

vordere Randleiste [R] (paracristid)—**VIII**

vordere Trigonid-Hauptleiste [R] (cristid with buccal and labial parts transecting trigonid basin—not shown).

vordere Trigonid-Randleiste [R] (para-cristid)—**VIII**

wing [Vv]—incompletely modified cingular portion of a crista (-id).

zalambdocone [McDowell 1958, p. 151; Van Valen 1967, p. 276] (eocone) —1

zalambdodont—upper molar with main crest (eocrista) V or U shaped in horizontal outline; also the dental system characterized by one or more zalambdodont teeth as in Docodonta, Symmetrodonta, Pantotheria, many forms of Insectivora.

zalambdomorphic—of or pertaining to upper dental crowns with V or zalambdodont enamel pattern; used to avoid the taxonomic connotation of Zalambdodonta.

zentralmulde [R] (talonid basin)—β

ACKNOWLEDGMENTS
The research on New World monkeys on which this paper is based was supported by the National Cancer Institute under National Institutes of Health contract PH 43–65–1040. Identified fossil material used in this study was made available by my colleague Dr. William D. Turnbull, associate curator of fossil mammals at the Field Museum of Natural History. Dr. Turnbull also graciously placed at my disposal specimens of *Docodon* and *Melanodon* lent to him for examination by the Peabody Museum of Yale University, and specimens of *Nesophontes*, lent by the American Museum of Natural History. My appreciation is expressed to the authorities of these institutions for the opportunity to examine the fossils.

The drawings were executed by Miss Marion Pahl, and the photographs are the work of Homer V. Holdren and John Bayalis.

REFERENCES
Aulerich, R. J., and Swindler, D. S. 1968. The dentition of the mink (*Mustela vison*). *J. Mammal.* 49:488–94.

Bensley, B. A. 1903. On the evolution of the Australian Marsupialia: With remarks on the relationships of the marsupials in general. *Trans. Linnaean Soc. London, Series 2,* 9:83–217.

———. 1906. The homologies of the stylar cusps of the upper molars of the Didelphyidae. *Univ. Toronto Studies, Biol. Ser.* 5:13.

Butler, P. M. 1937. Studies on the mammalian dentition. I. The teeth of *Centetes ecaudatus* and its allies. *Proc. Zool. Soc. London, Ser. B* 107:103.

———. 1939a. Studies on the mammalian dentition: Differentiation of the post-canine dentition. *Proc. Zool. Soc. London, Ser. B* 109:1–36.

———. 1939b. The teeth of the Jurassic mammals. *Proc. Zool. Soc. London, Ser. B* 109:329–56.

———. 1941. A theory of the evolution of mammalian molar teeth. *Amer. J. Sci.* 239:421–50.

————. 1956. The ontogeny of molar patterns. *Biol. Rev. (Cambridge)* 31:30–70.

————. 1961. Relationships between upper and lower molar patterns. International Colloquium on the evolution of lower and nonspecialized mammals, *Kon. VI. Acad. Vetensch. Lett. Sch. Kunsten Belgie, Brussels, Kl. Wettensch.*, 1:117–76.

Cope, E. D. 1887. *The origin of the fittest: Essay on evolution.* New York: D. Appleton and Co.

————. 1893. Note on the trituberculate type of superior molar and the origin of the quadrituberculate. *Amer. Nat.* 17:407–8.

————. 1896. *The primary factors of organic evolution.* Chicago: Open Court.

Crompton, A. W., and Jenkins, F. A., Jr. 1968. Molar occlusion in late Triassic mammals. *Biol. Rev.* 43:427–58.

Gaunt, W. A. 1955. The development of the molar patterns of the mouse (*Mus musculus*). *Acta Anat.* 24:249–67.

————. 1959. The development of the deciduous cheek teeth of the cat. *Acta Anat.* 38:187–212.

————. 1961. The development of the molar pattern of the golden hamster (*Mesocricetus auratus* W.) together with a re-assessment of the molar pattern of the mouse (*Mus musculus*). *Acta Anat.* 45:219–51.

Gidley, J. W. 1906. Evidence bearing on tooth-cusp development. *Proc. Wash. Acad. Sci.* 8:91–110.

Glasstone, S. 1967. Development of teeth in tissue culture. *J. Dent. Res.* 46:858–61.

Gregory, W. K. 1916. Studies on the evolution of primates. *Bull. Amer. Mus. Nat. Hist.* 35:239–55.

————. 1920. On the structure and relations of *Notharctus,* an American Eocene primate. *Mem. Amer. Mus. Nat. Hist.* (n.s.), 2:49–243.

Gregory, W. K. 1922. *The origin and evolution of the human dentition.* Baltimore: Williams and Wilkens.

————. 1934. A half century of trituberculy: The Cope-Osborn theory of dental evolution, with a revised summary of molar evolution from fish to man. *Proc. Amer. Philos. Soc.* 78:169–317.

Hershkovitz, P. 1962. Evolution of neotropical cricetine rodents (Muridae) with special reference to the phyllotine group. *Fieldiana: Zool.* 46:1–524.

————. 1969. Notes on Tertiary platyrrhine monkeys and description of a new genus from the late Miocene of Colombia. *Folia Primat.* 12:1–37.

Hopson, J. A., and Crompton, A. W. 1969. Origin of mammals. *Evol. Biol.* 3:15–72.

Hürzeler, Johannes. 1948. Zur stammesgeschichte der Necrolemuriden. *Schweiz. Paleo. Abh.* 66:1–46.

Jenkins, Farish A., Jr. 1969. Occlusion in *Docodon* (Mammalia, Docodonta). *Postilla,* Peabody Mus., Yale Univ. no. 139.

Kälin, J. 1962. Über *Moeripithecus marcgrafi* Schlosser und die phyletischen Vorstuffen der Bilophodontie der Cercopithecoidea. *Bibl. Primat.* 1:32–42.

Kermack, D. M.; Kermack, K. A.; and Mussett, F. 1968. The Welsh pantothere *Kuehneotherium praecursorius. J. Linn. Soc. (Zool.)* 47:407–23.

Kraus, B. S. 1963. Morphogenesis of deciduous molar pattern in man. In *Dental anthropology: Symposia of the Society for the Study of Human Biology,* ed. D. R. Brothwell, 5:87–104.

Kraus, B. S. and Jordan, R. E. 1965. *The human dentition before birth.* Philadelphia: Lea and Febiger.

McDowell, S. B. Jr. 1958. The Greater Antillean insectivores. *Bull. Amer. Mus. Nat. Hist.* 115:113–214.

McKenna, M. C. 1969. The origin and early differentiation of therian mammals. *Ann. N.Y. Acad. Sci.* 167(1):217–40.

Osborn, H. F. 1888a. The evolution of the mammalian molars to and from the tritubercular type. *Amer. Nat.* 22:1067–79.

———. 1888b. The nomenclature of the mammalian molar cusps. *Amer. Nat.* 22:926–28.

———. 1888c. On the structure and classification of the Mesozoic Mammalia. *J. Acad. Nat. Sci. Philadelphia* 9:186–265.

———. 1893. Recent researches upon the succession of teeth in mammals. *Amer. Nat.* 27:493–508.

———. 1897. Trituberculy: A review dedicated to the late Professor Cope. *Amer. Nat.* 31:993–1016.

———. 1907. *Evolution of mammalian molar teeth to and from the triangular type.* Ed. W. K. Gregory. New York: Macmillan Co.

Parrington, F. R. 1967. The origins of mammals. *Adv. Sci.* 24:165–73.

Patterson, B. 1956. Early Cretaceous mammals and the evolution of mammalian molar teeth. *Fieldiana: Geol.* 13:1–105.

Remane, A. 1960. Zähne und Gebiss. In *Primatologia,* ed. A. Hofer, A. H. Schultz, and D. Starck, 3(2):637–846.

Romer, A. S. 1966. *Vertebrate paleontology,* 3d ed. Chicago: University of Chicago Press.

Röse, C. 1892a. Über die Entstehung und Formatänderungen der menschlichen Molaren. *Anat. Anz.* 7:392–421.

———. 1892b. Über die Zahnentwicklung der Beuteltiere. *Anat. Anz.* 7:693–707.

Scott, W. B. 1893. The evolution of the premolar teeth in the mammals. *Proc. Phil. Acad. Nat. Sci.* 1892:405–44.

Simpson, G. G. 1928. *A catalogue of the Mesozoic mammalia in the geological department of the British Museum.* London: British Museum (Natural History).

———. 1929. American Mesozoic mammalia. *Mem. Peabody Mus. Yale Univ.* 3:1–171.

———. 1933. Critique of a new theory of mammalian dental evolution. *J. Dent. Res.* 13:261–72.

———. 1936. Studies of the earliest mammalian dentitions. *Dent. Cosmos.* (Aug.–Sept.), pp. 2–24.

———. 1955. The Phenacolemuridae, new family of early Primates. *Bull. Amer. Mus. Nat. Hist.* 105:411–42.

Swindler, D. R., and McCoy, H. A. 1964. Calcification of deciduous teeth in rhesus monkeys. *Science* 144:1243–44.

———. 1965. Primate odontogenesis. *J. Dent. Res.* 44:283–95.

Szalay, F. S. 1968. The beginnings of Primates. *Evolution* 22:19–36.

———. 1969. Mixodectidae, Microsyopidae, and the insectivore-primate transition. *Bull. Amer. Mus. Nat. Hist.* 140:193–330.

Taeker, J. 1892. Zur Kenntnis der Odontogenese bei Ungulaten. Inaugural Diss. [original not seen, work cited from Röse 1892 and Osborn 1893.]

Tims, H. W. M. 1896. On the tooth-genesis in the Canidae. *J. Linn. Soc.* 25:445–80.

Vandebroek, G. 1961. The comparative anatomy of the teeth of lower and non-specialized mammals. Internat. Colloq. on the evolution of lower and nonspecialized mammals. *Kon. VI. Acad. Vetensch Lett. Sch. Kunsten Belgie, Brussels, Kl. Wetensch,* 1:215–313.

———. 1967. Origin of the cusps and crests of the tribosphenic molar. *J. Dent. Morph.* 46, suppl., 5:796–804.

Van Valen, L. 1966. Deltatheridia: A new order of mammals. *Bull. Amer. Mus. Nat. Hist.* 132:1–126.

———. 1967. New Paleocene insectivores and insectivore classification. *Bull. Amer. Mus. Nat. Hist.* 135:217–84.

Van Valen, L., and Sloan, R. E. 1965. The earliest Primates. *Sci.,* 150:743–45.

Voruz, C. 1970. Origine des dents bilophodonts des Cercopithecoidea. *Mammalia* 34:269–93.

Winge, H. 1882. Om Pattedgrenes Tandskitte isaer med Hensyn til Taendernes Former. *Vid. Medd. fra Dansk Naturhist Foren.,* Copenhagen, 1882, pp. 15–69.

Woodward, M. F. 1896. Contributions to the study of mammalian dentition. II. On the teeth of certain Insectivora. *Proc. Zool. Soc. London* 1896:557–94.

Wortman, J. L. 1902. Studies of Eocene Mammalia in the Marsh collection, Peabody Museum. *Amer. J. Sci.* 13:39–46.

———. 1903. Studies of Eocene Mammalia in the Marsh Collection, Peabody *Mus. Amer. J. Sci.,* 16:345–68.

———. 1921. Evolution of molar cusps in mammals. *Amer. J. Phys. Anthrop.* 45:177–88.

9   The Trinity Therians: Their Bearing on Evolution in Marsupials and Other Therians

William D. Turnbull

Field Museum of Natural History, Chicago, Illinois

This paper will consider four related matters. The first is a cursory review of marsupial evolution. The second is parallels in dental evolution of marsupials and placentals. The third and most important matter is our understanding of the origins of marsupials and placentals. I intend to review and document the dental features of the Trinity (Albian Age) therians of metatherian-eutherian grade (*Pappotherium pattersoni, Holoclemensia texana,* and other teeth yet unassigned). In conclusion I will propose a revision of certain aspects of mammalian classification based on these considerations.

Marsupial Evolution

The infraclass Metatheria of conventional classifications contains only the single order Marsupialia (see, for example, Simpson 1945). However, constituted in that way it is a very diverse order in terms of the number of genera it contains and the extent of the overall adaptive specializations represented. The approximately 180[1] known living and extinct genera of marsupials are comparable in number to those assigned to the placental orders Insectivora (which today is usually divided), Primates (each with about 165 genera), Edentata (about 140), and Cetacea and Perissodactyla (each about 180), and the adaptive spread is at least as broad as it is in any of these. As an order, Marsupialia is surpassed in number of genera by only four placental orders: Carnivora (about

---

[1] These are conservative counts which vary with a worker's tendency to split or to lump. They are based mostly upon Simpson (1945) and reflect subsequent additions and deletions.

380), Artiodactyla (about 420), Chiroptera (about 200), and Rodentia (about 650), and Marsupialia is nearly as diverse adaptively as Rodentia.

A few years ago Stirton (in Bergamini 1964) presented a marsupial family tree that conveys a reasonably adequate picture of the extent of marsupial diversity and indicates the known or presumed family relationships. He encompassed marsupials within eighteen families, six of which comprise a New World group that, except for its North American Cretaceous origin and a very limited Old World offshoot, is essentially South American. The other twelve families of Stirton's tree radiated during the Tertiary in Austrialia where no native placental mammals occurred except bats, some peripheral marine mammals, and, beginning in Late Tertiary, a few murid rodents.

The earliest unequivocal record of marsupials (North American Cretaceous) has been documented by Clemens (1966, 1968, and this volume) and augmented and reviewed by Lillegraven (1969). It appears that at the end of the Cretaceous, following a limited adaptive radiation, marsupials verged on extinction. The didelphoid *(Alphadon)* line survived into the mid-Tertiary in North America without undergoing a major adaptive radiation. Members of the same line which had trickled into Europe during the Early Tertiary disappeared in the mid-Tertiary, also without having radiated. Other branches of this stock entered two of the southern continents, South America and Australia, where the two major, nearly simultaneous, Early Tertiary adaptive radiations occurred. Hence in the northern hemisphere marsupial history has been marked by early success, followed by a fading away presumed to be the result of an inability to compete with the full spectrum of evolving placentals.[2] In the southern hemisphere the histories appear to reflect greater success resulting from reduced exposure to placental competition. In Australia, where isolation was nearly complete, marsupial adaptive radiation was greatest. In South America, where there was placental competition, but where this was notably limited (especially by the lack of placental carnivores), there was a considerable adaptive radiation of both placentals and marsupials, and the latter occupied the canivore niche. However, in South America marsupial radiation never approached the diversity it attained in Australia.

Recently Patterson and Pascual (1968) reviewed the South American record in detail (recognizing seven marsupial families) drawing upon their own studies and the works of Simpson (1939, 1948, 1967) and Paula Couto (1952,[3]

---

[2] The living North American *Didelphis* is a notable exception. Since its invasion of temperate North America from Middle America it has successfully competed with placentals, and is now rapidly expanding its range. Apparently man, by eliminating the natural predators and by inadvertently offering the shelter of his buildings, is aiding the spread.
[3] A subsequent version appeared in 1961, containing additional material.

1962). In a similar way Keast (1968) reviewed the Australian record (recognizing nine families) relying heavily on works of Ride (1964, 1968), Stirton, Tedford and Woodburne (1968), Tate (1945*a,b,c,* 1947, 1948*a,b,* 1952) and Tedford (1966). Together with their main supporting sources, these review papers offer full access to the literature covering our current understanding of marsupial evolution.

Marsupial-Placental Dental Parallels

Marlow (1960) has reviewed a number of the structural convergences and habitus parallels of marsupials and placentals. Although he noted the dietary basis for many of these, he did not stress the dentition, but instead emphasized body form and ecological niche parallels. Keast (1968) has discussed a few such cases for which ecological, cranial, and dental parallels exist, placing somewhat greater stress on the dental parallels than Marlow did. The most extensive broad comparative dental study of marsupials is that of Bensley (1903), which mentions, but does not stress, placental parallels. Thus I believe it will be useful to tabulate broadly significant types of marsupial-placental dental parallels. These may be categorized as general comparisons and as molar tooth comparisons (see table 1).

TABLE 1

COMPARISON OF MARSUPIAL AND PLACENTAL DENTAL FEATURES

Marsupial		Placental
In marsupials nearly the entire dentition belongs to the first series. Only the last premolar of series 1 is replaced by a series 2 tooth, which is usually a very specialized "premolarized" tooth that replaces a very "molarized" one.	*General Comparisons* Both groups have two functional dental series. These are very differently developed within the two lines, but the so-called permanent molars in both lines are delayed members of the first series. Both groups inherited a dentition that was already serially differentiated, that was fundamentally alternate, and that had a developed embrasure shear mechanism. Early in their histories both showed a strong tendency for fixing the maximum number of postcanine teeth at seven, but the premolar-molar division was different. The primitive adult dental formulas show evident	In placentals the two series are more equally developed. The second series replaces all antemolars of the first, and the replacement teeth function along with the molars. There is less tendency for the last premolar to be so specialized.

TABLE 1—*cont.*

$I\frac{5}{4}, C\frac{1}{1}, P\frac{3}{3}, M\frac{4}{4} = 50$

$I\frac{3}{3}, C\frac{1}{1}, P\frac{4}{4}, M\frac{3}{3} = 44$

Molar Tooth Comparisons
Both groups appear to be composed mainly of forms with euthemorphic to dilambdamorphic, tribosphenic upper molars, but both appear to have had a zalambdamorphic (pretribosphenic?) heritage, and by most classifications both also include zalambdamorphic lines. These may be holdovers from the ancient common heritage. In both, the lower molars are more conservative structurally than the upper molars: there is only one basic tribosphenic type, and it has shown itself to be capable of forming a functional unit with each of the kinds of tribosphenic upper molars. This ability appears to derive from the mobility of the lower jaw. Whereas the upper molars evolved from the primitive buccal crown stage of the pre-Cretaceous mammals to the buccolingual one, and on to the predominantly lingual one (see Vandebroek 1967; Hershkovitz, this volume), the mobile lower molars were able to accommodate in large part by positioning the jaw so as to maintain a functional occlusal relationship.

Examples of forms with zalambdamorphic molars are:

Notoryctes, Necrolestes

Zalambdalestes, Deltatheridium, Oryzoryctes, Palaeoryctes, Chryso-

TABLE 1—*cont.*

		chloris, Tenrec, Nesogale, Setifer, Solenodon, Potomogale
Holoclemensia	The primitive euthemorphic type of molar is found in the Trinity therians (whether they are assigned to Marsupialia or Placentalia or left unassigned). They are:	*Pappotherium*
Pediomys, Didelphis, Dasyurus, Marmosa, Phascogale, Sarcophilis, Thylacinus, Peroryctes, Macrotis	Later examples of euthemorphic molars are numerous and intergrading; they range from the basically tritubercular to the more specialized incipiently quadritubercular and the fully quadritubercular (euthemorphic and dilambdamorphic) types. Examples of forms with simple tritubercular molars are:	*Gypsonictops, Cimolestes, Procerberus, Batodon, Palaechton, Nesophontes, Tupaia, Purgatorius, Euroscaptor, Condylura, Talpa, Scapanus, Cynocephalus, Galeopterus, Eptisicus*
Pediomys, Perameles	Forms with the incipiently quadritubercular molars are:	*Mixodectes, Paromomys, Omomys, Tricentes, Notharctus, Tarsius, Ictops, Paleosinopa, Europsilus, Rhinolophus, Urogale, Paramys*
Echimypera, Isoödon, Caenolestes, Petaurus, Burramys, Trichosurus, Wallabia	Examples of forms with quadritubercular molars are:	*Erinaceus, Echinosorex, Esthonyx, Sorex, Elephantulus, Nasilio, Perodictis, Nycticebus, Crocidura,*

TABLE 1—*cont.*

Suncus, Blarina, Hemiechinus, Hylomys, Hyopsodus

Within both marsupials and placentals it is common to find other specializations superimposed upon these major levels of molar specialization (including many of the examples given). This is especially true at the quadritubercular level. Features such as crest proliferation (with the accompanying valleys and pits), or loph specialization that may be found in one group often have remarkably exact equivalents in the other. Crenulation (or other enamel ornamentation), hyposodonty, secondary proliferation or reduction of the number of teeth in the molar series, and tooth simplification and degeneration are all features found in both groups.

Examples are:

Crest proliferation

phascolarctines and pseudocheirines

many selenodont artiodactyls, perissodactyls, and notoungulates

Loph specialization

macropodids and diprotodontids

tapiroids and some mastodonts

Crenulation

phascolarctines, some pseudocheirines, some species of *Phalanger*

some paramyid rodents, as *Thisbemys,* also some primates

Advanced hypsodonty
(but with pattern simplification)

wombats

Stylinodon, many edentates, and various rodents

(Advanced hypsodonty without pattern simplification is not found in marsupials, but is common in many placental orders; it occurs in many pe-

TABLE 1—*cont.*

	rissodactyls, artiodactyls, and rodents.)	
	Secondary additions to the primitive tooth number (usually accompanied by tooth simplification)	
Myrmecobius		many of the toothed whales (*Inia, Tursiops, Sotalia*)
	Secondary reduction of the primitive tooth number (usually accompanied by tooth simplification or degeneration, sometimes by extreme specialization of one or a few teeth)	
several pygmy possums (phalangerids)		many carnivores, some rodents
	Simplification and degeneration	
Tarsipes, Myrmecobius		some rodents, such as *Rhynchomys,* orycteropids, the carnivore *Proteles,* many cetaceans, myrmecophagids, pholidotids

This listing should suffice to point up the great potential of marsupials for providing a varied basis for dental morphological study which is remarkably comparable to that of the placentals. This and the ease of obtaining early developmental stages (pouch young) make marsupials ideally suited for tissue culture studies as well as for natural developmental and morphogenetic work.

It is possible, of course, to extend this sort of comparison to dental regions other than the molar field, and there follows one example pertaining to each of the other three dental regions:

Premolar region. The last premolar, which is commonly specialized in marsupials, is much less apt to be specialized in placentals, and yet there are a number of cases where placental tendencies in this direction are apparent. The multituberculate-like sectorial found in one of the early primate lines (carpolestid) is a good example.

Canine Region. Here the range of adaptations parallel in the two groups. The most striking example is the saber of the placental sabertooth cat *Smilodon* and that of the sabertoothed marsupial *Thyacosmilus.*

Incisor region. The parallels here are usually associated with rodentlike or ungulatelike diastemal developments, involving the canine area and often portions of premolar and incisor fields adjacent to it. In the former case wombats and rodents are examples, and in the latter macropods and many advanced ungulates will serve, *Macropus* and *Myotragus* being striking examples.

The considerable marsupial diversity prompted Ride (1964) to divide the classic Marsupialia into four orders: Marsupicarnivora (superfamilies Didelphoidea, Borhyaenoidea, and Dasyuroidea),[4] Paucituberculata (Caenolestidae and Polydolopidae), Peramelina (only Peramelidae), and Diprotodonta (Phalangeridae, Wynyardiidae, Vombatidae, Diprotodontidae, and Macropodidae). This was a logical and, I believe, justifiable move in the face of the generic and specific diversity, and the kind and degree of morphological differentiation, evidenced by the marsupials. It has the great advantages of putting marsupial and placental lines on a more comparable basis, of giving formal recognition to the known marsupial diversity, and hence of improving the perspective of our overall view of the mammalia—all needs pointed up by Cain (1959) in a discussion of phylogenetic weighting.

Recently Kirsch (1968), using serological data, has put forth a proposal similar to Ride's, in which he too agrees in principle that the marsupials represent several orders—he thinks three. The major difference[5] between his classification and Ride's is in ranking of the peramelids. Kirsch considers them as a suborder of his O. Polyprotodonta (essentially Ride's O. Marsupicarnivora), whereas Ride gave them full ordinal status. There appears to be agreement about their occupying an intermediate position between the Australian dasyuroid marsupicarnivorans and the Diprotodonta. I tend to favor Ride's scheme because it emphasizes the differences between peramelids and dasyuroids and because it is more broadly based. The current approximate counts of genera and species (living and extinct) for Ride's four marsupialian orders are as follows: O. Marsupicarnivora, 80 genera, 178 species; O. Paucituberculata, 21 genera, 44 species; O. Peramelina, 10 genera, 22 species; and O. Diprotodonta, 70 genera, 152 species. The list reflects a significant increase over Ride's list, owing to recent reports of Australian fossils.

Both this amount of diversity within marsupials and the many accompanying parallelisms and convergences that have evolved between Marsupialia and Placentalia appear to be the result of three primary factors: (1) their similar genetic base resulting from their common origins; (2) the vast amount of time

[4] He excluded Notoryctidae, which he left *incertae sedis* within the superorder Marsupialia.
[5] Other differences suggested on serological grounds are (*a*) that Phascolarctidae (s.s.) is near Vombatidae and is removed from the pseudocheirines and (*b*) that Pseudocheirinae and Petaurinae are close, comprising Petauridae, and (*c*) that *Tarsipes* is well removed from the other phalangeroids. Wegner (1964) revived the old notion of wombat-koala relationship on morphological grounds, but the dental and general cranial morphology argue against this; hence the serological evidence is of interest, but I am uncertain about the interpretation of it.

available (over 60 MY since separation of the stocks); and (3) the continental, or greater, scale of the geographic ranges open to each group. Throughout the Tertiary the placentals dominated the holarctic continents and Africa almost exclusively because of their superior competitive abilities or, in parts of this range, through isolation, and the marsupials dominated Australia, also almost exclusively, because of the protection of their nearly complete isolation there. Only in South America did a more nearly equal sharing of the environment long endure.

Evidence of the Trinity Therians

The therian mammals of the Trinity formation Albian (Early Cretaceous) Age of North Texas were originally described as being at metatherian-eutherian grade by Patterson (1956). He chose this procedure because collectively they represented a stage of therian evolution more advanced than that shown by the Jurassic eupantotheres, but not yet specialized enough for metatherian or eutherian distinctiveness to have become apparent. Patterson demonstrated two basic morphological types of upper therian molars and three of lower molars. For nearly a decade his work, based upon a score of specimens, stood as the sole published record of these important therians. Slaughter (1965), working on similar material from a nearby locality of equivalent horizon (eight additional specimens), continued this procedure. He described and named one taxon, *Pappotherium pattersoni,* based upon a single specimen (SMP-SMU 71725), a maxillary fragment with the last two molar teeth in position. For this specimen he erected a new family, Pappotheriidae, which he left unassigned at the ordinal and infraclass levels, and he indicated that one of Patterson's upper molar types (represented by PM 884, PM 999, PM 1075) corresponded morphologically with the type of *P. pattersoni.* At the same time he demonstrated that his material represented three additional types of lower molars. Hence there are now described two kinds of upper and six kinds of lower molars belonging to Trinity therians.

At about the same time, Clemens (1966) was further considering the original Albian therians as being very nearly ideal probable ancestors (i.e., protomarsupials) of the as yet undiscovered oldest (he presumed Mid-Cretaceous) marsupials and the known Late Cretaceous and Tertiary marsupials. Critical to this interpretation was his analysis of the trends and developments of the stylar shelf of the upper molars of the Albian therians compared with the Late Cretaceous marsupials under study. In addition to placing the Trinity therians at the base of the marsupial radiation, he implied that they could almost as well serve the placental radiation as protoplacentals. Thus the first three workers have substantially agreed that the Trinity therians are at a metatherian-eutherian grade.

Since then, Van Valen (1966) and Romer (1966) have both assigned the Pappotheriidae to the Insectivora, without commenting on the status or position of those Trinity therian teeth that have not been assigned. Recently Slaughter (1968*a*) described some premolars which, on the basis of their submolariform morphology, he assigned to the Eutheria, noting that they were too large to belong to *P. pattersoni*. Later in the year (1968*b, c*) he described and named *Holoclemensia texana*, based upon further new materials, two isolated upper molars (SMP-SMU 61997 and 62009) and a referred lower of the type 5 configuration. These he assigned to the marsupial family Didelphidae, largely on the basis of features of the stylar shelf. Subsequently Hopson and Crompton (1969) have apparently accepted Pappotheriidae (without commenting on what if anything beyond *Pappotherium* is encompassed within that family) as basal to both meta- and eutheria (p. 59). Most recently McKenna (1969) has cautiously treated *Holoclemensia* and *Pappotherium* as early precursors of Metatheria and Eutheria respectively; yet his phylogenetic chart implies an acceptance of that dichotomy by Albian time (p. 230).

Now that criteria for differentiating the two groups at this early evolutionary stage have been proposed and we are beginning to see assignments for certain of the Trinity therians to Metatheria or Eutheria, it seems appropriate and necessary to reconsider the original collection in the light of these assignments. In so doing I shall try to determine a broader set of criteria for distinguishing early metatherians from early eutherians, if indeed this is possible at this time.

Recalling that two types of upper molars and six types of lowers have been recognized by Patterson and Slaughter, I have critically reexamined all the Field Museum specimens, figures 2, 3, 5, 6, (those available to Patterson in 1956, and a few recovered since then) and have compared them in detail with Slaughter's published descriptions. As a result, I have made a generic assignment for each tooth, but in most cases have left the species indeterminate. An amended set of diagnostic criteria follows:

Upper Molars (figs. 1*a, b,* 2, 3)

Fig. 1. Schematic outline diagrams of the Trinity therian upper molar teeth. Standard outline patterns are used for all such teeth assigned to *Holoclemensia* and *Pappotherium* except last upper molars. This is done to connote the basic similarity of these teeth in both taxa. With the last molars, the differing outlines used indicate consistent differences between the two taxa. Cross-hatching marks areas missing on a specimen because of breakage. Ridges, valleys, and cusps shown within hatched areas are hypothetical and are dotted. They conform with the pattern suggested by the other teeth. The ancient eocrista (*heavy black line*) and its associated ancient cusp, the paracone, or eocone (*large black circle*), and the ancient terminal styles (*small black circles*) which are common to metatherian and eutherian lineages (as well as to others—see Vandebroek 1961, and summary by

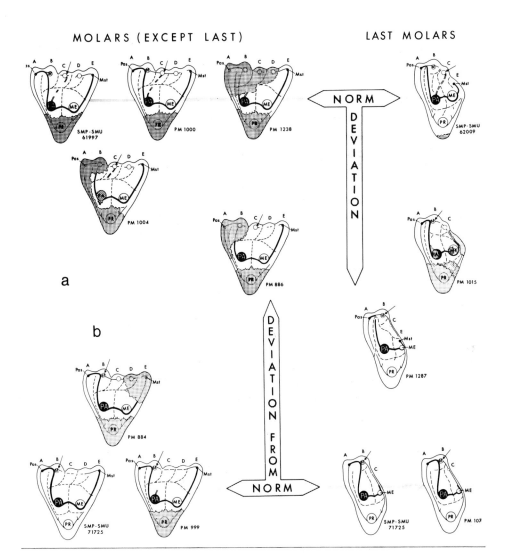

Hershkovitz, this volume) are indicated. Note especially the relationship of the anterior portion of the eocrista to the stylocone. Open circles represent cusps: those of the trigon (*PA, ME, PR*) are labeled and the stylar cusps are lettered *A* thru *E* (following Simpson and Bensley). In addition, parastyle, stylocone, and metastyle are labeled. Stylar cusp equivalents in the Hershkovitz terminology are: $A = a$, $B = j(+k)$, $C = l$, $D = m$, and $E = b$. Variability of stylar cusps *B*, *C*, and *D* is indicated as follows: *o* indicates only a trace of a cuspule present; *O*, a moderately well-developed cusp; and $\rightarrow O$, a hyperdeveloped cusp. Thin lines within the outlines indicate crests or ridges, and dashed thin lines denote valleys. Dashed double lines mark a particular crest referred to in the text. Variations from the normal condition are shown; the more extreme are farther from the norm line. Specimens reversed in the diagrams are indicated by (*R*) in the listing below.

(*a, top*) *Holoclemensia*. SMP-SMU 61997 (*R*) (type of *H. texana*); PM 1000; PM 1238; PM 1004 (*R*); PM 886 (*R*); SMP-SMU 62009 (*R*); and PM 1015 (7 teeth).

(*b, bottom*) *Pappotherium*. SMP-SMU 71725 (*R*) (type of *P. pattersoni*); PM 999 (*R*); PM 884; PM 1075; and PM 1287 (6 teeth).

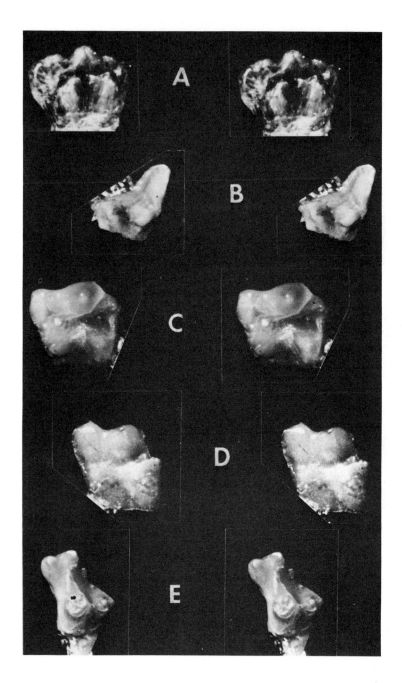

Fig. 2. Stereoscopic photo pairs of the Field Museum's Trinity therian upper molar teeth referred to *Holoclemensia* are shown in crown view, buccal edge at the top: *a*, PM 1000; *b*, PM 1238; *c*, PM 1004; *d*, PM 886; and *e*, PM 1015. Scale approximately × 20.

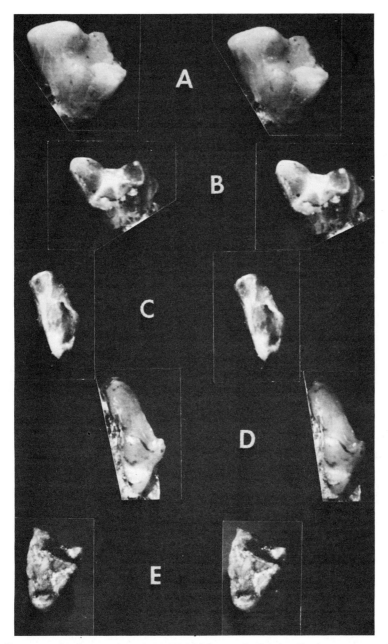

Fig. 3. Stereoscopic photo pairs of the Field Museum's Trinity therian upper molar teeth referred to *Pappotherium* (*a-d*), and to an indeterminate specimen (*e*), shown in crown view, buccal edge at the top: *a*, PM 884; *b*, PM 999; *c*, PM 1075; *d*, 1287; *e*, PM 1325, indeterminate therian upper molar fragment. Specimen consists of the protocone and proto- and metaconules. Scale approximately × 20.

Unifying criteria, features shares by both *Pappotherium pattersoni* and *Holoclemensia texana* and the other teeth referred to these genera, which are presumed to be archaic features common to the metatherian-eutherian grade.

1. Principal cusps of trigon are always present, but are variably developed. Paracone or eocone[6] (PA) and metacone (ME) usually tend to be subequal. The size gradient nearly always is PA > ME > PR (protocone). A parastyle is always developed; metastyle is usually so, but is small.

2. Eocrista is well defined. It is continuous both anteriorly and posteriorly from the apex of the paracone; anteriorly, it extends sharply buccally to the stylocone (or at least to the region immediately anterior to the stylocone) and then turns sharply anteriorly and runs to the parastyle; posteriorly, it runs nearly straight (euthemorphically) from the tip of the paracone to tip of the metacone across the intervening valley and then turns to take a mostly buccal course to the metastyle (or to metastylar area if no metastyle is developed, as may be the case in the last molar).

3. The protocone is lower than paracone and metacone, and appears as a well-developed, lingual cingular outgrowth. It is almost always connected by a cingular ridge to the parastyle. The presence of protoconule and metaconule is somewhat variable on last molars; presumably they are both present on all other molars and they are always small. (In *P. pattersoni,* the penultimate molar of the type and PM 1287, a last molar, both have conules whereas the last molar of the type has only a metaconule, and PM 1075, also a last molar, has only a protoconule. In *H. texana,* the only teeth preserving the area are the paratype, which has both, and PM 1004, which shows a trace of a metaconule. One isolated indeterminate therian tooth fragment, PM 1325 (fig. 3), that consists of protocone and a portion of the region labial to it has both conules. These indications plus the wide occurrence throughout Metatheria and Eutheria from Late Cretaceous onward are the basis for this presumption).

4. There is a wide stylar shelf, but its component cusps vary. Much of this variation suggests a metatherian-eutherian separation. The dividing line between anterior and posterior moieties of the stylar shelf lies between stylar cusps B (stylocone) and C.

Distinguishing criteria, features separating *Pappotherium pattersoni* from *Holoclemensia texana,* which may be indicative of archaic molar differences between Metatheria and Eutheria, can be paired as follows (table 2):

---

[6] I have used the long accepted Cope-Osborn-derived cusp and crest terminology as far as possible, but I combine it with some of the more useful newer terms, chiefly those of Vandebroek (1961); see the thorough summary of terms given by Hershkovitz in this volume.

TABLE 2

DISTINGUISHING FEATURES OF *H. texana* AND *P. pattersoni*

Feature	*H. texana* (fig. 1*a*)	*P. pattersoni* (fig. 1*b*)
Stylocone = stylar cusp B of Bensley (=j of Hershkovitz)	well formed, but only moderately large	well formed and hyperdeveloped, usually with a posterior ridge
Degree of compression of last molar	Compressed: posterior moiety of stylar shelf drastically reduced, but metacone still well formed, though crowded	extremely compressed: both posterior moiety of stylar shelf and metacone are drastically reduced
Stylar cusp C (=1 of Hershkovitz) and associated ridge to PA (eocone)	Hyperdeveloped, usually with a weak accessory ridge leading to paracone which is variably developed.	Distinct and small to moderately well developed, usually without trace of accessory ridge to paracone that is found in *H. texana*
Stylar cusp D (=m of Hershkovitz)	Usually moderately well developed but small	Always small to minute, or almost absent

Figure 1*a, b* illustrates diagrammatically all of these features for each of the known upper molars of Trinity therians. The figures also show the variations observed. Those which are considered minor are the metastyle and conule variations listed above, and the following: *Holoclemensia:* PM 1004 has an incomplete accessory (paracone-stylar cusp C) ridge, lacking the usual paracone portion. PM 886 lacks development of stylar cusp D and lacks the accessory ridge. PM 1015 also lacks this ridge, and has stylar cusp C only moderately well developed. *Pappotherium:* PM 999 shows a trace of an accessory ridge on paracone. PM 884 has its stylar cusp C developed beyond the normal condition for the species *P. pattersoni.*

Variations of perhaps greater significance are seen in two of the last molars, one of each species, PM 1015 and PM 1287. The tooth referred to *Holoclemensia,* PM 1015, has its stylar cusp C less hyperdeveloped than those of the other molars of the specimens assigned to the genus, including the paratype of *H. texana,* and the stylocone is the major stylar cusp. Its outline, which shows the anterior-posterior compression to be comparable to that of the paratype, allows for a nearly normal-sized metacone rather than a drastically reduced one such as is found in last molars of *Pappotherium.* In PM 1287, a specimen of *Pappotherium,* the eocrista is interrupted in the region of the stylocone, and the protocone-parastylar cingular ridge is interrupted buccad to the protoconule.

The range of variation among these upper molars is restricted enough to suggest that we are dealing with only a few, probably two, taxa, *H. texana* and

TABLE 3

MEASUREMENTS OF UPPER MOLARS
(in mm)

Specimen	Length	Width
Holoclemensia		
Molars other than last molars		
SMP-SMU (type *H. texana*)	1.73	——
PM 1000	1.55	——
PM 1238	>1.00	——
PM 1004	>1.40	——
PM 886	>1.30	——
Averages	>1.40 (N = 5)	——
Last molars		
SMP-SMU 62009 (ref. *H. texana*)	1.38	2.55
PM 1015	1.02	1.65
Averages	1.20 (N = 2)	2.10 (N = 2)
Pappotherium		
Molars other than last molars		
SMP-SMU 71725		
(type *P. pattersoni*—		
penultimate molar)	1.43	1.80
PM 999	1.28	——
PM 884	>1.40	——
Averages	>1.37 (N = 3)	1.80 (N = 1)
Last molars		
SMP-SMU 71725		
(type *P. pattersoni*—		
last molar)	0.88	1.75
PM 1075	0.60	1.48
PM 1287	0.92	1.76
Averages	0.80 (N = 3)	1.66 (N = 3)

NOTE: Values for SMP-SMU specimens are from measurement of Slaughter's scaled illustrations. Other measurements were made directly on Field Museum specimens. The differences from Patterson's published list result from different measures.

P. pattersoni, and that these two species belong to similar, related genera. The greater part of the observed variation is interpreted as being individual or serial in nature, but it might be argued that in each genus those specimens which deviate the most from the norm may represent other unnamed species. Because of this possibility I have not attempted to make positive specific assignments but instead allocate them as follows (see fig. 1*a*, *b*):

Holoclemensia texana SMP-SMU 61997, SMP-SMU 62009
H. cf. *texana* PM 1000, PM 1238, PM 1004
H. sp. PM 886, P. 1015
Pappotherium pattersoni SMP-SMU 71725
P. cf. *pattersoni* PM 999, PM 1075, PM 884
P. sp. PM 1287

There are two reasons for believing that these genera are very closely related: (1) the overall basic similarities in morphology; and (2) that the variations from the norm of one group trend toward features more characteristic of the other taxon.

Lower Molars (figs. 4*a*, *b*, 5, 6)

TABLE 4

MEASUREMENTS OF LOWER MOLARS
(in mm)

Specimen	Length	AW	PW
Holoclemensia			
SMP-SMU 62131			
(cf. *H. texana*)	1.95	1.25	0.90
PM 1005	1.93	1.41	1.06
SMP-SMU 61727	1.85	1.18	1.03
SMP-SMU 61735	——	——	——
PM 966	——	1.26	——
PM 965	1.78	1.16	0.88
PM 1119	——	0.94 (est.)	——
PM 1249	——	0.97	——
PM 948	1.46	0.99	0.89
PM 930	——	0.91	——
PM 887	——	1.44	——
PM 660	——	1.15	——
Averages	1.79 (N = 5)	1.15 (N = 11)	0.95 (N = 5)
Pappotherium			
PM 1046	——	0.60	——
SMP-SMU 61726	1.76	1.10	0.80
PM 1245	1.40	0.70	0.58
PM 922	1.29	0.68	0.58
PM 1120	——	>0.68	——
SMP-SMU 61728	1.35	0.80	0.55
Averages	1.45 (N = 4)	>0.76 (N = 6)	0.63 (N = 4)

NOTE: Values for SMP-SMU specimens are from measurement of Slaughter's scaled illustrations. Other measurements were made directly on Field Museum specimens. The differences from Patterson's published list result from different measures.

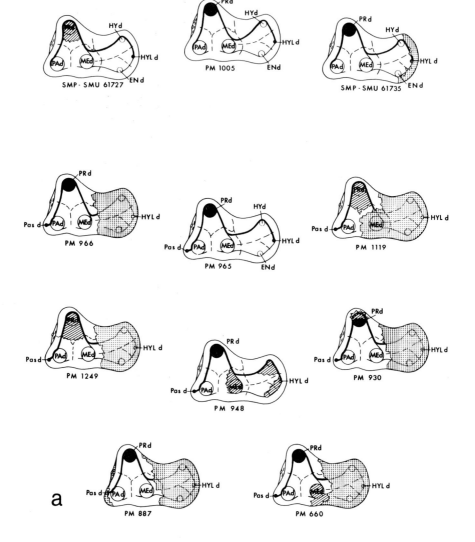

Fig. 4. Schematic outline diagrams of the Trinity therian lower molar teeth. Standard outline patterns of the teeth, one for each taxon, connote the differences between them. Teeth lacking parastylids are shown at the top; presumably these are M₁s. Trigonid (*PRd*, *PAd*, and *MEd*) and talonid (*HYd*, *HYLd*, and *ENd*) cusps are labeled. The eocristid and its associated ancient primary cusp, the protoconid or eoconid, and its terminals (*PASd* and *HYLd*), and the other features are shown in a manner comparable to that used for the eocrista, paracone, etc. in fig. 1. Other differences and variations are discussed in the text, but the latter are not ordered as was done in fig. 1.

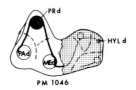

PM 1046

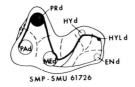

SMP-SMU 61726

SMP-SMU 61728

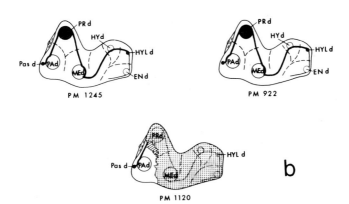

PM 1245

PM 922

PM 1120

b

(*a, left*) *Holoclemensia.* SMP-SMU 61727 (*R*); PM 1005; not shown, but nearly identical to PM 1005, SMP-SMU 62131 (*R*); SMP-SMU 61735 (4 teeth presumed to be M_1s).
PM 966 (*R*); PM 965; PM 1119 (*R*); PM 1249; PM 948; PM 930; PM 887; PM 660 (8 teeth, all presumed to be molars posterior to M_1).
(*b, right*) *Pappotherium.* PM 1046 (*R*); SMP-SMU 61726 (*R*); SMP-SMU 61728 (*R*) (3 teeth presumed to be M_1s).
PM 1245; PM 922; PM 1120 (*R*) (3 teeth presumed to be molars behind M_1).

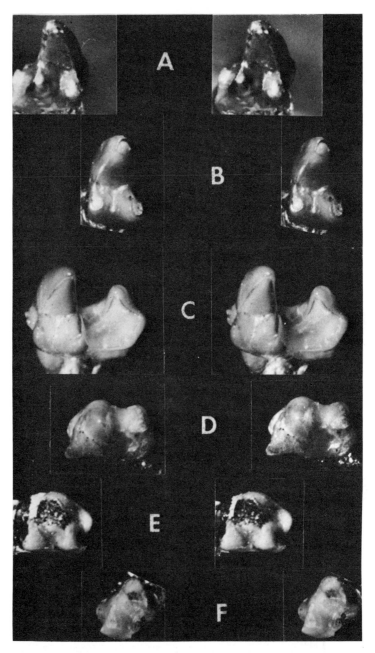

Fig. 5. Stereoscopic photo pairs of the Field Museum's Trinity therian lower molar teeth referred to *Holoclemensia* are shown in crown view, buccal edge at the top: *a*, PM 966; *b*, PM 887; *c*, PM 1005; *d*, PM 948; *e*, PM 1249; and *f*, PM 1119. Scale approximately × 20.

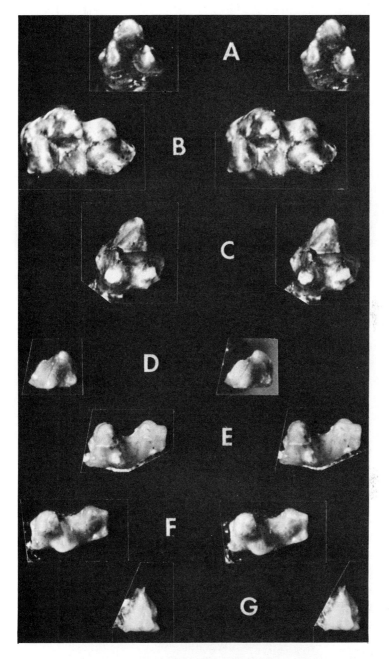

Fig. 6. Stereoscopic photo pairs of the Field Museum's Trinity therian lower molar teeth referred to *Holoclemensia* (*a-c*) and *Pappotherium* (*d-g*) are shown, crown view, buccal edge at the top: *a*, PM 930; *b*, PM 965; *c*, PM 660; *d*, PM 1046; *e*, PM 1245; *f*, PM 992; and *g*, PM 1120. Scale approximately × 20.

Unifying criteria, shared by the six previously designated types of lower therian molars are: (1) each has a trigonid that stands high above the talonid and is made up of the three major cusps (protoconid or eoconid, paraconid, and metaconid) that grade in size from PRd $\geqq$ MEd > PAd. (2) Each has an eocristid that is well defined. It runs in two directions from the primary cusp, the protoconid, anterolingually in the forward part and posterolingually behind. The anterior portion of the eocristid is deeply notched by the valley between the protoconid and the paraconid, and it always reaches the paraconid. If a parastylid is present, the eocristid turns sharply and runs forward to that stylid which is its usual anterior terminus; otherwise it does not go beyond the paraconid. The posterior segment of the eocristid is more complex. It extends from the protoconid toward the metaconid, crosses the intervening valley between these cusps where it is clefted, then turns sharply posteriorly in the region of the metaconid ,and leaving the metaconid area gradually swings in a posterobuccal direction to reach the hypoconid. From the hypoconid, the eocristid turns posterolabiad to reach its posterior terminus, the hypoconulid. (3) Each has a well-developed talonid that is nearly as long as the trigonid, if not somewhat longer, and its three cusps are usually present, or at least suggested by cresting. (4) Each has an obliquely inclined, transverse anterior cingulum with one (or more) low, centrally placed cuspule.

Distinguishing criteria tend to be masked by numerous variations, but there are three (perhaps related) that are consistent, and which therefore appear to be of significance: (1) crown view outline, (2) path of eocristid in metaconid region, and (3) position of talonid cusps.

The larger teeth, all presumably referrable to *Holoclěmensia* (either to the species *H. texana* or as *H.* sp. indet., fig. 4a) have a trigonid that is usually compressed anteroposteriorly, and an eocristid that usually does not quite reach as far lingually as the top of the metaconid. In them the relatively wide talonid extends straight back behind the trigonid, and the hypoconid (HYd) and entoconid (ENd) are equally spaced from the hypoconulid (HYld), the latter being the most posterior cusp. The size grading is HYd $\geqq$ HYLd $\geqq$ ENd.

The smaller teeth (one of which is *Peramus*-like, according to Butler, personal communication), all presumably referrable to *Pappotherium* (either as *P.* cf. *pattersoni,* or *P.* sp. indet., fig. 4b) have a trigonid that is usually compressed anteroposteriorly, and an eocristid that usually extends to the posterolingual side of the metaconid. In them the talonid is relatively long and narrow and is bent buccally so that the entoconid and hypoconulid lie at the posterior corners of the tooth on a line transverse to the axis of the tooth at its back edge, and the hypoconid is located more anteriorly. The hypoconulid is about equidistant from the other talonid cusps, and the size gradient is HYd $\geqq$ HYLd $>$ ENd. In addition to the cristid obliqua portion of the eocristid (crista obliqua of some—see Szalay [1969] or Hershkovitz [this volume]), there may be an additional axial crest developed on the talonid which alters that region as is seen in the type 6 tooth.

Each of these two basic kinds of therian lower molars (*Holoclemensia* and *Pappotherium*) shows variation in the presence of a parastylid. Possibly those that lack it are first molars, as in some living marsupials and placentals. A gradient is present in the degree of expression of this stylid in *Didelphis marsupialis* and *Echinosorex gymnurus,* where all molars have at least a trace of it, and where the weakest expression is in M_I. A closer parallel is seen in some phascogales (*Antechinus* and *Sminthopsis*) and some peramelids (*Perameles* and *Echimypera*), and in the placental *Elephantulus,* in which M_I appears to lack the stylid, whereas the rest of the molars have one.

Size and form differences of the lower molars readily permit one to assign them generically, either to *Holoclemensia* (types #1 & #2 of Patterson and #5 of Slaughter, fig. 4*a*) or to *Pappotherium* (types #3 of Patterson and #4 & #6 Slaughter, fig. 4*b*), but specific assignment is a somewhat less certain matter. The genotypes of both are species based upon specimens consisting only of upper molars: the only lower molar thus far definitely assigned is SMP-SMU 62131, which Slaughter referred to *H. texana.* As with the upper molars, I consider the variations found within the lower molars of *Holoclemensia* all to be most reasonably interpreted as differences that might be expected to occur along a toothrow and from individual variation. However, I cannot exclude the possibility that some of them may be indicative of specific differentiation. Therefore I designate them as follows:

Holoclemensia cf. *texana.* SMP-SMU 62131, PM 1005

H. sp. (probably *H. texana*). SMP-SMU 61727, SMP-SMU 61735, PM 966, PM 965, PM 1119, PM 1249, PM 948, PM 930, PM 887, PM 660

With regard to *Pappotherium,* the arguments are much the same. I believe that the lower molars, except possibly for SMP-SMU 61728, belong to the one named species, *P. pattersoni,* and that the one exceptional specimen could represent an unnamed related species. However, as with most deviant of the last upper molars assigned to this genus (PM 1287), I prefer to look upon such a case as representing an example of rather extreme variation. The reason for this is that the overall outlines and proportions of these teeth conform to a common pattern, and this suggests that we are dealing with a single specific taxon, for I weight these likenesses as having greater significance than the crest deviations observed within the pattern. The *Pappotherium* lower molars are thus designated as follows:

Pappotherium cf. *pattersoni*. PM 1046, SMP-SMU 61726, PM 1245, PM 992, PM 1120

P. sp. SMP-SMU 61728.

Conclusions

The Trinity therians afford dental evidence that bears directly upon our understanding of the marsupial-placental dichotomy. This dichotomy has recently been thoroughly reviewed by Lillegraven (1969), who, in addition to presenting the paleontological, dental, and skeletal evidence, gave considerable stress to the comparative anatomical evidence of the reproductive physiology within the two groups. In general he found these two sorts of evidence to be in harmony. The further point not stressed by Lillegraven, but which this study sets forth, and which I believe also to be in harmony with the physiological evidence, is drawn from the Cretaceous and Early Tertiary record, especially that of the Trinity therians. It is that both the marsupial and placental lineages appear to have inherited developed tribosphenic lower molars, and that both inherited at least incipiently tribosphenic upper molars. Moreover, the upper molars in both lines show decided trends leading toward the ultimate reduction of the stylar shelf, the area which comprised virtually all of the upper teeth of most ancestral (premarsupial-preplacental) Jurassic forms, and correlated with this they show an expansion of the lingual shelf. These trends are further borne out by the subsequent Tertiary record. However, the important point is that these trends are by no means equally pronounced, uniform, or consistent within the various branchings of either of the two lineages. In the main, the placentals appear to have led in the abandonment of the ancient stylar shelf in favor of a more developed, modern lingual one (*Gypsonictops, Procerberus, Mixodectes, Protungulatum, Palaeosinopa, Paromomys*, etc.), but some lines, on the other hand, did not (*Nyssodon, Didelphodus*). In marsupials similar, if less pronounced, trends are apparent in some lines (*Pediomys, Glasbius*), but a little if at all evident in others (*Didelphodon, Alphadon, Peratherium*). Thus within both groups there are lines that show trends that run counter to the ultimate successful general trends of their own group. Both lineages, it seems, were "experimenting" with the same kinds of dental modifications, much as both were simultaneously "experimenting" with refinements of a reproducitve development, placentation (see Lillegraven 1969, pp. 99–104). Ultimately lines within each group arrived at different solutions to the problems within each of these areas.

Therefore it seems to me to be premature, possibly even erroneous, to attempt to force the Trinity therians into the metatherian-eutherian dichotomy. Instead, I believe it is more defensible to erect a new metatherian-eutherian grade, primitive euthemorphic, stem group taxon for them. Coordinate with this new stem taxon, I tentatively also include another one to encompass the zalambdamorphic forms, O. Zalambdadonta (in the sense of Vandebroek 1961, but with the addition of the zalambdamorphic marsupials). Therefore I take the formal step of proposing a new order, Tribosphena, to include the pre-metatherian, preeutherian, primitive euthemorphic stem group forms such as the Trinity therians, *Aegialodon*, and *Peramus*, and I group together the orders Zalambdadonta and Tribosphena into a cohort Tribosphenata. The Tribosphenata are assumed to have evolved from somewhere within the Dryolestoidea. The basis for this placement of the expanded O. Zalambdadonta derives from my giving greater weight in this case to the dental evidence than I do to reproductive (placental) development. Attainment of an incipient tribosphenic dentition I take to indicate relationship to orders whose members have the more advanced tribosphenic dentition (Tribosphenata, and all metatherian-eutherian orders), even though the details of that relationship are vague and uncertain. This much does seem clear—the zalambdamorphic forms are more primitive dentally than are the fully tribosphenic forms, since in them the upper molars usually consist of little more than the primitive stylar shelf, as with symmetrodonts and pantotheres.

The following classification expresses these apparent relationships. Its basis is much broader than mere dental similarities and differences, of course, but these are nevertheless the most consistently used basic criteria for the suggested change.

This classification is much like Vandebroek's of 1964; however, he grouped Triconodonta and Symmetrodonta together into Péneclass Triconotheria, a relationship long out of vogue but which may be correct. Parrington (1967), Crompton and Jenkins (1968), Hopson and Crompton (1969), and McKenna (1969) each suggested reasons that argue for a reconsideration of a "cusp rotation" hypothesis for deriving the Symmetrodent-Therian lineage from an ancestral triconodont stem. And the Hopson and Crompton phylogenetic chart (pp. 58–59), without using the Péneclass Triconotheria by name, in effect would accommodate such a grouping (Küehneotheriidae and Eozostrodontidae) at the very base of the mammals. Inasmuch as the dentitions of triconodonts and symmetrodonts were evolving in different directions, I tentatively retain an expression of the uncertainty as to subclass assignment for the former group. The Vandebroek assignment that I find hard to accept is that of close relationship of Docodonta and Dryolestoidea. I had been convinced by Patterson's (1956) argument that this then widely held notion was erroneous, but since I have no studied basis for rejection or acceptance of the Vandebroek assignment other than Patterson's argument, I prefer the noncommittal uncertain subclass treatment of O. Docodonta.

Class Mammalia
    Subclass Prototheria
        O. Multituberculata   Cope 1884
    Subclass Allotheria
        O. Multituberculata   Cope 1884
    Mammalia of uncertain subclass
        O. Triconodonta   Osborn 1888
        O. Docodonta   Patterson 1956
    Subclass Theria
      Infraclass Pantotheria
        O. Symmetrodonta   Simpson 1925
        O. Dryolestoidea   Vandebroek 1964
Infraclass Eutheria (*sensu* Vandebroek 1961, 1964, and Hershkovitz, this volume)
    Cohort Tribosphenata nov.
        O. Zalambdadonta   Gill 1884 (with additions)
        O. Tribosphena nov.
    Cohort Marsupiata (= Old Metatheria or Marsupialia)
        O. Marsupicarnivora   Ride 1964
        O. Paucituberculata   Ameghino 1894
        O. Peramelina   Gray 1825
        O. Diprotodonta   Owen 1866
    Cohort Placentata (= Old Eutheria or Placentalia)
      Cohort Division Unguiculata (= Old Cohort of the same name)
        O. Insectivora   (or O's Menotyphla and Lipotyphla)
        O. Dermoptera
        O. Chiroptera
        .... etc.   (Rest of placental orders and superorders. grouped within the several divisions of the cohort Placentata: Glires, Mutica, and Ferungulata).

In this classification cohorts are employed throughout the infraclass Eutheria. This act necessitated the use of an additional category within the cohort Placentata, termed cohort division, where it seemed reasonable to retain the usual groupings of orders and superorders.

ADDENDA

Since this paper was submitted two works bearing on the subject have appeared. One of these, J. A. Hopson, The classification of nontherian mammals (*J. Mamm.* 51 [1970]:1–9) encompasses all pretherian mammals within an expanded subclass Prototheria. Although the Prototheria by this scheme (or its equivalents in the scheme I used) are peripheral to my focus on parts of the subclass Theria, the implication for monophyly, or at least for a reduced degree of polyphyly within Mammalia is commendable. I tentatively accept it for this reason. It provides a solution to the complaint voiced by C. A. Reed, which is aptly summed up in the title of his paper, Polyphyletic or monophyletic ancestry of mammals; or, What is a class? (*Evolution* [1960]:314–22), and it is more acceptable a solution for mammalian classification than Reed's was.

The other recent paper, by B. G. Sharman, is a comprehensive review of a complex and fascinating subject (Reproductive physiology of marsupials, *Science* 167 [1970]:1221–28). However, I feel that Sharman's conclusion that "the many unique features of marsupial reproductive physiology suggest that viviparity evolved separately in eutherian and marsupial stocks after that derivation from a common oviparous ancestor," neglects the greater number of common features of the two groups. The point that the separation is an ancient one (perhaps within the Tribosphenata) is well taken, but that it preceeded viviparity seems to me to be unlikely.

ACKNOWLEDGMENTS

The schematic drawings (figs. 1 and 4) are the work of Dr. Ribor Perenyi, artist on the Field Museum staff. The stereoscopic photos (figs. 2, 3, 5, 6) were taken by me with the help and advice of Homer Holdren and John Bayalis of the Museum's Division of Photography. Fred Huysmans, also of that division, printed the enlargements from my negatives. I am indebted to Philip Hershkovitz and my wife Priscilla for many discussions and for reading the manuscript drafts, and to Miss Jeanette Forster for typing.

REFERENCES

Bensley, B. A. 1903. On the evolution of the Australian Marsupialia: With remarks on the relationships of the marsupials in general. *Trans. Linnean Soc. Lond., Ser. 2, Zool.* 9:83–217.

Bergamini, D. 1964. *The land and wildlife of Australia.* Life Nature Library. New York: Time.

Cain, A. J. 1959. Deductive and inductive methods in post-Linnean taxonomy. *Proc. Linnean Soc. Lon.* 170:185–217.

Clemens, W. A., Jr. 1966. Fossil mammals of the Type Lance Formation Wyoming. Part II. Marsupialia. *Univ. Calif. Pubs. Geol. Sci.* 62:1–122.

———. 1968. Origin and early evolution of marsupials. *Evolution* 22:1–18.

Crompton, A. W., and Jenkins, F., Jr. 1968. Molar occlusion in late Triassic mammals. *Biol. Rev.* 43:427–58.

Hopson, J. A., and Crompton, A. W. 1969. Origin of mammals. *Evol. Biol.* 3:15–72.

Keast, A. 1968. Evolution of mammals on southern continents. IV. Australian mammals: Zoogeography and evolution. *Quart. Rev. Biol.* 43:373–408.

Kirsch, J. A. W. 1968. Prodromus of the comparative serology of Marsupialia. *Nature* 217:418–20.

Lillegraven, J. A. 1969. Latest Cretaceous mammals of upper part of Edmonton formation of Alberta, Canada, and review of marsupial-placental dichotomy in mammalian evolution. *Univ. Kansas Paleont. Contrib.,* art. 50 (Vert. 12):1–122.

Marlow, B. J. 1960. The evolution and radiation of mammals. *Austral. Mus. Mag.* 13:184–90.

McKenna, M. C. 1969. The origin and early differentiation of Therian mammals. *Ann. N.Y. Acad. Sci.* 167:217–40.

Parrington, F. R. 1967. The origins of mammals. *Adv. Sci., Lond.* 24:1–9.

Patterson, B. 1956. Early Cretaceous mammals and the evolution of mammalian molar teeth. *Fieldiana: Geol.* 13:1–105.

Patterson, B., and Pascual, R. 1968. Evolution of mammals on southern continents. V. The fossil mammal faunas of South America. *Quart. Rev. Biol.* 43:409–51.

Paula Couto, C. d. 1952. Fossil mammals from the beginning of the Cenozoic in Brasil. Marsupialia: Polydolopidae and Borhyaenidae. *Amer. Mus. Novit.* 1559:1–27.

———. 1961. Marsupiais fósseis do Paleoceno do Brasil. *Acad. Brasileira Ciencias. Anais.* 33:321–33.

———. 1962. Didelfídos fósiles del Paleoceno do Brasil. *Rev. Museo Argent. Cienc. Natur.* 8:135:66.

Ride, W. D. L. 1964. A review of Australian marsupials. *J. Roy. Soc. W. Austral.* 47(16):97–131.

———. 1968. The past, present, and future of Australian mammals. *Austral. J. Sci.* 31:1–11.

Romer, A. S. 1966. Vertebrate paleontology. 3d ed. Chicago: University of Chicago Press.

Simpson, G. G. 1939. The development of marsupials in South America. *Physis* 14:373–98.

———. 1945. The principles of classification and a classification of mammals. *Bull. Amer. Mus. Nat. Hist.* 85:1–350.

———. 1948. The beginning of the Age of Mammals in South America. Part I. Introduction, systematics: Marsupialia, Edentata, Condylarthra, Litopterna, and Notioprogonia. *Bull. Amer. Mus. Nat. Hist.* 91:1–232.

———. 1967. The beginning of the Age of Mammals in South America. Part II. Systematics: Notoungulata concluded (Typotheria, Hegetotheria, Toxodonta, Notoungulata incertae sedis); Astrapotheria; Trigonostylopoidea; Pyrotheria; Xenungulata; Mammalia incertae sedis. *Bull. Amer. Mus. Nat. Hist.* 137:1–260.

Slaughter, B. H. 1965. A therian from the Lower Cretaceous (Albian) of Texas. *Postilla* 93:1–18.

————. 1968a. Earliest known Eutherian mammals and the evolution of premolar occlusion. *Texas J. Sci.* 20:3–12.

————. 1968b. Earliest known marsupials. *Science* 162:254–55.

————. 1968c. Holoclemensia instead of Clemensia. *Science* 162:1306.

Stirton, R. A.; Tedford, R. H.; and Woodburne, M. O. 1968. Australian Tertiary deposits containing terrestrial mammals. *Univ. Calif. Pubs. Geol. Sci.* 77:1–30.

Szalay, F. S. 1969. Mixodectidae, Microsyopidae, and the Insectivore-Primate transition. *Bull. Amer. Mus. Nat. Hist.* 140:193–330.

Tate, G. H. H. 1945a. The marsupial genus Phalanger. *Amer. Mus. Novit.* 1283: 1–41.

————. 1945b. The marsupial genus *Pseudocheirus* and its subgenera. *Amer. Mus. Novit.* 1287:1–24.

————. 1945c. Notes on the squirrel-like and mouse-like possums (Marsupialia). *Amer. Mus. Novit.* 1305:1–12.

————. 1947. On the anatomy and classification of the Dasyuridae (Marsupialia). *Bull. Amer. Mus. Nat. Hist.* 88:97–156.

————. 1948a. Studies on the anatomy and phylogeny of the Macropodidae (Marsupialia). *Bull. Amer. Mus. Nat. Hist.* 91:233–352.

————. 1948b. Studies in the Peramelidae (Marsupialia). *Bull. Amer. Mus. Nat. Hist.* 92:313–46.

————. 1952. Mammals of Cape York Peninsula, with notes on the occurrence of rain forest in Queensland. *Bull. Amer. Mus. Nat. Hist.* 98:563–616.

Tedford, R. H. 1966. A review of the macropodid genus *Sthenurus*. *Univ. Calif. Pubs. Geol. Sci.* 57:1–72.

Vandebroek, G. 1961. The comparative anatomy of the teeth of lower and non-specialized mammals. Int. Colloq. on the Evolution of Lower and Non-specialized Mammals. Kon. Vl. Acad. Wetensch. Lett. Sch. Kunst. België, Brussels, K1. Wetensch. 1:215–320; 2:1–181.

————. 1964. Recherches sur l'origine des mammifères. *Ann. Soc. Roy. Zool. Belgique* 94:117–60.

————. 1967. Origin of the cusps and crests of the tribosphenic molar. *J. Dent. Res.* 46 (supplement, part 1):796–804.

Van Valen, L. 1966. Deltatheridia: A new order of mammals. *Bull. Amer. Mus. Nat. Hist.* 132:1–126.

10 Mesozoic Evolution of Mammals with Tribosphenic Dentitions

William A. Clemens

Department of Paleontology,
University of California, Berkeley

With the exception of the platypus and echidna, all living mammals are descendants of a common stock characterized by a tribosphenic dentition. A few modern mammals, *Tupaiia* and *Marmosa* for example, have dentitions little modified from the basic tribosphenic pattern, but in most the dentition has been extensively altered during the 100 million years or more since their lineages started to diversify.

In contrast, the tribosphenic dentition is not found in any of the earliest mammals that appear in the fossil record of the late Triassic, approximately 190–180 M.Y.B.P. (million years before the present). The fossil record of the Jurassic, 180–135 M.Y.B.P., documents instances of convergence in form or function and the evolution of the ancestral stock (fig. 1). But only in the earliest Cretaceous, approximately 135–125 M.Y.B.P., is there a definite record of a mammal with a tribosphenic dentition. Not until the middle of the Cretaceous, approximately 100–110 M.Y.B.P., does the fossil record document a major evolutionary radiation of mammals with this kind of dentition—a group including the ancestors of modern marsupials and placentals.

Here I shall attempt to review the evolution of mammals with tribosphenic dentitions during the Cretaceous, emphasizing their adaptive radiation and extinctions of various lineages at the close of the period. Radiometric age determinations indicate that the Cretaceous was a relatively long segment of geological time, approximately 71 million years in duration (135–64 M.Y.B.P.). This is fully one-third of the total history of the class Mammalia and is longer than the Cenozoic (64 M.Y.B.P. to the present), when mammals evolved without dinosaurian contemporaries.

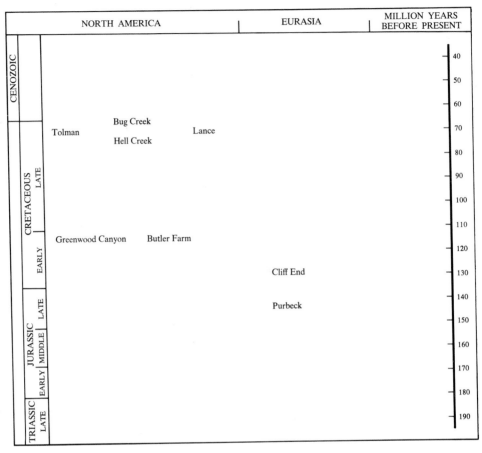

	NORTH AMERICA	EURASIA	MILLION YEARS BEFORE PRESENT

CENOZOIC

CRETACEOUS — LATE

CRETACEOUS — EARLY

JURASSIC — LATE

JURASSIC — MIDDLE

JURASSIC — EARLY

TRIASSIC — LATE

Tolman   Bug Creek   Lance
          Hell Creek

Greenwood Canyon   Butler Farm

Cliff End

Purbeck

40
50
60
70
80
90
100
110
120
130
140
150
160
170
180
190

Fig. 1. Stratigraphic chart showing relative positions of local faunas mentioned in the text.

The Tribosphenic Dentition

From their reptilian ancestors the earliest mammals inherited dentitions clearly subdivided into incisiform, caniniform, and, with few exceptions, premolariform and molariform teeth. Although morphologically differentiated, the ontogeny of the postcanines, where known, differs from that found in marsupials and placentals (Crompton and Jenkins 1968). Anterior postcanines were lost and not replaced, and molariform teeth appear to have been added to the distal end of the dental arcade.

Other dental characteristics frequently thought to be typical of mammals are not found in their earliest representatives. In the late Triassic mammal *Megazostrodon*, for example, extensive wear occurred as the postcanines came into function (Crompton and Jenkins 1968). Unlike teeth of a tribosphenic pattern (Marshall and Butler 1966), their occluding surfaces required a significant amount of abrasion before they matched and, presumably, reached their maximum functional efficiency. Also, all the earliest mammals investigated to date lack the prismatic structure of the enamel (Moss 1969; Poole 1967) seen in later mammals.

During the Jurassic the stage was set for evolution of the tribosphenic, or trituberculosectorial, dentition. This type of dentition is distinguished by the morphology and function of the molariform teeth (fig. 2). Upper molars have

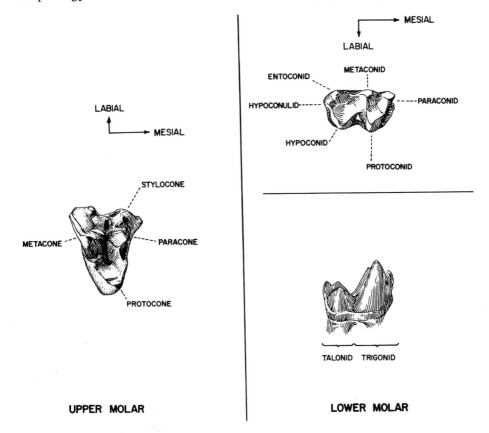

Fig. 2. Principal morphologic features of tribosphenic molars.

a basic trigon consisting of paracone, metacone, and protocone. Subsequent discoveries substantiate Patterson's (1956) view that a broad shelf labial to the paracone and metacone, carrying a stylocone and other stylar cusps, characterizes primitive tribosphenic upper molars. The lower molars are divided into a higher, mesial trigonid formed of three major cusps and a lower talonid, a cusp-encircled basin receiving the protocone.

Unlike their ancestors, the earliest mammals with tribosphenic molars could produce two different actions during mastication. Their dentitions can be occluded in patterns producing shear between crests of the trigon and stylar shelf and those of the trigonid and talonid. In addition, because of the opposition of the protocone and talonid, food could be crushed between major segments of the crowns of the molars. In *Didelphis*, the modern opossum, which has a slightly modified tribosphenic dentition, mastication begins with crushing of the food, abetted by the puncturing action of high, conical cusps. Once sufficiently reduced, the food is cut between the shearing crests of the molars (Crompton and Hiiemae 1969).

The combination of crushing and shearing functions of the tribosphenic dentition provided the opportunity for a wide variety of adaptive modifications. A brief survey of the dentitions of modern mammals ranging from those of felids, with their emphasis on shearing, to ungulates and rodents, in which crushing and grinding are the dominant functions, demonstrates how this potential was exploited in the later radiations of mammals.

Earliest Tribosphenic Dentitions

To date no Jurassic mammals with tribosphenic dentitions have been discovered, but probably their ancestry is to be found within the eupantotheres (sensu Kermack and Mussett 1958). Among the eupantotheres the genus *Peramus*, a member of the late Jurassic Purbeck local fauna of England, has been suggested to be representative of the stock ancestral to mammals with tribosphenic dentitions (Mills 1964). Subsequent studies of new and better-prepared material have brought me to a slightly different conclusion. The small size of the stylocones of its upper molars and other characters appear to rule *Peramus* out of the direct ancestry of mammals with tribosphenic dentitions. However, among the late Jurassic mammals so far discovered, it remains as probably the closest representative of the eupantotherian ancestral stock.

Aegialodon, from the early Cretaceous Cliff End local fauna of England, is known from only one fossil. The slightly basined talonid of this lower molariform tooth bears a wear facet probably produced by a protocone, a character diagnostic of the tribosphenic dentition (Kermack, Lees, and Mussett 1958).

By the close of the early Cretaceous, 100–110 M.Y.B.P., mammals with fully tribosphenic dentitions were in existence and had begun to diversify. This radiation is documented in North America by fossils from the later early Cretaceous Greenwood Canyon and Butler Farm local faunas of Texas described by Patterson (1956) and Slaughter (1965, 1968).

Probably the initial radiation of mammals with tribosphenic dentitions was not limited to North America, but conclusive evidence from other continents has yet to be recovered. A Mesozoic Asian mammal, *Endotherium*, clearly has a tribosphenic dentition, but its geological age is open to question. Although it was first considered to be late Jurassic, Kermack, Lees, and Mussett (1965) have argued that the age of *Endotherium* is post-Jurassic and possibly as recent as the later part of the early Cretaceous.

Comparisons with dentitions of modern mammals indicate that the first mammals with tribosphenic dentitions were small carnivores or omnivores. None show modifications of the dentition characteristic of mammalian herbivores. However, circumstantial evidence suggests that origin of the tribosphenic dentition was one of the mammailan adaptations to a major change in the terrestrial flora during the early Cretaceous.

Unequivocal records of angiosperms have yet to be found in Jurassic or older strata. They are also lacking in floras of the Wealden Series (Watson 1969) of England from which *Aegialodon* was recovered, but approximately contemporaneous floras containing flowering plants are known from the east coast of North America. Allen (1969) and others have suggested that in the early Cretaceous these sites in Europe and North America were in much greater geographic proximity, perhaps within the same rift valley, and were not separated by a major ocean basin. After making their appearance in early Cretaceous deposits now in middle latitudes, angiosperms underwent both an evolutionary diversification and a poleward extension of range. By the middle of the Cretaceous, floras at high latitudes were angiosperm dominated and mammals with tribosphenic dentitions had begun their evolutionary radiation.

The tribosphenic dentitions of early Cretaceous mammals were not adapted to cope with the demands of a herbivorous diet. The contemporaneous mammalian herbivores were the rodentlike multituberculates, a lineage that branched off the earliest mammalian stocks before origin of the tribosphenic dentition. Possibly, terrestrial invertebrates formed the link between origin and diversification of both mammals with tribosphenic dentitions and angiosperms. Although it is not yet documented in the fossil record, certainly insects, arachnids, and other kinds of terrestrial invertebrates must have diversified and increased in numbers amid the plants and litter of the angiosperm-dominated forests. These terrestrial invertebrates could have provided an expanding source of food for mammals with dentitions capable of crushing and shearing.

Late Cretaceous Radiation of Marsupials

Marsupials and placentals differentiated from a common ancestral stock of mammals possessing tribosphenic dentitions (Lillegraven 1969). Large collections of fossils from later Cretaceous sites demonstrate that this had occurred by approximately 80 M.Y.B.P. From his studies of material found in Texas, Slaughter (1965, 1968) concludes that the differentiation took place earlier, before the end of the early Cretaceous, approximately 100 M.Y.B.P. The early

Cretaceous fossils thought to represent a marsupial are placed in the genus *Holoclemensia*.

Marsupials are diverse and abundant in North American late Cretaceous faunas (Clemens, 1964). Their oldest records are from North America and they are not present in the few collections of late Cretaceous mammals from other continents. Apparently the origin and first adaptive radiation of the group was centered in, if not restricted to, North America. Indirect evidence suggests that by the end of the Cretaceous marsupials had dispersed toward or into South America and Australia.

The late Cretaceous marsupial radiation gives evidence of several patterns of dental modification (fig. 3) that were independently paralleled during the

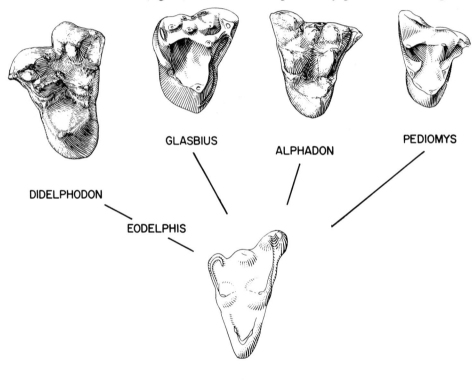

Fig. 3. Occlusal views of upper molars of the Late Cretaceous marsupials *Didelphodon*, *Glasbius*, *Alphadon*, and *Pediomys*, and a restoration of an upper molar of *Holoclemensia* from the Early Cretaceous.

Cenozoic by the evolution of American and Australian stocks (Clemens 1968). For example, in most late Cretaceous lineages the primitively broad stylar shelf of the upper molars is maintained or enlarged. Only in the pediomyids does in undergo reduction. This pattern of reduction is found in the evolution of both the South American marsupial carnivores, the borhyaenids, and the ancestors of the Tasmanian wolf, *Thylacinus*. Also, the paracone and metacone of Cretaceous marsupials were maintained at approximately equal height except in the lineage including *Didelphodon*, in which the paracone was reduced. The modification was paralleled later in the Cenozoic evolution of the New World didelphids and, independently, Australian dasyurids.

In the samples of each genus of late Cretaceous marsupials a few upper molars have a small, sometimes irregular precingulum, postcingulum, or both. These structures are neither as large nor as constant as the cingula of some placental mammals, and none of the Cretaceous marsupials exhibit even incipient evolution of a distinct hypocone.

The lower molars of late Cretaceous marsupials show a stricter adherence to a basic morphological plan. Characteristic alignment of paraconid, metaconid, and entoconid, and close approximation of the entoconid and hypoconulid appear to have evolved early and undergone little change (Slaughter 1965). Two extremes in variation are the development of a prominent labial cingulum on all lower molars of *Glasbius* and a borhyaenid-like reduction of the metaconid of the molars of *Didelphodon* (Clemens 1966).

Near the close of the Cretaceous, approximately 64 M.Y.B.P., marsupials were diverse and abundant in North American local faunas. For example, with an approximately equal number of the rodentlike multituberculates they make up 80 to 90% of the type Lance mammalian fauna.

Late Cretaceous Radiation of Placentals

Placentals—eutherian mammals—although rarer than marsupials in most late Cretaceous, North American local faunas, have a wider zoogeographic range. They are also known from late Cretaceous sites in Mongolia, Europe, and possibly South America. Slaughter (1968) suggested that *Pappotherium*, from the early Cretaceous of Texas, is the oldest eutherian yet recovered. Morphological characters and the diversity of Mongolian Cretaceous placentals (Kielan-Jaworowska 1969) have prompted the suggestion that eutherians had Asian or Eurasian origins (Lillegraven 1969), even though the Asian fossils are more recent than those from Texas.

North American Cretaceous placentals are members of two major lineages. One is represented by the leptictid insectivore *Gypsonictops* (fig. 4). Its molars differ from the primitive tribosphenic pattern in the presence of precingulum and postcingulum, reduction in width of the stylar shelf, and loss of stylar cusps. Lower molars differ in the greater breadth of the talonid basin and the small size and position of the paraconid.

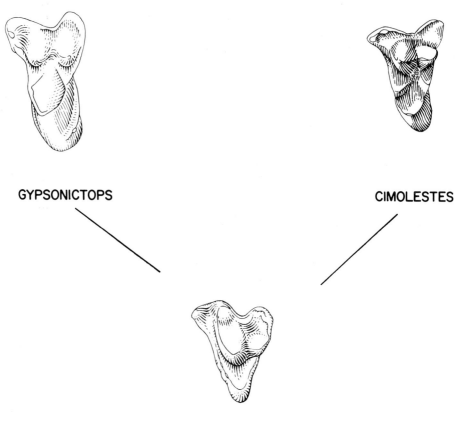

GYPSONICTOPS   **CIMOLESTES**

PAPPOTHERIUM

Fig. 4. Occlusal views of upper molars of the Late Cretaceous eutherians *Gypsonictops* and *Cimolestes*, and *Pappotherium* from the Early Cretaceous.

The posterior two premolars of *Gypsonictops* are noteworthy for their high degree of molariformity. P^4 differs from M^1 only in the slightly closer approximation of its paracone and metacone and relatively larger parastyle. Likewise P_4 clearly differs from M_1 only in absence or small size of the paraconid and, on some teeth, presence of less than three talonid cusps. The postcanine dentition consisted of three molars and four or five premolars. The mandibular angle is long and slightly inflected, a characteristic formerly regarded as indicative of marsupial affinities.

Gypsonictops is a member of the stock suggested to be ancestral to primates, rodents, and many of the modern insectivores. Of these and other descendant groups only the primates, represented by *Purgatorius*, are known to have originated by the end of the Cretaceous.

Cimolestes is representative of the second major late Cretaceous placental lineage. Upper molars of this palaeoryctid differ from those of *Gypsonictops* in having relatively wider stylar shelves and, on the molars of some species, a minute stylocone. Lingual cingula are missing from the upper molars of some species but had evolved in others. Although protocones are present on P^{3-4}, these teeth, like the distal lower premolars, are not as molariform as their homologues in the dentition of *Gypsonictops* (Lillegraven 1969).

By the end of the Cretaceous, the evolutionary radiation of North American palaeoryctids had gone farther than that of the leptictids. *Protungulatum*, a palaeoryctid descendant present in some late Cretaceous local faunas, can be allocated to the Condylarthra, the group ancestral to the various orders of Cenozoic ungulates. Also, the numerous species of *Cimolestes* appear to document the beginnings of the radiation that gave rise to the Carnivora and other placental orders (Lillegraven 1969).

A third major late Cretaceous placental lineage is represented by *Zalambdalestes*, a Mongolian mammal unknown in North American local faunas. Unless related to the ancestry of lagomorphs (Van Valen 1964), it apparently lacks descendants in the modern mammalian fauna.

Mammalian Extinctions at the Close of the Cretaceous

Summaries of vertebrate evolution during the Cretaceous tend to dwell on the radiations of dinosaurs and other reptiles. They frequently give the impression that mammalian evolution came near to stagnation until after the extinction of the dinosaurs at the end of the Cretaceous. This interpretation is now known to be erroneous. By the end of the Cretaceous, marsupials and placentals, as well as the rodentlike multituberculates, had undergone evolutionary radiations. Some groups that were to rapidly diversify in the early Cenozoic, primates and condylarths for example, had already differentiated from their ancestral stocks.

Although much has been written about the cause of dinosaurian extinction, a complete explanation eludes us. Whatever the causal factor or factors were, they must have been of worldwide efficacy and, as is now clear, had an impact on the mammalian as well as the reptilian faunas. Directly applicable information about the nature of mammalian extinctions at the close of the Cretaceous comes only from North America. This is the only continent in which both latest Cretaceous and earliest Cenozoic faunas are known from a limited geographic area, the Rocky Mountains and western High Plains. The data show that multituberculates, marsupials, and placentals suffered different fates at the close of the Cretaceous.

Multituberculates were mammalian herbivores that differentiated from the earliest mammalian stocks in the Jurassic and never evolved a tribosphenic dentition. The order lasted on into the Cenozoic until the late Eocene when they were finally fully displaced by a combination of placental herbivores (Van Valen and Sloan 1966). Of the slightly more than a dozen species now recognized in North American latest Cretaceous local faunas, only approximately 25% appear to lack descendants in Paleocene local faunas of the same areas (data from Van Valen and Sloan 1966 and unpublished sources). Those that survived underwent a significant evolutionary radiation in the earliest Cenozoic.

A broadly similar pattern pertains to the evolution of placentals (data from Lillegraven [1969] and unpublished sources). A few, 25% or less, of the latest Cretaceous placental species appear to lack Cenozoic descendants. Most are known to have survived the close of the Cretaceous; they then underwent an evolutionary radiation of greater magnitude than that of the multituberculates.

In clear contrast to these two groups, most of the lineages of Cretaceous marsupials became extinct at the close of the period. Only one, derived from *Alphadon*, is known to have survived into the Cenozoic. In North America the descendants of *Alphadon* did not undergo a major evolutionary radiation during the Cenozoic. Major Cenozoic marsupial radiations took place only in South America, where the diversity of contemporaneous placentals was limited, and Australia, where terrestrial placentals appear to have been excluded until the later Cenozoic (Clemens 1968).

Further collecting will certainly modify and refine knowledge of mammalian extinctions and survival at the close of the Cretaceous, but it probably will not invalidate the basic pattern described here. Many mammalian lineages, most of them marsupial, became extinct at the end of the Cretaceous. Survival or extinction of a species at this time does not appear to have been directly correlated with the presence or absence of a tribosphenic dentition. This suggests that the cause of the mammalian extinctions was not the loss of an accustomed source of food.

Summary

Although mammalian in many respects, the dentitions of the earliest mammals lacked, for example, the precision of occlusal pattern, the ontogeny, and the enamel structure characteristic of most modern mammals. Excluding the platypus and echidna, all living mammals descended from an ancestral stock characterized by a tribosphenic dentition.

The tribosphenic dentition evolved in eupantotherian mammals during the early Cretaceous, before differentiation of marsupials and placentals. The functions of this kind of dentition and the time and place of its origin suggest that its evolution was one of the adaptations of a group of mammals to a diet based on the expanding fauna of terrestrial invertebrates in the rapidly evolving angiosperm-dominated floras.

During late Cretaceous time, adaptive radiations increased the diversity of modifications of the tribosphenic dentition. The radiation of marsupials appears to have been limited to North America until the latest Cretaceous, when they possibly dispersed to South America and Australia. Placentals had a wider geographic range, including both the Old and the New World.

The wave of extinction at the close of the Cretaceous included many mammalian lineages. Extinction or survival of these mammals does not appear to be correlated with type of dentition, suggesting that the causal factors did not include restriction of preferred or requisite sources of food.

ACKNOWLEDGMENTS
I am indebted to Professor P. M. Butler and Professor D. E. Savage for long discussions of aspects of Mesozoic mammalian evolution and for their comments on this paper. Some of the research of the author cited here was carried out with the support of a National Science Foundation postdoctoral fellowship and grant GB 5121, which are gratefully acknowledged.

REFERENCES
Allen, P. 1969. Lower Cretaceous sourcelands and the North Atlantic. *Nature* 222: 657–58.

Clemens, W. A. 1964. Fossil mammals of the type Lance formation, Wyoming. Part I. Introduction and Multituberculata. *Univ. Calif. Publ. Geol. Sci.* 48:1–105.

———. 1966. Fossil mammals of the type Lance formation, Wyoming. Part II. Marsupialia. *Univ. Calif. Publ. Geol. Sci.* 62:1–122.

———. 1968. Origin and early evolution of marsupials. *Evolution* 22:1–18.

Crompton, A. W., and Hiiemae, K. 1969. Functional occlusion in tribosphenic molars. *Nature* 222:678–79.

Crompton, A. W., and Jenkins, F. A., Jr. 1968. Molar occlusion in Late Triassic mammals. *Biol. Rev.* 43:427–58.

Kermack, K. A.; Lees, P. M.; and Mussett, F. 1965. *Aegialodon dawsoni,* a new trituberculosectorial tooth from the Lower Wealden. *Proc. Roy. Soc., Ser.* B 162:535–54.

Kermack, K. A., and Mussett, F. 1958. The jaw articulation of the Docodonta and the classification of Mesozoic mammals. *Proc. Roy. Soc. Ser.* B 149:204–15.

Kielan-Jaworowska, Z. 1969. Preliminary data on the Upper Cretaceous eutherian mammals from Bayn Dzak, Gobi Desert. *Palaeont. Polonica* 19:171–91.

Lillegraven, J. A. 1969. Latest Cretaceous mammals of upper part of Edmonton formation of Alberta, Canada, and review of marsupial-placental dichotomy in mammalian evolution. *Univ. Kansas, Paleont. Contrib.,* art. 50 (vert. 12):1–122.

Marshall, P. M., and Butler, P. M. 1966. Molar cusp development in the bat, *Hipposideros beatus,* with reference to the ontogenetic basis of occlusion. *Archs. Oral Biol.* 11:949–65.

Mills, J. R. E. 1964. The dentitions of *Peramus* and *Amphitherium. Proc. Linn. Soc. Lond.* 175:117–33.

Moss, M. L. 1969. Evolution of mammalian dental enamel. *Amer. Mus. Novit.,* no. 2360.

Patterson, B. 1956. Early Cretaceous mammals and the evolution of mammalian molar teeth. *Fieldiana: Geol.* 13:1–105.

Poole, D. F. G. 1967. Phylogeny of tooth tissues: Enameloid and enamel in recent vertebrates, with a note on the history of cementum. In *Structural and chemical organization of teeth,* ed. A. E. W. Miles, 1:111–49. New York: Academic Press.

Slaughter, B. H. 1965. A therian from the Lower Cretaceous (Albian) of Texas. *Postillia* 93:1–18.

———. 1968. Earliest known marsupials. *Science* 162:254–55.

Van Valen, L. 1964. A possible origin for rabbits. *Evolution* 18:484–91.

Van Valen, L., and Sloan, R. E. 1966. The extinction of the multituberculates. *Syst. Zool.* 15:261–78.

Watson, J. 1969. A revision of the English Wealden flora. I. Charales-Ginkgoales. *Bull. Brit. Mus. (Nat. Hist.)* 17:207–54.

11

A Current Review of the Interrelationships of Oligocene and Miocene Catarrhini

E. L. Simons   *Department of Geology and Geophysics, Yale University*

Summary

New evidence on the nature of earliest Old World Hominoidea has been recovered by seven Yale expeditions to the Oligocene beds of the Fayum province, north of Lake Qarun, Egypt, UAR. The continental riverine deposits of the Jebel el Qatrani formation contain three faunal horizons. These faunas are primarily from the quarry sites designated by symbols A through U. The classic Fayum faunas described by Beadnell, Andrews, Schlosser, and others are from quarries A, B, C, D, and E, representing the lowest faunal zone. About 140 feet above these horizons the middle faunal sample has been obtained at quarry G, and about 165 feet above this quarry the uppermost faunal sample has been found primarily at localities I, J, N, and O.

Earliest undoubted Anthropoidea from these levels include in the upper level two fossil apes, *Aegyptopithecus zeuxis* and *Aeolopithecus chirobates*, as well as two parapithecid primate species, *Apidium phiomense* and an undescribed large species of *Parapithecus*. At quarry G occurs a small species of *Apidium*, *A. moustafai*, which is perhaps ancestral to *A. phiomense* of the upper level. Isolated teeth from quarry G resembling those of the types of *Pro-*

This paper, presented at the second symposium on dental morphology at Royal Holloway College, England, in September 1968, constituted an updating of a review presented in Paris in 1966 which was published by the Centre National de la Recherche Scientifique in "Evolution des Vertébrés," no. 163, pp. 597–602.

Inasmuch as that article is not widely available to students of primate dental evolution, the editors of this volume have asked me to publish here the revision of the earlier text. This occasion also makes it possible to publish new and better illustrations of some of the fossils discussed.

193

pliopithecus haeckeli and *"Moeripithecus" markgrafi* indicate that these species may have been recovered at about this level or perhaps in the lowest level of quarries A, B, C, D, and E. Study of the whole series of teeth from quarry G shows that the genus *Moeripithecus* is a junior synonym of *Propliopithecus*. The shallow jaw of the type is due to its having been a juvenile, as is also indicated by the nearly complete lack of wear on M_{1-2} and the longitudinally striated nature of the bone of the ramus. *Aeolopithecus* from the upper level could be related to the later apes of the *Pliopithecus* group, whereas *Aegyptopithecus* is more demonstrably related to the ancestry of *Dryopithecus* (particularly to subgenus *Proconsul*). New finds of *Dryopithecus* from Uganda and the Siwaliks reinforce the idea that this latter genus is ancestral to the living great apes. Moreover, at the end of the Miocene some individual dryopithecines had jaw and face proportions within the size range of the living gorilla.

Oligocene Primates

Many recent discoveries have added greatly to our knowledge of the relationships of Oligocene and Miocene higher primates of the Old World, particularly in the case of the Hominoidea. Together with these finds, a number of new studies have been published in the last few years which are based on material found long ago. The conclusions indicated by these various lines of evidence and the opinions of the scientists concerned are not always clear-cut. Therefore it seems appropriate at this time to undertake a brief survey of the several separate lines of evidence on early phyletic relationships among catarrhine primates.

The main sources of new evidence on Oligocene Anthropoidea come from discoveries made during seven Yale winter expeditions, under my direction, to the Fayum Oligocene continental sediments in the badlands north of Lake Qarun, Egypt. The last five of these were supervised in the field by G. E. Meyer of Yale. From quarries in the upper part of the stratigraphic section exposed there, in the Jebel el Qatrani formation, come the oldest undoubted Old World Anthropoidea. Finds made over a half century ago in this formation were the basis for establishment of four genera of Early Oligocene primates. These are: *Apidium* Osborn 1908; and *Parapithecus*, *Propliopithecus*, and *Moeripithecus* Schlosser 1910, 1911. All the early discovered mandibular material of these primates was reviewed in 1961 by Josef Kälin in a well-illustrated monograph.

The new finds from the Fayum Oligocene demonstrate the existence of three additional primate genera in these beds: *Oligopithecus* Simons 1962; *Aegyptopithecus* and *Aeolopithecus* Simons 1965. They also provide evidence that the genus *Moeripithecus* is a junior synonym of *Propliopithecus*, although the species *M. markgrafi* is apparently distinct specifically from *P. haeckeli*. It differs principally in its slightly larger size and more expanded or rounded lower molar cusps with slightly smaller occlusal fovea. Thus, to the three valid early de-

scribed genera, with four contained species, must be added the three species
of the above new monotypic genera, together with a second species each of
Apidium and *Parapithecus, A. moustafai* Simons 1962 and *Parapithecus* sp.
nov. This brings the known Fayum primate fauna to a total of nine species, the
last of which is represented in the Yale and Cairo Museum collections, but has
not yet been described. Since this may seem to be a rather large number of
primate genera and species to be found from one area, it should be stressed
that not all the species are contemporaneous.

The Jebel el Qatrani formation, containing the continental vertebrate faunas
of the Fayum, according to recent studies by Vondra (in prep.) is about 940 feet
thick in the center of the fossil fields in a section running from Garat el Esh
through Wadi Granger and Tel Beadnell to the top of Jebel el Qatrani. In fact,
the Jebel el Qatrani formation could be subdivided into two or more members
or even into two separate formations in his opinion (see Simons and Wood
1968). The sediments of this formation probably represent at least two deposi-
tional cycles, each consisting of a sequential development of channel-flood
plain complex climaxed by formation of ponds and lakes that deposited fresh-
water limestones. The time involved in building up this varied sequence of
sediments must have been considerable, and the faunas contained in these deposits could conceivably represent samples of time-successive faunas covering
a period of time perhaps comparable to that elapsed during the Wasatch
provincial age in North America (five to seven million years). Our collections
come from three faunal zones and have been recovered primarily from a series
of quarries designated A through O. Quarries A, B, and C were named and
worked by the American Museum expedition in 1906/7, while the remainder
have been located and worked by the Yale expeditions. The early or "classic"
Fayum faunas described by Andrews (1901*a, b;* 1906), Beadnell (1905),
Schlosser (1910, 1911), and others are from the "Lower Fossil Wood Zone"
of Osborn (1908).

Quarries A, B, C, D, and E are all in this zone. It is not certain at what level
the types of the early discovered Fayum primates, *Apidium phiomense, Parapithecus fraasi, Propliopithecus haeckeli,* and *"Moeripithecus" markgrafi,* were
found. Since the early collectors in the Egyptian Fayum concentrated their
quarrying in this lower zone, these species may have been recovered in the
Lower Fossil Wood Zone, but our new evidence does not entirely corroborate
this possibility. About 140 feet above the level of quarries A through E a second faunal sample from Yale quarry G has been obtained and about 165 feet
above this single, but productive, quarry the uppermost faunal zone occurs.
The bulk of the fossil material at this level comes from Yale quarries I, J, N,
and O.

In the lower Fossil Wood Zone there is only one demonstrable occurrence of a primate: that of *Oligopithecus savagei*, figure 1, from Yale quarry E. This very small primate has the dental formula 2? 1.2.3., typical of later Catarrhini. There is some anteroposterior elongation of P_3 and the mandibular ramus is comparatively deep, as in many pongids. The molars of *Oligopithecus* show a crown pattern that is about equally similar to the Eocene Holarctic Omomyidae and to the other Fayum primates. On the basis of observable morphology in this one specimen it is not possible to allocate this species taxonomically with certainty, but it may be that this form represents a type close to the basal separation of Cercopithecoidea and Hominoidea (Simons 1962). More recently I have come to the view that it may be closer to the Hominoidea—a possibility also suggested by P. M. Butler (personal communication). The gap between canine and P_3 seen in figure 1 has been produced by postmortem anterior rotation of the canine. In life there was no alveolus or diastema in this position.

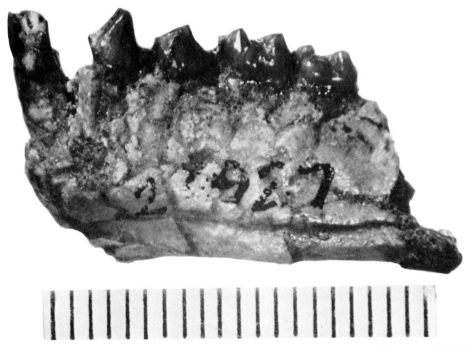

Fig. 1. The oldest undoubted member of Anthropoidea from the Oligocene, Jebel el Qatrani formation of Egypt. *Oligopithecus savagei* type, C.G.M. 29627. (Photographs in figs. 1–7 are by A. H. Coleman; in fig. 8, by J. Howard.)

The many newly recovered jaws of *Apidium phiomense*, of *Apidium moustafai*, and of an undescribed large species of *Parapithecus* show clearly that these two genera are closely related and both should be grouped together as conceptualized by Kälin (1961). Although he gave the group family status these animals should probably more properly be considered a primitive subfamily of Cercopithecidae. *Apidium phiomense* is the commonest mammal found at Yale quarry I in the Upper Fossil Wood Zone, and it is probable that the majority of primate postcranial bones (of proper size) in this quarry belong to this species. In addition an isolated frontal of a size suitable to belong to *Apidium phiomense* has been recovered from quarry I. Although showing juvenile striated bone, this specimen exhibits complete fusion of the frontals, a feature atypical of juvenile Prosimii but characteristic of young Anthropoidea. Anthropoidean relationship for parapithecines is also indicated by the complete symphyseal fusion of the mandibular horizontal rami seen in juvenile jaws of both *Apidium* and *Parapithecus* from quarry I. Such an allocation of this family is further suggested on grounds of dental morphology, as has been observed in a number of earlier papers including Simons (1963).

In 1967 in quarry I the author discovered shattered remains of a cranium and dentition of *Apidium phiomense* at one single spot no more than six inches wide. This specimen includes upper teeth definitly identifiable as *A. Phiomense* together with basicranial fragments and a piece of the central part of the frontal in the region of the interorbital septum. This frontal fragment also shows complete closure of the metopic suture. It is of the same absolute size as and has identical morphology to the same region of the more complete frontal from the Fayum described by Simons in 1959. Thus, all these small frontals apparently belong to *A. phiomense*. They confirm that closure of the metopic suture was in a preadult stage and that a catarrhine grade of advance, both in this metopic closure and in the presence of postorbital plates, had been attained. In view of these findings it is somewhat amusing that as recently as 1968 (p. 36) Hürzeler chose to publish the remark: "C'est pourquoi je ne suis pas du tout persuadé de la nature 'primate' du genre *Apidium*."

There can no longer be any such doubt that *Apidium* is a primate and that it shows significant dental and mandibular resemblances to both cercopithecids and to *Oreopithecus*. Over sixty upper and lower jaws of this genus are now known. In consequence it was misleading in 1968 for Hürzeler (p. 36) to have written that: "La prudence veut que l'on ne se serve pas de formes aussi mal connues et aussi controversées que *Apidium* . . . pour la reconstitution de l'histoire des Anthropomorphes. La même aventure que celle d'*Hesperopithecus* pourrait leur arriver."

Controversies about fossil primates arise not so much because the fossils cannot be understood as because some workers, such as Hürzeler or Osborn, *will* make controversial statements about them. *Hesperopithecus* was based on a single broken, heavily worn upper tooth of a peccary, of which essentially no structural details could be determined. It was controversial for Osborn in 1922 to have stated that such a find was a pongid, a position he was advised against taking before his publication and one from which he later had to back down. Knowledge of *Apidium* was never as inadequate as that of *Hespero-pithecus*. When only one specimen with four lower teeth was known, it was possible to demonstrate that it was a primate (Simons 1960). After five Yale expeditions I was able to report in the first version of this paper that *Apidium* was known from many new jaws and was the most abundant mammal at quarry I. Inasmuch as Dr. Hürzeler was then present, I am surprised that he can consider *Apidium* as poorly known as *Hesperopithecus*. In 1967 a maxilla of *Apidium* was found in quarry M which preserved much of the ventral and lateral orbital wall. This specimen, together with the American Museum frontal, allows for reconstruction of the face of *Apidium* (fig. 2).

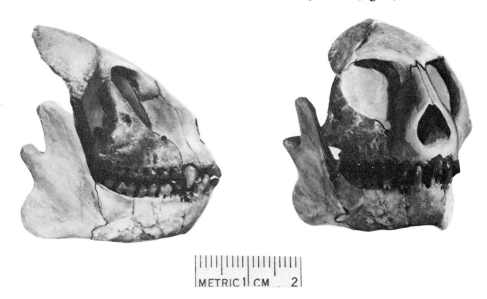

Fig. 2. Reconstructed model of the face of *Apidium phiomense*, based on A.M.N.H. 14556 frontal, C.G.M. 26929 maxilla, Y.P.M. 21016 mandible; upper canines and incisors isolated finds known to be from *Apidium* by other associations. Rostrum, orbits, and ascending mandibular ramus restored.

It shows that, unlike *Aegyptopithecus,* the face of this parapithecine was very short and rather marmosetlike. New parapithecid mandibles from quarry I also demonstrate that in both *Parapithecus* and *Apidium* the dental formula below was 2.1.3.3., the same as that of New World monkeys. Several maxillae of *Apidium* indicate that the same formula occurred above also. Judging from alveoli, the lower lateral incisors were larger than the central. Only one of the new specimens of *Apidium phiomense* retains incisors and in this only the central pair; see figure 3 (center). Presumably this specimen was fossilized in a

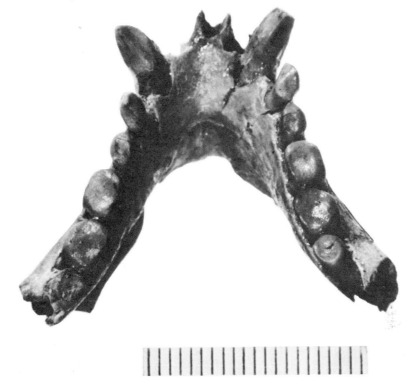

Fig. 3. A gibbonlike primate from the Egyptian Oligocene, *Aeolopithecus chirobates* type C.G.M. 26923, which, although much smaller, resembles various members of the Miocene subgenera of *Pliopithecus*.

state similar to that of the type of *Parapithecus fraasi* studied in detail by Kälin (1961). He noted that there was a break or, as he assumed, a suture at the symphysis between the mandibular rami of the type and only specimen of *Parapithecus fraasi*. Several jaws we now have show that even in juvenile parapithecines the symphysis is fused. When considerations are made in the light of the new parapithecid mandibles preserving this region, it appears that during collection of the type specimen of *P. fraasi* the exceedingly fragile anterior mandibular border and alveolar margins were lost. The two central incisors set in the reconstructed specimen are not in their natural alveoli but are glued on the anterior face of the mandible, and the rims of the lateral incisor alveoli are lost, so that the specimen now reconstructed gives an erroneous impression of the dental formula, suggesting only one incisor pair. Moreover, because of the missing bone in the symphyseal region, the converging angle of the jaw rami is too acute, or V-shaped as restored. This has also created a false resemblance to the V-shaped dental arcade of *Tarsius*. The new parapithecid mandibles which preserve the symphysis show a more parabolic or U-shaped tooth row.

The question of the relationship of Parapithecidae to later primates now seems more understandable, as primitive allies of the cercopithecid monkeys may have had no later descendants; but it still appears, of course, that the species we know, with minimal modification of tooth crown patterns and anterior teeth, could have given rise to cercopithecids or oreopithecids (Simons 1960). This would, however, require that loss of $P_{\frac{2}{2}}$ be an independent event in Hominoidea and Cercopithecoidea.

In regard to the long-known Fayum ape species *Propliopithecus haeckeli*, our expeditions have recovered only one molar tooth that seems identical in size and morphology with those of the type of this species. This isolated lower M_1 or M_2 was found in quarry G with the middle faunal sample. No data exist with the type of this species as to its locality in the Jebel el Qatrani formation. Teeth from this same quarry provisionally referred to *Pliopithecus* are more or less intermediate between the molars of *P. haeckeli* and *Aegyptopithecus zeuxis* from the upper faunal zone, figures 2 and 4. These finds from quarry G

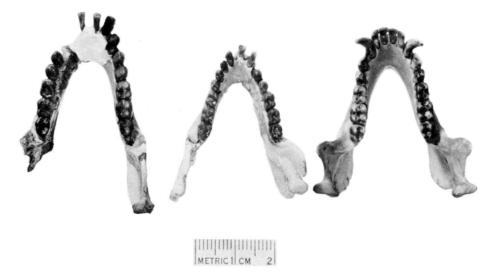

Fig. 4. Two Fayum parapithecines, compared with a modern cercopithecine monkey: *left*, two disassociated rami and four unassociated teeth of a new species of *Parapithecus; center*, mandible of a new *Apidium phiomense*, with ascending rami restored from other specimens; *right*, mandible of modern African *Miopithecus talapoin*.

suggest that the genera *Propliopithecus* (including *Moeripithecus*) and *Aegyptopithecus* could be phylogenetically interrelated.

In the upper level but only at quarry I, a distinctive small, gibbonlike ape,

Aeolopithecus chirobates Simons 1965, is known (fig. 4). This ape is distinctly different from its contemporary *Aegyptopithecus zeuxis* and shows a number of features (apart from small size) which suggest a relationship with the later, lesser apes of the genera *Pliopithecus* and *Hylobates*. Primary among these features of resemblance is the conformation of symphysis, which is deep and gibbonlike and becomes markedly shallow posteriorly, unlike mandibular rami in the remainder of Fayum primates, in which the mandibular ramus is relatively deeper to the rear. The molars do not increase in size posteriorly as is typical of the pongids other than *Hylobates* and some *Pan* and *Pliopithecus*.

At present, the best known and largest of the Fayum apes is *Aegyptopithecus zeuxis* Simons 1965. In addition to the mandibles illustrated here in figures 5 and 6 and skull figure 7, there are a number of isolated upper and lower teeth, so that at present nearly the whole dentition is known. On grounds of detailed resemblance in the upper and lower molar crown patterns between this species

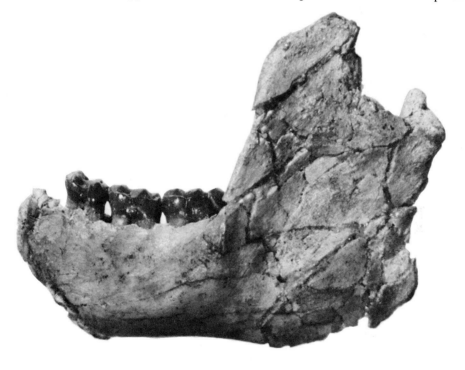

Fig. 5. An Oligocene dryopithecine. Lateral view of the left lower jaw of *Aegyptopithecus zeuxis*, Y.P.M. 21032.

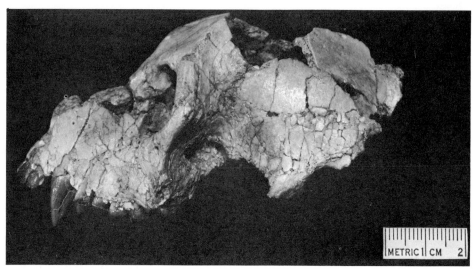

Fig. 6. Lateral view of the skull of *Aegyptopithecus zeuxis* Y.P.M. 23975, incisors unassociated.

and those of *Dryopithecus* (subgenus *Proconsul*) from the early or middle Miocene of East Africa, it seems most likely that *Aegyptopithecus* is in or near the ancestry of the dryopithecine subfamily of apes. Nevertheless, it is considerably smaller than even the smallest described East African Miocene dryopithecine species *Dryopithecus africanus*.

New studies or discoveries of materials that could be compared with these Fayum Oligocene Anthropoidea have been made in the past five years. These include the recovery by Dr. Wilson of the University of Texas, in 1964, of a virtually complete, uncrushed skull of an early Oligocene omomyid primate from West Texas. Wilson (1966) published a preliminary description of this skull for which he has established a new genus and species *Rooneyia viejaensis*. Although more primitive in the relevant cranial features than any known Anthropoidea, this skull suggests relationships to the undoubted earliest catarrhines of the Fayum, and to the microhoerine prosimians of the European Eocene. It is close to the borderline between Prosimii and Anthropoidea in observable cranial features. Other possible related forms have either been found or redescribed in recent years. These include redescription of the materials of *Pondaungia* and *Amphipithecus* from the Late Eocene Pondaung sandstone of Burma, which have been recently restudied by Simons (1963) and by von Koenigswald (1965). Von Koenigswald has concluded that *Ponduangia* is a condylarth and *Amphipithecus* a prosimian, basing this argument in part on the observation that "there are no signs of a faunal exchange between Africa and the rest of the Old World before the Miocene." He therefore concludes that, since early Anthropoidea definitely do occur in the Fayum Oligocene, if there was no

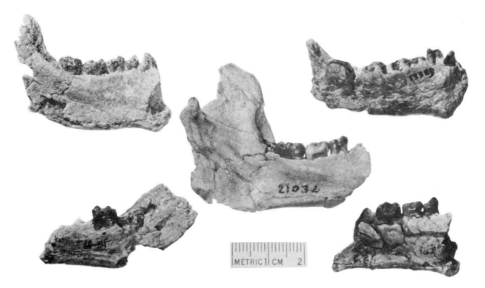

Fig. 7. Lateral views of five fragmentary mandibular rami of *Aegyptopithecus zeuxis*. *Upper left,* Y.P.M. 23944; *upper right,* A.M.N.H. 13389; *center,* Y.P.M. 21032; *lower left,* C.G.M. 29135; *lower right,* type C.G.M. 26901.

pre-Miocene faunal exchange between Eurasia and Africa the Burmese forms cannot be higher primates. However, there *is* evidence of early faunal exchange. My comparisons suggest that anthracotheres of the Pondaung sandstone are almost certainly congeneric with those of the Fayum. Moreover, an undescribed carnivore from the Fayum in the Yale collections is probably at least congeneric with one of the European Eocene proviverrine genera (Van Valen, personal communication) but, as this group has not been adequately revised, the generic name with priority is uncertain. *Metasinopa* Osborn 1909 is in the opinion of Van Valen (1966, p. 75) not clearly separable from European *Paracynohyaenodon.* In addition, the Fayum carnivore genera *Apterodon* and *Pterodon* have European Eocene genotypes. A species of *Rhagatherium,* a Swiss Eocene artiodactyl, is also reported from the Fayum by Andrews (1906).

Consequently, there is clear evidence that pre-Miocene faunal exchange between Africa and Eurasia did occur, probably in the late Eocene. Because of their fragmentary nature, the types and only specimens of *Amphipithecus* and *Pondaungia* are difficult to classify, but the preserved parts are more like primates than like members of any other order. If not Anthropoidea, it is just possible that they may be advanced omomyid prosimians.

Miocene Primates

Turning to the primates of the Miocene age, a number of relatively recent finds have been made which provide new evidence on the extent and interrelationships of the catarrhine radiation. Among these new discoveries is the report by Leakey (1962) of a fauna of late Miocene age on the Wicker farm near Fort Ternan, Kenya. This site has been dated by the potassium-argon method of geochemical dating as about fourteen million years old. This is an age estimate about two million years greater than is commonly given for rocks of earlier Pliocene age in North America. In his 1962 publication and at the Chicago conference on "The Origin of Man" in April 1965, Leakey has now reported from this one small site fauna which includes species apparently belonging to three hominid primate genera, including *Dryopithecus* and *Ramapithecus,* an oreopithecid (Leakey 1968*b*), and cercopithecine monkeys. The remainder of this fauna has not been fully reported, but the potassium-argon date and the degree of morphological difference from species in the older Rusinga Island series suggest a later age. Moreover, the many new faunal elements seen at Fort Ternan strengthen the probability that the new site is of Miocene age. The other primates correlate well with the late Miocene appearances of *Dryopithecus sivalensis* and *Ramapithecus punjabicus* in the Chinji zone of the Siwaliks (Simons and Pilbeam 1965). A specimen which cannot be separated taxonomically from the Indian materials of *R. punjabicus* has been found in the Fort Ternan locality (Simons 1964). Moreover, the Leakeys have continued collecting in the Rusinga Miocene sites known to them, and Leakey has announced recently (Chicago conference) the discovery of an almost complete mandible of the largest species of subgenus *Proconsul, Dryopithecus major.* This is a welcome new addition to knowledge of this largest African Miocene ape. This find is particularly relevant at this time since it can be compared and contrasted with the relatively complete palate of the same species, first reported in 1961 by Allbrook and Bishop of the Uganda Museum, which was found near Moroto, Uganda. In 1964, on another visit to this site, Bishop's party recovered in three portions an isolated lower jaw which may belong to the same individual and most of the upper teeth of the palate other than right central upper incisor which had been lost in life. Parts of the facial bones were also recovered. Although he had not seen this new material, Leakey (1965) was prepared to state that this palate could not be *Dryopithecus (Proconsul) major.* Through the kindness of Dr. Bishop, I have studied the original palate at Yale, together with the mandible from the same site, Moroto II, Karamoja District, Uganda, and these two specimens do belong to *Dryopithecus major.* These specimens exhibit fully the most characteristic defining features of subgenus *Proconsul.* In the mandibular ramus, the P_3 is placed directly posterior to the canine and separated from it by a gap instead of being located posterolateral and close to the canine as in many modern African apes. In addition, the M_3 is triangular in outline, a feature that is common in *Proconsul* from Kenya. The most backwardly projecting region of the symphyseal cross section is midway up and the preserved part of the symphyseal cross section is just as it is in the Kenya *D. major* jaws. In showing comparatively well-developed hypocones and large, crenulate lingual cingula on upper molars the Moroto II upper dentition also falls within subgenus *Proconsul*. Moreover, this maxillary dentition occludes perfectly with that of the type mandible of *Dryopithecus (Proconsul) major*, partly because the two specimens were from individuals with faces of very comparable size. Reconstructions of the palates of two Miocene apes *Dryopithecus africanus* and *D. major* are contrasted in figure 7 with a reconstructed palate of the earliest known possible hominid *Ramapithecus punjabicus*. Recently Pilbeam (1970) has published an exhaustive review of the Miocene apes of Uganda. These have been carefully compared with the contemporary fossil apes of Kenya. Pilbeam concludes that *D. africanus* may be in or near the ancestry of the chimpanzee and *D. major* of the gorilla. He concurs with my view that *"Kenyapithecus africanus"* (Leakey 1967, 1968a) is not a hominid. Actually, most and possibly all of the specimens allocated to it belong to the three East African species of *Dryopithecus*.

A further study of African Miocene primates consists of an analysis of the monkeys of the Rusinga and Maboko Island faunas of the Kenya Miocene by von Koenigswald (1969).

Having located in the Cairo Museum the type specimens of *Dryopithecus? mogharensis* and *Prohylobates tandyi* from a Miocene fauna in Wadi Moghara, Egypt, I have only recently completed a restudy of these materials (Simons 1969). Neither of these specimens is an ape and both of these "specimens" from Wadi Moghara represent only one species of cercopithecoid monkey. This has to be called, rather inappropriately, *Prohylobates tandyi,* an unfortunate name since it is not a gibbon. The faunal correlations suggest an age similar to or somewhat younger than that of the Rusinga Island monkeys. The question of generic identity between these two African samples of earliest known Old World monkeys can now be considered since the publication of von Koenigswald's study of the East African Miocene monkeys. Unlike the Kenya Miocene cercopithecoid, in which molar size increases posteriorly, the Wadi Moghara cercopithecoid had an M_3 smaller than M_{1-2}. Consequently it is probably a distinct genus.

Turning to discoveries from the European Miocene, recent searching for pre-Pontian pongids in northern Spain under the direction of Dr. Crusafont has yielded a total of about fifty specimens of fossil apes. Perhaps the most significant of these is the first *Dryopithecus* maxillary recovered in Europe. This find has been under study by Dr. Hürzeler in Basel. In Asia Minor a large *Dryopithecus* mandible was described by Ozansoy (1957). According to Ozansoy this

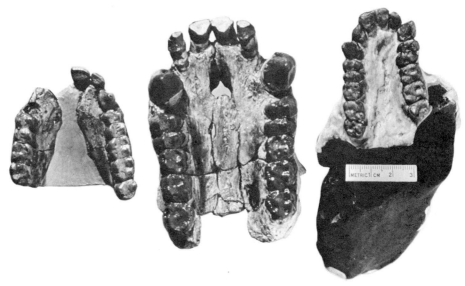

Fig. 8. Comparison of casts of the palates of three kinds of Miocene Hominoidea. *Left*, *Ramapithecus punjabicus* from Haritalyangar, Himachal Pradesh, India, right P³–M² Y.P.M. 13799; and left, the same mirror image, left M³ G.S.I. 18068, left I²⁻³ and C hypothetically restored on the basis of alveolar and root size and in harmony with the C and I² of *Ramapithecus* from Fort Ternan, Kenya. *Center, Dryopithecus (Proconsul) major*. Middle palate from Moroto, Uganda with right I² restored and parts of other teeth restored. *Right*, palate of *Dryopithecus (Proconsul) africanus* (1948 skull).

jaw is associated with a fauna of apparent Pontian age, but although it was given a new name the specimen appears to be taxonomically indistinguishable from the Siwalik species *Dryopithecus indicus*. Discoveries in the coal fields near Keiyuan, China, reported in 1957 and 1958 by Woo have extended the range of Siwalik primates eastward. Chow (1958) has stressed that one of the Yunnan finds is like *Dryopithecus indicus* and the other close to, or the same as, *Ramapithecus* (non *Dryopithecus*) *punjabicus*. Other kinds of mammals found as fossils in the Yunnan coal fields also correlate with various elements of the Siwalik Chinji-Nagri zones. In India itself twelve new finds of *Dryopithecus* and *Ramapithecus* from the region of Haritalyangar, Hemichal Pradesh, have been published, in 1962 and 1964 by K. N. Prasad of Calcutta. More recently he (1969) has reviewed the Siwalik apes and has argued for the validity of a small extinct Indian ape species originally named by Pilgrim (1927), *Dryopithecus (= Sivapithecus) chinjiensis*. In April 1968 the Yale expeditions under my direction secured a remarkably well preserved mandible of Middle Pliocene *Gigantopithecus* (about 6 million years) from Dhok Pathan horizons east of Haritalyangar, India (see Simons and Chopra 1969). This specimen apparently links in morphology and is intermediate in time between 10 and 12 million year old *Dryopithecus indicus* and the much younger 1–5 million-year-old *Gigantopithecus blacki* from South China.

REFERENCES

Andrews, C. W. 1906. *A descriptive catalogue of the Tertiary vertebrata of the Fayum, Egypt.* London: Brit. Mus. Nat. Hist.

Chow, M. C. 1958. Mammalian faunas and correlation of the Tertiary and early Pleistocene of South China. *J. Paleont. Soc. Ind.* 3:123–29.

Crusafont, M. 1965. El desarrollo de los caninos en algunos Driopithecidos del Vallesiense en Cataluña. *Notas y Comuns. Inst. Geol. Min. España.*

Hofer, H. O., and Wilson, J. A. 1967. An endocranial cast of an early Oligocene primate. *Folia Primat.* 5:148–52.

Hürzeler, J. 1968. Questions et réflexions sur l'histoire des Anthropomorphes. *Ann. Paléontol.* (Vertébrés) 54 (fasc. 2):11–41.

Kälin, J. 1961. Sur les primates de l'Oligocène Inférieur d'Égypt. *Ann. Paléontol.* 47:1–48.

Koenigswald, G. H. R. von. 1965. Critical observations upon the so-called higher primates from the Upper Eocene of Burma. *Proc. Koninkl. Nederl. Akademie van Wetenschappen, ser. B,* 68:165–67.

———. 1969. Miocene Cercopithecoidea and Oreopithecoidea of East Africa. In *Fossil vertebrates of Africa,* ed. L. S. B. Leakey, 1:39–51. New York: Academic Press.

Leakey, L. S. B. 1962. A new Lower Pliocene fossil primate from Kenya. *Ann. Mag. Nat. Hist.,* ser. 13, 4:689–96.

———. 1965. Remarks on hominid and pongid evolution. In *The origin of man: A symposium,* ed. P. L. DeVore. New York: Wenner-Gren Foundation Anth. Res.

———. 1967. An early Miocene member of Hominidae. *Nature* 213:155–63.

———. 1968a. Lower dentition of *Kenyapithecus africanus. Nature* 217:827–30.

———. 1968b. Upper Miocene primates from Kenya. *Nature* 218:527–28.

Osborn, H. F. 1908. New fossil mammals from Fayum Oligocene of Egypt. *Bull. Amer. Mus. Nat. Hist.* 24:265–72.

———. 1909. New carnivorous mammals from the Fayum Oligocene, Egypt. *Bull. Amer. Mus. Nat. Hist.* 26:415–24.

———. 1922. *Hesperopithecus,* the first anthropoid primate found in America. *Amer. Mus. Nat. Hist. Novit.* 37:1–5.

Ozansoy, F. 1957. Faunes des mammifères du Tertiare de Turquie et leurs revisions stratigraphiques. *Bull. Min. Res. Exp. Inst. Turkey* 49:29–48.

Pilbeam, D. R. 1970. Tertiary Pongidae of East Africa: Evolutionary relationships and taxonomy. *Bull. Peabody Mus. Nat. Hist., Yale Univ.* 31:1–185.

Pilgrim, G. E. 1927. A *Sivapithecus* palate and other primate fossils from India. *Palaeont. Ind.* 14:1–24.

Prasad, K. N. 1962. Fossil primates from the Siwalik beds near Haritalyangar, Himachal Pradesh, India. *J. Geol. Soc. Ind.* 3:86–96.

———. 1964. Upper Miocene anthropoids from the Siwalik beds of Haritalyangar, Himachal Pradesh, India. *Palaeontology* 7:124–34.

———. 1969. Critical observations on the fossil anthropoids from the Siwalik system of India. *Folia Primat.* 10:288–317.

Schlosser, M. 1910. Über einige fossile Säugetiere aus dem Oligocän von Ägypten. *Zool. Anz.* 35:500–508.

———. 1911. Beiträge zur Kenntnis der Oligozänen Landsäugetiere aus dem Fayum (Ägypten). *Beitre Paläont. Österreich-Ungarns* 24:51–167.

Simons, E. L. 1959. An anthropoid frontal bone from the Oligocene of Egypt: The oldest skull fragment of a higher primate. *Amer. Mus. Nat. Hist. Novitat.* 1976: 1–16.

———. 1960. *Apidium* and *Oreopithecus*. *Nature* 186:824–26.

———. 1962. Two new primate species from the African Oligocene. *Postilla, Peabody Mus. Nat. Hist. Yale Univ.* 64:1–12.

———. 1963. A critical reappraisal of Tertiary primates. In *Genetics and evolutionary biology of primates,* ed. J. Buettner-Janusch, pp. 65–129. New York: Academic Press.

———. 1964. On the mandible of *Ramapithecus*. *Proc. Nat. Acad. Sci.* 51:528–35.

———. 1965. New fossil apes from Egypt and inital differentiation of Hominoidea. *Nature* 205:135–39.

———. 1969. Miocene monkey (*Prohylobates*) from northern Egypt. *Nature* 223: 687–89.

Simons, E. L., and Chopra, S. R. K. 1969. *Gigantopithecus* (Hominoidea), a new species from North India. *Postilla, Peabody Mus. Nat. Hist., Yale Univ.* 138: 1–18.

Simons, E. L., and Pilbeam, D. R. 1965. Preliminary revision of the Dryopithecinae (Pongidae, Anthropoidea). *Folia Primat.* 3:81–125.

Simons, E. L., and Wood, A. E. 1968. Early Cenozoic mammalian faunas, Fayum Province, Egypt. *Peabody Mus. Nat. Hist. Yale Univ. Bull.* 28:1–105.

Van Valen, L. 1966. Deltatheridia, a new order of mammals. *Bull. Amer. Mus. Nat. Hist.* 132:1–126.

Wilson, J. A. 1966. A new primate from the earliest Oligocene, West Texas, preliminary report. *Folia Primat.* 4:227–48.

Woo, J. K. 1957. *Dryopithecus* teeth from Keiyuan, Yunnan Province. *Vert. Palas.* 1:25–32.

———. 1958. New materials of *Dryopithecus* from Keiyuan, Yunnan. *Vert. Palas.* 2:31–43.

Part III

Morphology

12 A Systematic Description of Dental Roots

I. Kovacs   *Brussels, Belgium*

Introduction

The study of the morphological characteristics of dental roots is of great interest in the fields of descriptive anatomy, anthropology, comparative anatomy, phylogenetics, the study of sexual dimorphism, and dental anomalies, let alone parodontosis and dental prothesis.

However, when reviewing the various studies dealing with the morphology of teeth, their variations, anomalies, and morphological aspects, one notices that most of the studies deal with the dental crown and that only a minority relate to the root.

This disproportion in the number of studies dealing with crowns and roots also results from the fact that the latter have diverse aspects which make them difficult to describe. The difficulty arises because, apart from the number of roots and their length, there has been no guide for the systematic description of root morphology. In this presentation each feature is described in sufficient detail to allow the study of the microevolution of the dental root.

Species are generally divided into three main groups: Carnivora, Herbivora, and Omnivora, according to the gnathos function and foods used. Apart from the features pertaining to these three groups there must also exist intermediate features. Results of several experiments are described. The observations made would seem to indicate that dental roots of man are closer to those of the carnivora than to those of the omnivora.

This paper is meant to serve as a guide for root studies. The reader is also referred to the works of Brabant, Klees, and Werelds (1958), Taviani (1953), and Visser (1948), and also to those of Jorgensen (1956), Pedersen (1949), and Tratman (1950).

211

Material and Method

Preparation of the tooth for investigation of roots is very important, especially for modern teeth. For instance, at the level of the neck of the tooth are found traces of circular ligaments which must be removed. These are not present in ancient teeth. Moreover, roots of teeth from excavations have become slightly colored, whereas the color of enamel on the crown remains rather unchanged. However, sometimes enamel of ancient teeth has cracked off because of dryness. In such cases a magnifying glass (10 ×) with light was used.

The teeth were carefully cleaned and soaked in a 30% solution of Oxygenol for several hours. They were then colored with a 2.5% methylene blue solution and, when dry, were rubbed with a moist chamois. This procedure brings out markings caused by forceps or other abrasions.

Comments on the Ontogenetic Morphology of Dental Roots

During development, an organ undergoes "dynamic" transformations, and in ontogenetic-morphologic study these transformations must be followed and registered. Since organs successively take various shapes, some well-determined stages in development can be observed and recorded. These observations are easier on teeth because they are easily isolated.

Ontogenetic studies offer answers to numerous questions relating to the morphology of roots (Kovacs 1963, 1964, 1967).

This paper will be directed toward summarizing the stages in root development and the morphologic findings obtained by macrophotography, particularly at the level of the interradicular bifurcation of multirooted teeth (fig. 1).

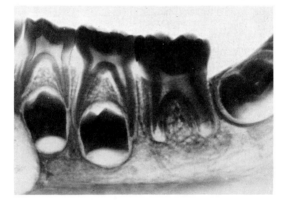

Fig. 1. Radiograph of a human mandibular first molar, at the time it is in occlusion, showing the root at two thirds of its development. At this time, the root comes against the compact bone part at the base of the roots and, before its apical part can form, alveolar resorption must occur.

Development of Dental Roots. There are two phases in the development of roots, the eruptive and the penetrative (fig. 2).

The *eruptive phase* starts when the root begins to develop and ends when the tooth is in occlusion. At that time about two-thirds of the root is developed. This proportion can vary, however, according to individual species and type of tooth.

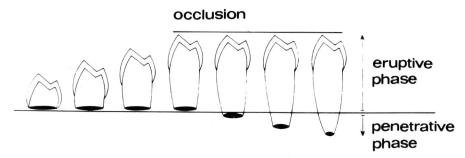

Fig. 2. Diagram of Root Formation. Two phases in the development of the root can be distinguished on the basis of the anatomical stages in the jaw during its formation: the eruptive phase and the penetrative phase. The eruptive phase goes on until the time when the tooth is in occlusion. During the eruptive phase the level of the diaphragm remains constant; during the penetrative phase, it is displaced toward the alveolar base.

During the eruptive phase, the level of the diaphragm (Orban 1962) remains constant. The diaphragm consists of an internal layer of odontoblasts and an external layer of primary cementoblasts; it is, in fact, the diaphragm of a two-dimensional organ. The apposition of dentin and cementum always occurs at the same level; that is, the space between the diaphragm and the bone wall of the germ remains identical. This is contingent on the alveolar resorption above the crown being sufficient to provide for eruption.

The *penetrative phase* begins when the tooth is in occlusion. During this phase the level of the diaphragm is displaced toward the alveolar base. This phase can be seen on the root, which shows on the apical third (fig. 3) an irregular rough and corrugated surface contrasted to the smooth, crack-free surface of the eruptive phase. These two phases in root development can also be seen on deciduous teeth.

In impacted or embedded teeth, the penetrative phase often starts at a higher level on the root when contact is made with another tooth or object.

The pathological mechanism of ankylosis in embedded teeth during the disappearance of periodontal tissue has the characteristic of intermediary tissue resulting in the diaphragm's penetrating into the bone.

The mechanism of accessory canals can also be explained by a modification

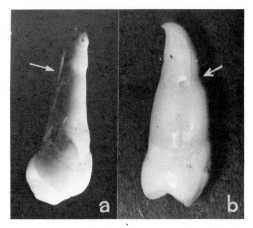

Fig. 3. (*a*) Maxillary second premolar of man shows the characteristic aspects of the two parts of the root, the apical third and the two-thirds located toward the crown. The surface of this latter part of the root is polished and has a clear-cut outline. The surface of the apical third of the root shows small undulations and circular pleating. (*b*) The division between the two phases is sometimes shown on the teeth by a pronounced break.

in the level of the diaphragm. Similarly, tooth concrescence occurs during the penetrative phase.

Comparative Study. The ontogenetic-morphologic study is also interesting from the viewpoint of comparison between species. We have had the opportunity to study the development of multirooted teeth in Carnivora (lions), Herbivora (horse), and Omnivora (chimpanzees, gorilla). Preliminary investigations on ten jaws per species seem to indicate that the proportion of root developed during each phase, that is, the proportion between "smooth" surface and "rough" surface, varies according to the species. In carnivores the penetrative phase seems to start later than in other orders and the smooth surface part of the root is proportionately greater. The proportion of smooth surface part of the root seems to decrease from carnivore to omnivore and to herbivore.

Root Bifurcation. Histologic investigation makes it possible to understand rather well the various stages in the development of the roots of teeth. Macroscopic and microscopic sections alone, however, generally are not sufficient to allow morphologic syntheses because they are limited in dimension. The same applies to radiographs.

Combining macroscopic study with macrophotography can effectively help interpret the radicular bifurcation, because this method facilitates the observation of details.

On the subject of root bifurcation, reference is made to Siffre (1921), Sicher and Tandler (1928), Meyer (1951), Orban (1962), Alexandersen (1962), Jorgensen (1950), and Carlsen (1967).

I have also dealt with this subject in earlier works (Kovacs 1963, 1967), which gave the following conclusions:

In multirooted teeth, development of roots begins with the narrowing of the epithelial diaphragm at the level of the tooth neck. From this diaphragm, horizontal processes begin to develop; these have a tendency to meet and to penetrate the pulp. After the various processes have met in the center of the interradicular bifurcation, the junction and complete closing of the various radicular rings occurs. Therefore two, three, or more diaphragms of the roots are constituted from the original diaphragm which is at the base of the crown, determining the number of roots (fig. 4).

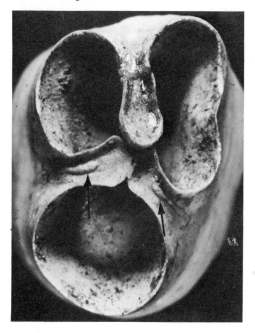

Fig. 4. Germ of a human maxillary first molar; the three diaphragmatic processes are about to meet. In the axes of these processes, there are elongated protuberances that correspond to primary filaments.

The length of the tooth root depends on the narrowing of the diaphragm. If the diaphragm narrows rapidly, the root will be shorter. If the narrowing occurs more slowly, the root will be longer.

The level, direction, length, and number of the transverse processes of the diaphragm determine the morphologic characteristics of the future root. The diaphragmatic processes, in the beginning, are limited to promontories that prepare the room for their future development. When the calcified transverse processes of the diaphragm are ready to unite, they take the shape of an arrowhead. In place of a process, a longitudinal fold sometimes appears under the root. This peculiarity suggests that root formation represents the product of a radicular fusion (fig. 5).

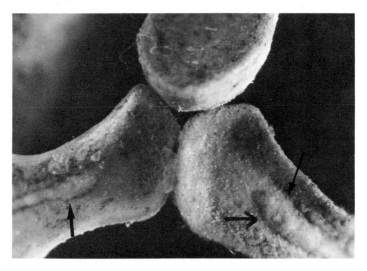

Fig. 5. Enlargement of fig. 4 showing that the protuberances on the three processes are enamel.

At the point where the processes meet, a perfect obturation is realized by a dental proliferation, a ridge which has the appearance of a cicatrix or callus. This callus can be found not only on the tooth germ at this stage, but also at the top of the interradicular bifurcation of formed teeth. This callus also can be found in deciduous, multirooted teeth at the point where the diaphragmatic processes meet (fig. 6).

Macrophotography shows that on the edge of the diaphragm, mineralization is produced by small processes (fig. 7). These processes may be important not only in tooth eruption but in the change of position of the tooth germ.

No accessory canal has been observed at the point where the diaphragmatic processes meet. Accessory canals occasionally have been observed at the point where the promontory develops; that is, at the top of the interradicular bifurcation.

In the maxillary and mandibular first molars, the transverse processes always develop in a typical manner, but the second molar shows a tendency to polymorphism. This tendency is even more pronounced in third molars.

Comparative Study. We have had the opportunity to examine several dozen tooth germs from gorillas, chimpanzees, horses, and lions. The processes of determination of the bifurcation occur the same way as in human teeth. The

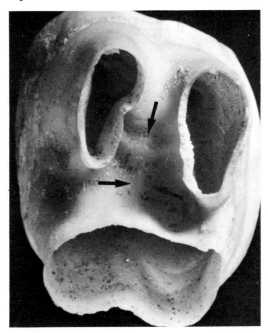

Fig. 6. Germ of a gorilla beringei's first maxillary molar. Ontogenetic development seems identical to that in man. A ridge in Y form is also found in the interradicular area.

processes, as well as the interradicular ridge, can be seen on the fully developed teeth.

Actual Length of Roots

The majority of books on anatomy give the actual length of dental roots but very few of them give detailed information on the number of roots, races, and so on, nor do they always describe the way measurements were made. This lack of information makes the figures given less valuable. The height of the crown in human teeth varies from side to side, and the length of the roots will be different as it is measured on one side or the other. It is not always clear in the accounts which root the measurements relate to, though each of the roots frequently differs in length.

On the other hand, the question of actual measurement of the root length is very complex because the root does not always lie in prolongation of the axis of the crown but, according to Muhlreiter (1920), it shows a tilting on the distal side of about 18°. Measurement is even more complicated in animal teeth, for instance rodents, since the roots are curved and look like the arc of a circle (fig. 8).

Measuring the root is not difficult if it is in prolongation of the axis of the crown and if it is straight. However, when the root forms an angle with the

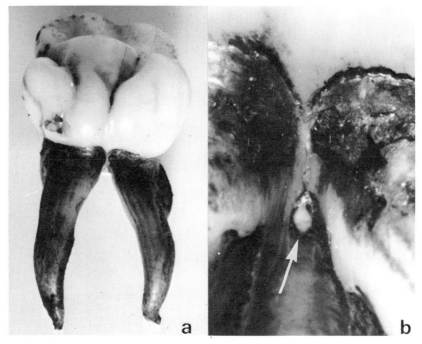

Fig. 7. Deciduous maxillary second molar—human tooth: (*a*) macrophotographs showing a supernumerary root on palatine side; (*b*) enlargement (× 20) showing interradicular
extension with an enamel pearl. This enamel interradicular extension was noticed in all
seven teeth in our collection that had a supernumerary root.

crown or when it is curved its length will be different according to whether
measurement is made on the whole tooth or on the crown and root separately.

We suggest two ways to measure curved roots: divide the root into small
straight parts which are measured separately and then add the results together;
or use a tin wire (because of its pliability) which is applied to the root, cut to
exact dimensions, and then measured.

When we do not find in a tooth an anatomically differentiated crown covered
with enamel and a root covered with cement, such as the hypsodont teeth, we
recommend using the words "root in function" and "crown in function" when
comparing them. The limit between the root in function and crown in function
would be the dentogingival junction, and the root would comprise that part
which is embodied in the alveolar bone of the jaw and the circular ligaments
up to the epithelial junction. This level is often recognizable by the pigmenta-
tion of the crown, that is, the functional part.

The length of the root can be modified as a result of pathological influences
which give rise to either resorption, which may shorten the root, or hyper-
cementosis, which may increase the length of the root.

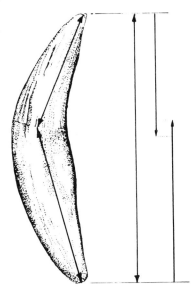

Fig. 8. This drawing of a mandibular canine of a lion (*Felis leo*) shows how results are affected by how measurements are made: the length will be different when the entire tooth is measured and when the crown and root are measured separately.

Consideration should be given to anomalies related to excessive or reduced lengths. It is suggested that the degree of deviation and the statistical implications from the normal range be assessed.

Relative Length of the Root

The relative length of the root is the proportion of the real length of the root to that of the total tooth.

The importance of that information is that it enables comparative study better than the actual length, especially in the case of an anomaly and in pathological cases, or when comparison with teeth of different zoological species is desired.

On the other hand, we are of the opinion that the relative length of the root and its surface are the most important features from a morphologicofunctional viewpoint. There is a correlation between the biological processes and the basic laws of physics and engineering. From the viewpoint of gnathodynamics, anchorage plays an important part by its depth, its surface, and its relationship with superstructure.

To express the relative length of the root we need a formula which simply shows a proportion:

$$\frac{\text{length of root} \times 100}{\text{length of tooth}} = \text{index of relative length of root.}$$

For hypsodont teeth we recommend considering the root and the crown "in function" in order to figure out the index.

Here are the normal indexes for an incisor calculated from the dimensions given by:

a) Lenhossek:

> Lenth of root   : 16 mm
> Total length of tooth : 28 mm   Index : 57.14

b) De Jonge:

> Length of root   : 13.4 mm
> Total length of tooth : 24.0 mm   Index : 55.83

Among anomalies, we took an interest in extremely short roots. In our collection of 500 maxillary central incisors we looked for three teeth having the shortest roots and determined the relative length of the roots:

	Length of Root	Total Length	Index
a)	6.2 mm	16.5 mm	37.57
b)	8.0 mm	20.0 mm	40.00
c)	7.8 mm	18.9 mm	41.27

(These three teeth had been extracted because of their excessive migration linked to alveolysis and considerable mobility. We were able to determine the hereditary character of such short teeth in one family where the father and two daughters showed the same anomaly.)

Excessively short roots and rootless teeth have been discussed in several studies among which are those of De Jonge (1958), Ballschmiede (1922), Massler and Schour (1941), Zellner (1957), Wegner (1939), and Brabant (1969a).

Let us mention also that the difference in index between permanent teeth and deciduous teeth seems to be about 10% in favor of the latter. Deciduous teeth would, therefore, seem to be better anchored in the jaw than permanent teeth.

As a preliminary investigation we compared the relative length of *canines* from different zoological species. Sampling comprised eight to twenty-one teeth per animal. To make the comparison with human teeth we used the average dimensions of canines given by Muhlreiter (1920):

	Human Beings	Lion	Chimpanzee	Gorilla
Relative root length index:	55.11	59.35	66.92	71.41

For first mandibular *molars* the results are as follows for a sampling of between seven and twenty teeth. For human teeth we also used the dimensions given by Muhlreiter (1920).

	Human Being	Lion	Chimpanzee	Gorilla	Horse
Relative root length index:	63.59	66.15	73.69	77.19	78.20

These preliminary results seem to us very surprising and we believe that a more elaborate study and statistical calculations will show highly significant differences between the various zoological groups.

When a more direct comparison between the length of the root and that of the crown is desired it may be interesting to divide the length of the root multiplied by 100 by the length of the crown instead of that of the whole tooth.

Cementoenamal Junction

At first sight the cementoenamel junction does not seem to fit into the frame of this study on the root proper, since it is only a boundary between the crown and the root. However, we are of the opinion that it is a determining factor in the formation of the root and we have tried to find on the cementoenamel junction several features appearing on the root.

General Comments. Anatomic description of human teeth has shown that the cementoenamel junction line is not regular on the whole periphery of the tooth. On the mesial side of the tooth a bend toward the crown can be seen which is more pronounced than that on the distal side. This feature seems to be common among the primates. It also makes it possible to distinguish the mesial side of a tooth and, therefore, to tell whether it comes from the right side or the left side of the jaw. On the distal side, the junction line is sometimes rather straight or is bent toward the root. On the buccal and lingual sides alignment varies according to individuals, species, and teeth.

The distribution of enamel on the root in the interradicular area is of interest from the viewpoint of periodontal disease because epithelial attachment on enamel definitely has less value than epithelial attachment on cement. When interradicular extension of enamel is present there is a predisposition to the formation of a pathological pocket.

Only one feature of the junction, interradicular extension at the level of bifurcation, has been dealt with statistically from a racial viewpoint, by Pedersen (1949), Tratman (1950), Brabant and Sahly (1962), and Twiesselman and Brabant (1960). Other studies dealing with this subject are Jørgensen (1956), Carlsen (1968), Moeschler (1968), and Sakai (1967). Some writers set up a classification of the outline of the junction, such as Watson and Woods (1926), Pedersen and Thyssen (1942), Jørgensen (1956), and Carlsen (1968).

Method of Study. To study the cementoenamel junction, Sakai (1967) dissolved the enamel with acids.

After several tests, we recommend as the best procedure the coloring of the teeth with methylene blue, which shows a greater affinity for cement than for enamel and consequently creates a contrast of colors against which islands and pearls of enamel stand out. The presence of little islands of cement on enamel has been discussed by Euler and Brabant (1954).

The cementoenamel junction exhibits three types of relationship, according to Noyes, Schour, and Noyes (1943) and Krebel (1964).

1. The most common arrangement is an overlapping of the cementum over a small part of the enamel (65%).
2. Enamel and cementum meet end to end in about 30% of cases.
3. In a smaller number of cases (5%) enamel and cementum do not touch, exposing dentin surface in this region.

Before our study, we tried to determine how to obtain an image of the junction. The junction can be examined: (a) on the entire periphery of the tooth; (b) on one whole side of the tooth; or (c) on a length of 2 mm on one side.

The pantograph helps obtain a somewhat enlarged graph. We also examined the junctions with the help of a magnifying glass equipped with a light, which enlarges the picture about ten times. We then used macrophotographs, either snapshots or slides, which enlarge the pictures about three hundred times.

The study of lengths of about 2 mm on the junction line, enlarged 30 to 300 times, allowed us to observe various types of lines:

straight line
slightly undulated line
very undulated line
circuitous line
broken line
line with one or more trigonid notches
complex line.

Examination of the junction line on whole sides of the tooth showed extremely complex lines and though we would have liked to classify them we consider that this requires a much more thorough investigation than we have been able to make.

One important point when examining the cementoenamel junction is *enamel extension at the level of bifurcation*. This extension can vary greatly in length and is often present, even in the case of fused roots. Very narrow interradicular extensions prolonging the notches were found much more often than we had expected. Sometimes there was a break between the notch and its extension; the latter is then called an island. These extensions are hardly visible and generally appear on the buccal side of maxillary molars, the frequency of occurrence increasing from the first to the third molar.

On thirty-one *mesiodens* that were studied it was observed that the line of the cementoenamel junction shows a bend toward the crown that is more pronounced on one side and that it is on that same side that the pointed part of the tooth tips. On the other side the line is concave, convex, or straight.

The same universal feature was observed on *supernumerary teeth* and *teeth* found in *dermoid cysts.*

We also investigated other anomalies such as *fossacoronoradicular* (figs. 9 and 10) and the *syndesmocoronoradicular tooth* (fig. 11).

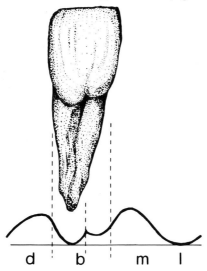

Fig. 9. Central maxillary incisor—human tooth. This drawing of the buccal side of a tooth shows a "fossacoronoradicular" anomaly. In such cases a hollow is found on the crown and is also noticed on the root in a more or less pronounced form. The diagram shows this irregularity.

In the former we noticed that the junction line, instead of showing a bend toward the crown as it generally does, was divided into two often unequal parts and showed at that place a hollow which was nearly always present in the crown and very often in the root and can also continue on the latter up to the apex. Observation on macrophotographs showed that the junction line was rarely clear-cut, and it seems that cement overlaps enamel. In our collection of five hundred incisors we found fifteen such teeth. On the other teeth we very often found this feature, but it was less pronounced. According to Brabant and Sahly (1962) it can sometimes be found on teeth dating back to prehistoric and medieval eras.

The second anomaly mentioned above, syndesmocoronoradicular tooth, falls into the same category as the first one. In was described by Chompret, as cited by Dechaume (1959), and by Brabant, Klees and Werelds (1958). In this case, the junction looks like a broken line on the lingual side. We found one such case among the teeth of thirty-one gorillas (maxillary lateral incisor).

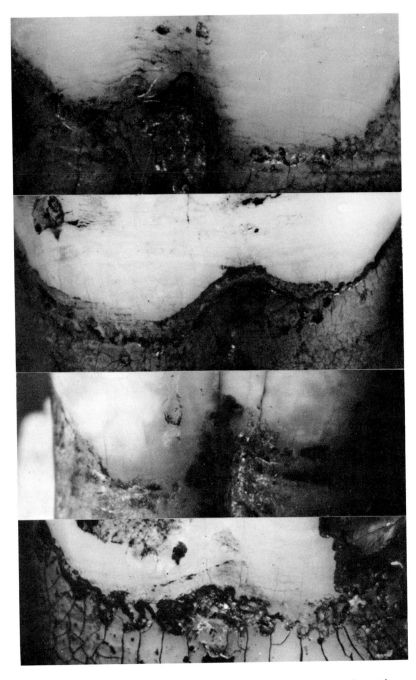

Fig. 10. Cementoenamel junction of various human central incisors. Macrophotographs enlarged 22 times—buccal side. Cases of "fossacoronoradicular" anomalies.

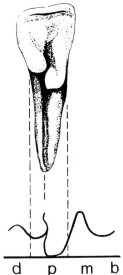

d   p   m   b

Fig. 11. Maxillary lateral incisor—human tooth. The drawing and diagram show the palatine side. A syndesmocoronoradicular anomaly can be observed which affects both the crown and the root and is clearly shown on the cementoenamel junction by a sudden lowering of its level.

Topography of the Bifurcation

In this section we will deal with two aspects of the bifurcation; vertical, the relative height of bifurcation, and horizontal, its location.

Relative Height of Bifurcation. By relative height of bifurcation we mean the distance between the cementoenamel junction and the summit of the bifurcation.

In the literature, a close relationship is drawn up between the height of the bifurcation and the height of the pulp chamber. When the height of the pulp chamber is extremely great the tooth is called *prismatic* (or in French *taurodonte*). This type of tooth was first described by Gorjanovic-Kramberger (1908). Since then, many writers have been interested in this question. When the height of the pulp chamber is small and even insignificant, it is called *cynodont.*

In an earlier work (Brabant and Kovacs 1964) attention was drawn to an important distinction which should be made in prismatic and cynodont teeth: the distinction between internal and external morphology. In that same work it was proved that the two did not always correspond and that, although the pulp chamber looks like that of a synodont tooth, external morphology of the tooth can show a very high bifurcation, that is to say, a prismatic character (fig. 12).

The height of the bifurcation is more important from the viewpoint of

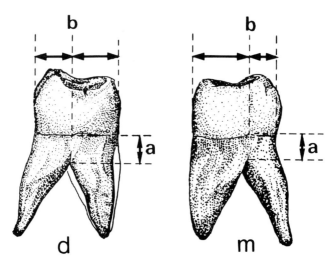

Fig. 12. This drawing of a first maxillary molar shows two aspects in the topography of the bifurcation: vertically, *a* shows the relative height of bifurcation, i.e., distance between the cementoenamel junction and the summit of the bifurcation; horizontally, *b* shows its location; *d* refers to distal side; *m* refers to mesial side.

pathology than many practitioners generally think it is. This is proved in periodontal disease when alveolysis is progressing and extends farther than the bifurcation. In such a case, in principle, the tooth is lost, since food is retained in the bifurcation. The wider the distance between the cementoenamel junction and the bifurcation, the later alveolysis will occur at the level of bifurcation (fig. 13). Therefore, in the prognosis of extension of the disease, the morphologic character of the tooth plays an important part. This applies to all teeth having two or more roots. A single-rooted tooth in this sense stands a better chance of preservation. This also holds for multirooted teeth with fused roots.

In the literature, numerous works deal with the height of the bifurcation in relation to prismatic teeth, but very few have used objective measurements as basis for their study. Shaw (1928) suggested a subjective classification of the various degrees of prismatism: hyper-, hypo-, and mesotaurodontism.

Jørgensen (1956) was the first to propose a study based on objective measurements of the bifurcation, in his very interesting work dealing with deciduous teeth. He considers the height normal when it is lower than 2.5 mm. There is an anomaly when it is higher than 2.5 mm.

Frederiksen and Hegdahl (1963) measured the height of the bifurcation of first and second permanent human mandibular molars and noticed that it was higher in second molars than in first molars, and also higher on the lingual side than on the buccal side.

In regard to prismatic teeth we suggest identifying the typical cases and in

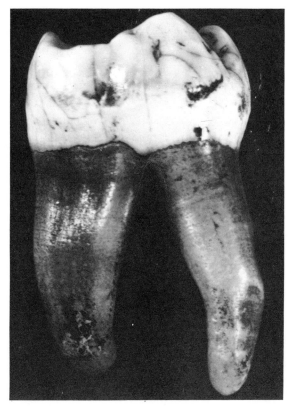

Fig. 13. Second maxillary—human tooth. The cementoenamel junction line shows a notch extending to the level of the bifurcation. Measurement showed that the height of bifucation is only 1 mm.

those cases not taking into account the size of the pulp chamber. Only external morphology should be considered; that is to say, the diagnosis should be related to the measured height of the bifurcation.

Measurement of the height of bifurcation sets a problem since the cemento-enamel junction is not always a straight line. We decided to use the method suggested by Jørgensen (1956), who drew a leveled line of junction, that is, a straight line which coincided on its greater length with the real line. Another possibility is to measure the height of the bifurcation between its summit and the occlusal plane. This type of measurement is recommended for hypsodont teeth, for instance those of the horse.

A condition for accurate measurements is the distinction between enamel and cement. To obtain this distinction we have colored the teeth as described in a previous section.

We made numerous measurements using slide calipers and then double-checked them for accuracy. This double check showed significant differences. We found out that the discrepancy was because the summit of the bifurcation is not always in the same plane as the cementoenamel junction. We therefore measured this distance with compasses with two points, one a sliding point, which helped us transcribe that distance on a sheet of paper where it was possible to measure it on a corrected plane with the slide calipers.

As an experiment, we calculated the relative height of the bifurcation of some human teeth in the Belgian population. The results of our investigation are given in tables 1 and 2. Table 1 shows a greater height of bifurcation on the distal side and a lower one on the buccal side. Table 2 shows a greater height of bifurcation on the lingual side than on the buccal side.

TABLE 1

HEIGHT OF BIFURCATION, MEAN VALUES, AND STANDARD DEVIATIONS OF HUMAN FIRST MAXILLARY MOLARS IN THE BELGIAN POPULATION (in mm)

Human First Maxillary Molars	Height of Bifurcation			
	Mean	Error	Standard Deviation	Error
Medial side	4.831	0.062	±0.763	0.043
Buccal side	4.049	0.054	±0.670	0.038
Distal side	4.903	0.079	±0.975	0.056

NOTE: N = 152.

Some measurements were also made on chimpanzee teeth as a comparison (see table 3).

The test of Student Fisher has been calculated for the comparison between human and chimpanzee teeth (see table 4). The results show that the difference observed between the first mandibular molars of human and chimpanzee are highly significant, for both the buccal and the lingual sides.

TABLE 2

HEIGHT OF BIFURCATION, MEAN VALUES, AND STANDARD DEVIATIONS OF HUMAN FIRST MANDIBULAR MOLARS IN THE BELGIAN POPULATION (in mm)

Human First Mandibular Molars	Height of Bifurcation			
	Mean	Error	Standard Deviation	Error
Buccal side	3.027	0.062	±0.695	0.044
Lingual side	4.198	0.065	±0.720	0.046

NOTE: N = 123.

TABLE 3

HEIGHT OF BIFURCATION, MEAN VALUES, AND STANDARD DEVIATIONS OF THE
FIRST MANDIBULAR MOLARS OF THE CHIMPANZEE (*Pan satyrus* Schweinfurti)
(in mm)

Chimpanzee First Mandibular Molars	Height of Bifurcation			
	Mean	Error	Standard Deviation	Error
Buccal side	2.154	0.283	±1.198	0.200
Lingual side	2.915	0.207	±0.949	0.146

NOTE: N = 22.

To make possible a true comparative study between human teeth and those of other zoological groups, we recommend the use of an index in which the distance between the bifurcation and the cementoenamel junction is related to the total length of the tooth. We call this the *height of bifurcation index,* and it is calculated as follows:

$$\text{Index} = \frac{\text{distance between cementoenamel junction and bifurcation} \times 100}{\text{total length of tooth}}.$$

We calculated this index for the teeth of chimpanzees, and the results obtained for the first mandibular molars are given in table 5. Sampling consisted of twenty-two teeth.

TABLE 4

TEST OF STUDENT FISHER CALCULATED BETWEEN THE FIRST
MANDIBULAR MOLARS OF HUMAN AND CHIMPANZEE

Height of Bifurcation	Human and Chimpanzee First Mandibular Molars	
	Test of Student (*t*)	Probability (*p*)
Buccal side	4.591	0.001
Lingual side	7.249	0.001

Horizontal Location of the Bifurcation. The horizontal location of the bifurcation is important from the viewpoint of periodontal prosthesis, since in some cases of alveolysis when a tooth is prepared for crown fitting this preparation must take into account the horizontal location of the bifurcation. It is also of interest in comparative anatomy.

In order to determine the horizontal location of the bifurcation on one side, one takes as ancillary line the cementoenamel junction and at the level of that junction draws a straight line from which a perpendicular is drawn to the sum-

TABLE 5

HEIGHT OF BIFURCATION INDEX, MEAN VALUES, AND STANDARD DEVIATIONS OF
THE FIRST MANDIBULAR MOLARS OF THE CHIMPANZEE
(in mm)

Chimpanzee First Mandibular Molars	Height of Bifurcation Index			
	Mean	Error	Standard Deviation	Error
Buccal side	11.270	1.375	±6.303	0.972
Lingual side	15.362	1.023	±4.688	0.723

NOTE: N = 22.

mit of the bifurcation. The parting point determined by this perpendicular line on the ancillary line shows the location of the bifurcation.

Morphology of the Bifurcation

The shape of the bifurcation can be an angle which is more or less sharp and varies from a few degrees to 60°. It can also look like an arcade which in its turn can be more or less round. For example, the shape of the bifurcation is different on the buccal side from the mesial side or the distal side.

It is sometimes noticed that the bifurcation seems to continue on the root toward the crown in the form of a ridge which can be more or less pronounced. This ridge can extend as far as the cementoenamel junction or even further on the crown. This is especially noted on first human premolars, on the mesial side, and also on the roots of multirooted teeth of anthropoids.

The outline of the bifurcation can be reproduced by means of a pantograph of precision.

Interradicular Area

Three points should be considered in relation to the interradicular area: its shape, the bifurcational ridge, and the accessory canal.

It has been observed that the interradicular surface of human teeth can be either concave, convex, or flat. Also, very often a *ridge* is found running across the bifurcation, its shape depending on the number of roots of the tooth. If there are two roots the ridge will join them together, though it does not always lie in the middle of the area. When there are three roots, the ridge is Y-shaped.

It seems that the ridge becomes less acute with age, probably as a result of superimposition of secondary cementum (fig. 14). A more thorough investigation may make it possible to evaluate the importance of this feature in determining the age of a person.

Everett et al. (1958) were the first to deal with this subject and to report the results of a histologic study regarding the interradicular area which allowed them to observe the presence of the bifurcational ridge in 73% of cases. They did not, however, relate this feature to age.

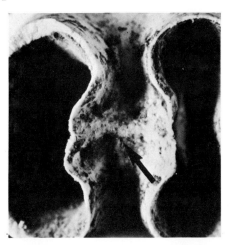

Fig. 14. At the point where the processes have met, there is hyperproduction of cementum. This constitutes the scar that ensures closing of the cavity at this point. This scarring always is found on the teeth at the level of the root bifurcation.

The bifurcational ridge forms during the development of multirooted teeth. At the meeting point of the interradicular processes there is hyperproduction of cementum that ensures closing of the cavity at this point. The rough surface of that ridge reminds one of a "callus."

We have already dealt with the bifurcational ridge in another work (Kovacs 1963, 1967) and are coming back to it in this study in the section dealing with ontogenetics, where details are given in relation to the formation and development of those ridges.

Comparative study in various species of animals showed that the bifurcational ridge can be found on the teeth of these species which have multirooted teeth. This was observed in lions (*Felis leo*), leopards (*Felis pardus*), Beringei gorillas, chimpanzees (*Pan satyrus* Schweinfurti), horses (*Equus caballus* Linné), and zebras (*Equus [hippotigris]* quagga crawshayi de Winton).

The accessory canal was studied on macrophotographs or direct enlargements of dental germs and of already developed teeth, the roots of which we had cut off. According to Orban (1962), an accessory canal can form between the crown and the interradicular space if the junction of the diaphragmatic processes is not complete (fig. 15). In our study, contrary to Orban's findings, an accessory canal was never found at the bifurcational ridge but only in the middle of the original diaphragmatic processes. Our investigation therefore confirms the histologic researches made by Klees (1956).

Root Diagram Characteristic of Tilting, Divergence, and Curvature of the Root
Studies made by various writers deal on the one hand with the anatomic description of the root in relation to the crown and to the occlusal plane, and on

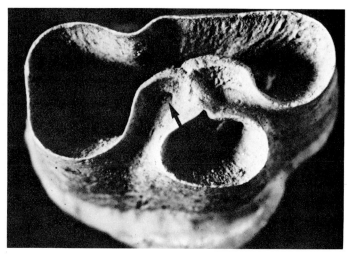

Fig. 15. Dental germ of a maxillary right second molar. The meeting of the vestibular and distal processes of the diaphragm is shown. In the middle of the distal process there is a pulpy communication (*arrow*). According to Orban (1962), an accessory canal can be constituted at the base of the dental crown if the diaphragmatic process is incomplete and does not meet its homologues. In our study, accessory canals were never seen at the point where the diaphragmatic processes meet, but they were found in the middle of a process.

the other hand with the arrangement of roots (either fused or extremely diverging) in ethnic groups. These various studies were made from the phylogenetic point of view.

In regard to the anatomic arrangement of roots, Muhlreiter (1920) was the first, in 1870, to describe root tilting and defined it as representing a prognath angle of 16° to 20°. According to De Jonge (1958), this is also a property of shape which is universal in character, since all roots are tilted distally. Divergence and convergence of roots in various ethnic populations were studied by Owen (1874), Pedersen (1949), Tratman (1950), Shaw (1928), Broca (1879), Campbell (1925), Jørgensen (1956), and Brabant (1967).

The significance of the arrangement of the roots, however, was seldom investigated. Let us mention Herpin (1928), Schroder (1926, 1963), and Brodie (1934). Jørgensen (1956) was the first to suggest actual measurement of the angle of divergence of the root. In his work dealing with deciduous dentition he drew their axes in pencil on the roots and then measured their devergence with the help of the Zeiss goniometer.

The arrangement of roots of human teeth in the maxillary bones was studied by Dempster et al. (1963), who measured statistically the direction of the roots and the degree of tilting.

The works of the writers mentioned above are worth discussing in depth because they expressed an assumption regarding the relationship between the crown and the root and root divergence or fusion, considered from the viewpoint of evolution or retrogression of the tooth; but their arguments are mainly based on subjective findings. There is no graph allowing the exact position of roots in space to be recorded, a graph which would put forward the differences between various individuals, species, and teeth.

For that reason, our aim in this section is to work out a diagram which allows us to record the direction of the root in relation to the crown and the occlusal plane, as well as its curvature, divergence, or convergence. This graph will also make it possible to distinguish individuals, races, species, and periods. We have given the collective name *root diagram* to this graph (figs. 16–20). It

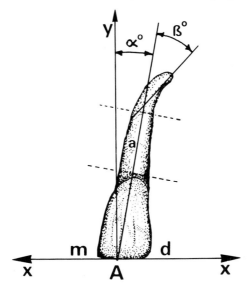

Fig. 16. Root diagram of a left maxillary lateral incisor. The tooth is set in a system of coordinates: *x* corresponds to the occlusal plane; *a* is the axis of the root which crosses *x* in the *A*; *b* is the axis of the curved part of the root; angle *α* expresses the distal tilting of the root; angle *β* indicates the curvature of the root; *m* indicates mesial side; *d* indicates distal side.

includes three detailed features of the root arrangement: (1) tilting of the root; (2) divergence or convergence of the roots; (3) curvature of the root.

The arrangement of the roots can be looked at in relation to the occlusal plane or in relation to the longitudinal axis of the crown. Since the axis of the crown is rather difficult to determine, the use of occlusal plane is recommended, though this does not prevent the longitudinal axis of the crown from also being used in particular cases.

Construction of the Diagram. In order to construct the diagram we set the tooth in a system of coordinates as follows:

1. A photograph is made of the tooth in the usual four planes: buccal, lin-

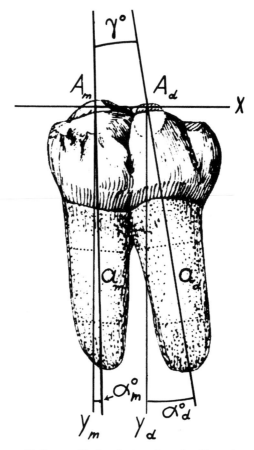

Fig. 17. Root diagram of left mandibular first molar of a *Sinanthropus pekinensis* (taken from Weidenreich 1937, figure 139).

gual, mesial, and distal. It is preferable to enlarge the photographs, as this makes it possible to get more accurate results. The root diagram will then be constructed on the photograph.

2. If the tooth is set in the jaw, one can use X rays or enlargements of X rays. This obviously limits the study to one plane only. In this case the condition of success is the good incidence of the rays.

3. In some cases it is possible to construct the graph on roots which are still in the jaw when the roots are sufficiently well exposed. We found such completely exposed roots in the skulls of gorillas.

4. The root diagram can sometimes be drawn directly on loose teeth. The axis is drawn in pencil and the angle formed with the occlusal plane is then measured.

Tilting of the Root. An auxilliary line *x* is drawn at the level of the occlusal plane. In the system it corresponds to the axis of the coordinates. The axis of

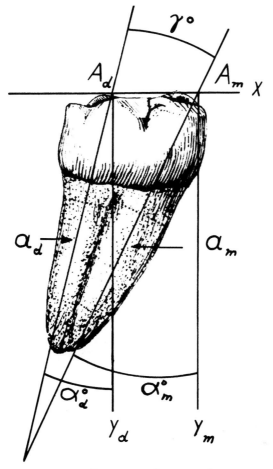

Fig. 18. In the literature, extreme divergence of roots and pronounced distal tilting are considered a primitive feature, as opposed to fusion, which is considered a sign of evolution. I believe this question is more complex and I am showing, as an example, this tooth of a *Sinanthropus pekinensis* bearing number 45. This figure was shown by Weidenreich (1937). This tooth shows nearly complete fusion of the roots and, at the same time, a very pronounced tilting. These are contrary features which are found on the same tooth. The root diagram shows: angle α mesial root, 27°; angle α distal root, 14.5°; convergent angle γ, 13°.

the root is then drawn without taking into account its curvature. To obtain the axis of the root of a single-rooted tooth (fig. 16), two transverse lines are drawn on the root, one at the level of the neck, the other at about two-thirds of its length toward the apex. The central points of the two lines are marked and the axis of the root is the line which crosses those two points. In multirooted teeth, the transverse line will be drawn at the level of bifurcation. Axis a of the root crosses the occlusal line x at a point of intersection A. From A, we draw a perpendicular line y to the occlusal line x. The angle formed at the

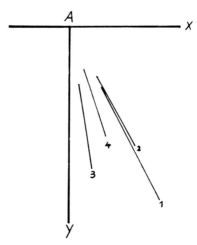

Fig. 19. The system of coordinates allows rather easy comparison of teeth in different species. For instance, the drawing above shows comparison between distal root of left mandibular first molars from (1) a gorilla; (2) the Meganthropus; (3) the Sinanthropus 36; (4) human tooth, present times. In the comparison, axis *x* and *y* and point *A* are used as a basis for reference.

meeting point of axis *a* and straight line *y*, or angle *a*, gives in degrees the tilting of the root. In the case of multirooted teeth, the system of coordinates is set out, in one plane, as many times as there are roots. One angle *a* is thus obtained for each root.

In a plane, three dispositions of the axis of the root or axis *a* in relation to *y* are possible. For instance, in the buccal plane:

a) The axis of the root tilts distally. This type of tilting is found in the majority of cases described by Muhlreiter (1920) as showing a prognath angle of 16° to 20°.

b) The axis of the root tilts mesially. This can sometimes happen in normal cases among central incisors and maxillary premolars and also in the mesial roots of molars, and with anomalies such as supernumerary roots. It can be found also in the roots of premolars of the Carnivora.

c) The axis of the root is identical to *y*. There is no distal or mesial tilting.

We have explained this tilting characteristic of the root in one plane, the buccal, but in order to obtain a clear picture of the root in space we have to determine this characteristic in the four planes usual in dentistry: mesial, distal, buccal, and lingual. The syntheses of those diagrams will give the exact position of the roots in space in relation to the occlusal plane.

Convergence and Divergence of Roots. This study is obviously limited to multirooted teeth. In such cases it is important to determine not only the tilting of roots independently of one another, but also the relationship between the

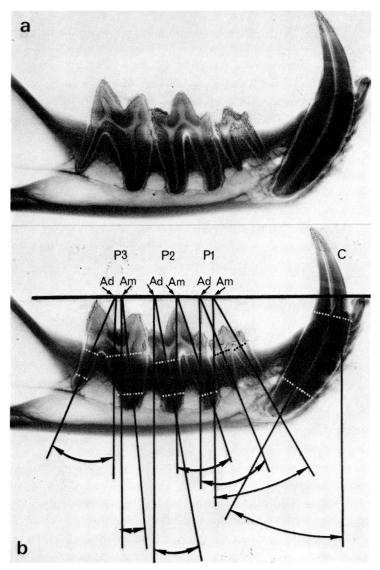

Fig. 20. (*a*) X ray of half of jaw of *Felis pardus*. The tilting of the three premolars is a typical features of the Carnivora. The roots tilt mesially in a very pronounced way; tilting decreases from the first premolar to the third. Only the distal root of the third premolar tilts distally; (*b*) root diagram drawn on the X ray.

roots. This relationship is shown by the angle formed by the axes of two roots. This angle, which we call γ, is already shown by the meeting of the two axes *a*. It only has to be measured. It expresses the divergence or convergence of the roots. In regard to the direction of the angle, there are three possibilities:

a) The angle diverges toward the apex of the roots. In this case there is a spreading out of the roots in the apical region. This arrangement is found in the majority of cases and mainly in the roots of mandibular first molars and the palatine root of maxillary first molars. This is considered by several writers mentioned above as a *primitive* feature.

b) The angle converges toward the apex of the roots. This is fusion or tendency to root fusion. This feature is considered by several writers as an indication of *evolution* of the roots.

c) The angle is nil. The two roots are parallel to each other. The distance between the two points *A* could be the subject of a further study.

These three possibilities express the relationship of the roots between themselves but not in relation to the occlusal plane. In order to determine this relationship we suggest drawing the bisecting line or convergent or divergent angle γ. The direction of the bisecting line will then be examined. In one plane, for instance the buccal plane, three alternatives are possible:

a) The bisecting line tilts on the distal side.

b) It tilts on the mesial side.

c) It is perpendicular to the occlusal plane.

Curvature of the Root. This characteristic shows the relationship between the axis of the root and the position of its apex.

The curvature of the root occurs about in its middle or two-thirds toward the apex. Sometimes this change of direction is barely noticeable, and sometimes the root curves at about 90°. These pronounced curves are mostly found in the region of the maxillary sinus, the dental canal, and the nasal cavities (Kovacs 1964).

To determine this characteristic, it is necessary to first determine the characteristic of tilting of the root which shows the relationship between the axis of the root and the occlusal plane.

To construct this diagram, one marks the ultimate parting point of axis *a* (i.e., the ultimate point on axis *a* toward the apex of the root, which divides the body of the root in two equal parts). From this point a straight line is drawn up to the pointed tip of the apex. The angle formed by axes *a* and *b* shows the degree of curvature of the root. We call it β.

In one plane, the position of axis *b* in relation to axis *a* can vary. For instance, in the buccal plane:

a) Axis *b* tilts distally. This happens in most cases.

b) Axis *b* tilts mesially. This is sometimes seen in maxillary premolars when the root adapted itself to the maxillary sinus during the penetrating phase.

c) Axis *b* coincides with axis *a*. This is often seen in central incisors and the palatine root of first maxillary molars.

The three characteristics described above can also be determined in fused roots when the roots are joined but a longitudinal groove, more or less deep, indicates the position of fusion. In this case, the characteristics can be determined for each fused root.

Apart from the constituents of the root diagram described above, the system also makes it possible to study other relationships between the roots (for instance the distance between points *A* in parallel roots) whose full significance is not yet known since such a study must be made on a wide sampling of teeth before any conclusions can be drawn.

Surface Area of the Root

In mastication, the important elements are the forces applied by the masticating muscles, the direction of the forces, which is determined by the joint, and the duration of the action.

The occlusal surface of the crown and its surface area is important since there is a biological relationship between that surface and the surface area of the root. In the Carnivora, premolars practically have no occlusal surface, the teeth being destined for shearing rather than milling. In the Herbivora, Omnivora, and Rodentia, on the contrary, there is a well-shaped occlusal surface.

In order to explain the biological relationship between the occlusal surface of the crown and the surface area of the root, let us give a very schematic example of this relationship, assuming the intensity and direction of the forces to be constant. This question is of course much more complex.

a) There is transmission of the forces when the surface area of the root is equal to the occlusal surface area.

b) there is distribution of the forces on the surface of the root when the latter is greater than the occlusal surface area of the crown.

c) There is concentration of the forces on the surface of the root when the latter is smaller than the occlusal surface area of the crown.

The surface area has a biomechanical importance, since during the action, in physiological cases, the force is distributed on the surface of the root. This question of surface also intervenes in the pathology of periodontium and in dental prosthodontics.

The direction of the forces is linked with the function, which varies according to the species. In the Carnivora the forces are vertical, whereas in the Herbivora and Rodentia they are horizontal. In the Omnivora the two types of forces are combined. Teeth which resist vertical forces will not necessarily resist horizontal ones, since in lateral movements there is an effect of leverage.

The knowledge of the above is useful in acute periodontal disease, when the extent of contact of the roots with the alveolar bone has diminished as a result of alveolysis. We would then apply permanent splinting by welding several teeth together with a fixed device. In this case all the roots participate in the action and the forces are shared among them. The distribution of the forces is therefore better.

The forces exerted on the crown are transmitted to the surface of the root which is in contact with the alveolar bone. The size of this bone is also important since the distribution of the forces depends on it. The size of the bone varies according to individuals, species, and age. It also varies according to the type of tooth.

The part played by the circular ligaments in the transmission, distribution, or concentration of the forces should also be mentioned, though it is known only to an extent. This remains an open question.

Teeth have a special mechanical character, since between the cementum on the root and the lamina dura one observes ligaments, the implantation of which allows the tooth to counteract the pressure of depression; the hydraulic lymph also acts as a protective measure to counteract the forces of mastication. (Weski 1959).

There are two ways to measure the surface area of the root: to measure the area limited by the cementoenamel junction, or to measure the area in contact with the bone. The latter area can be smaller than the former because the bone does not always extend up to the cementoenamel junction.

In order to make the comparison with hypsodont teeth we recommend taking the epithelial attachment as the boundary between the crown in function and the root in function. The root will comprise all that part of the tooth which is enclosed in alveolar bone and circular ligaments.

The aspects of the surface of the root can be considered: microscopic surface and macroscopic surface.

The microscopic aspect of the surface is dealt with in the section entitled "Relief of the Root Surface."

Literature on the root is mainly devoted to its macroscopic surface rather than its microscopic surface. Morelli, cited in Jespen (1963), was the first to draw attention to the surface area of the root, which he considered a geometrical form, and to compute its area by using the mathematical formula pertaining to its shape.

Brown (1950) studied the surface of the root in relation to osteolysis. He compared the length and shape of the root on nine teeth of different lengths and shapes (incisors). He also compared the surface of the whole root from the cementoenamel junction up to the apex; then, starting from a line drawn at 2, 4, or 5 mm from the junction up to the apex, he computed the percentage of decrease in surface in relation to the decrease in length. In a study dealing with prosthetics, Tylman and Tylman (1960) tried to find out the relationship between the applied forces and the root surface area of periodontal membrane attachments in 678 partially edentulous male patients. They do not, however, explain the method followed for the measurements. Kloehn (1958), in his study of the significance of root shapes determined by occlusal forces, tried to find out the relationship between the root surface area and the incisal surface in the Rodentia, the Carnivora and the Herbivora.

Muller (1959, 1963) studied the relationship between the surface area of crowns and roots and between the volume of crowns and roots with a view to applying his findings to periodontal diseases. Jespen (1963) measured 238 extracted maxillary and mandibular teeth of all types except third molars, with a view to finding a way to calculate the surface area of the root by applying the theory of mathematical probability. His process uses a membrane in polyvinyl baked at 130°. He suggests measurements be made on X rays of the root.

Another process, this time based on weight, consists in covering the root with metal by galvanoplasty or applying a metal foil on the root. This method was first described by Charon (1949), who used the double foil method to obtain the tooth contact surface: precious alloy—enamel and dentin. The surface is calculated as follows:

$$\frac{\text{weight of metal deposited}}{\text{specific gravity of metal} \times \text{thickness of foil}} \; .$$

The metal should be weighed on the analytical scale.

Kovacs and Kaan (1966) computed the surface area of roots of 1,440 teeth as well as the surface area of the crowns in order to make a comparative study of the surface of removable prosthesis. They also used the process based on weight for their measurements. The root was covered with a tinfoil 0.1 mm in thickness.

The advantage of galvanoplasty is that perfect covering of metal in hollows is possible. A disadvantage is that the layer of metal deposited on the surface is not regular in thickness when regular thickness is imperative for the accuracy of measurements.

To measure the surface area of the root, Brown (1950) used a "membrane." He covered the root with a latex solution which, when dry, is removed like a membrane. The latter is then laid on graph paper and the number of millimeter squares is counted. The same process was used by Boyd et al. (1958).

We ourselves used the following process: We applied on the root surface a foil of Staniol 0.02 mm in thickness; we then painted the foil with highly colored nail polish to obviate the inconvenience resulting from the folds on the Staniol foil. The colored foil was then divided into as many fragments as was necessary to be able to place them flat on the graph paper and then measure the surface area.

Index. The relationship between the surface area of the root and that of the other parts of the tooth is very interesting and we tried to consider it in two ways:

a) From the anatomical viewpoint. Here, we determine the relationship that exists between the surface area of the root and that of the crown or of the occlusal surface area, in the same tooth, in teeth of different types, and in teeth of different zoological species.

b) From the functional point of view. Here comes into account the height of the crown, the latter being considered as the arm of a lever. Its importance is obvious, notably in periodontal diseases.

We therefore tried to figure out for the root surface area an index which would allow study or comparison from the viewpoint envisaged. If the interest lies in anatomical relationship, the index could be as follows:

$$\frac{\text{surface area of root} \times 100}{\text{surface area of crown}}$$

or else

$$\frac{\text{surface area of root} \times 100}{\text{occlusal surface area}}.$$

When this relationship is looked at from a functional viewpoint, the index should register the decrease in the height of the crown caused by natural wear or selective grinding, which shortens the arm of the lever; it should also register the decrease in the surface area of root in function occurring in periodontal diseases. Such index might be:

$$\frac{\text{root surface area} \times 100}{\text{crown surface area} + \text{height of crown}^2}.$$

For hypsodont teeth or in periodontal diseases, epithelial attachment is used as boundary between crown and root.

As an experiment, we measured the surface root area of teeth by the method described earlier in this chapter, using Staniol foil. We computed the surface index with a view to comparing normal human teeth between themselves and also with other zoological species. On the other hand, we computed the root surface index of three central incisors having an extremely short root (anomaly) in order to compare them with other normal human incisors.

Comparison between Human Teeth and Teeth of Other Zoological Species

formula used: $\dfrac{\text{surface area of root} \times 100}{\text{surface area of crown}}$.

	Number of Teeth	Mean Index
Mandibular Canines		
Man	15	154.22
Lion (*Felis leo*)	9	155.94
Chimpanzee (*Pan satyrus* Schweinfurti)	17	217.16
Gorilla (Beringei)	7	285.65
Mandibular First Molar		
Man	15	128.31
Chimpanzee (*Pan satyrus* Schweinfurti)	18	158.34
Gorilla (Beringei)	7	166.40
Horse (*Equus caballus* Linné)	4	301.34

Comparison between Human Teeth (central incisors), normal and abnormal (the latter had extremely short roots)

formula used: Root surface area index $= \dfrac{\text{root surface area} \times 100}{\text{crown surface area} + \text{height of crown}^2}$

Results	*Index*
Normal teeth,	
mean index of 7 samples	56.00
Abnormal teeth	
sample 1	33.94
sample 2	28.16
sample 3	39.19

Relief of Root Surface

The relief of root surface is certainly important in relation to the decomposition of forces. The surface visible to the naked eye, which seems to be smooth, is in fact not as large as the actual surface area, since undulations and corrugations evidently increase the surface area.

There are several methods of observation of the surface: *a*) direct observation, i.e., macroscopic; *b*) observation with slight enlargement, on macrophotographs; *c*) microscopic observation; *d*) molecular specific surface.

Direct Observation. Observation of the roots shows several grooves and crevices, especially on the rather flat part of the root, which are always directed in the same direction as the applied forces. Very often those longitudinal grooves remind us of the fusion of roots which would have left its mark.

Careful study of the surface of the root also shows a constant morphological aspect, the division of the root into two parts: On the one hand, there is the third of the root toward the apex, the surface of which shows small undulations or circular or rough creases. This part of the root develops during the penetrative phase. On the other hand, there is the remaining two-thirds, the surface of which is smoother. This part develops during the eruptive phase.

This division of the root allows us to reconstitute the development of the root. This was dealt with in an earlier work (Kovacs 1963), to which those who are interested may refer.

Our study showed that at the time of occlusion two-thirds of the root of human teeth has developed. This proportion varies according to individuals and teeth. Study on X rays of the jaws of chimpanzees, gorillas, and lions shows a difference in the development of the root. In the anthropoid the part of the root which develops during the eruptive phase is smaller, whereas in the Carnivora most of the root develops before the tooth is in occlusion.

It seems that the roughness of the surface of the root helps distribute the forces of mastication. The direction of the forces is important and teeth with rougher roots respond better to transverse forces.

Observation on Macrophotographs. Macroscopic study combined with macrophotographs can be useful in the observation of the roots, since this makes it easier to study details which would be hardly noticed by the naked eye.

In order to better show the irregularities on the surface of the root we colored the tooth with india ink. We then rubbed it with a moist chamois, which removed the ink somewhat from the prominent parts, giving an effect of contrast.

The following were then observed on the surface:

a) Regular longitudinal or transverse *undulations* and irregular *corrugations*. On the roots of human teeth we found horizontal lines. These also appear on the roots of the Carnivora but are less pronounced. On the roots of the anthropoid we found horizontal and vertical lines, whereas in the Herbivora the lines were vertical.

b) *Resorptions*, which are very often found. Brabant (1969) reported that normal teeth and teeth in function show small radicular resorptions at those points where the pressure is applied, the ratio being 9 to 10. These resorptions, however, are rather limited.

c) *Rough spots,* which develop mainly during the eruptive phase, since they are generally found on the part of the root toward the apex.

Microscopic Observation. In industry the roughness of materials has been accurately studied, since the quality of the surface plays an important part in the sliding of two parts against each other.

The roughness can be looked at either longitudinally or on an area. Measurements can be made by feeling, optical means, or pneumatic means (Wiemer and Lehmann 1957).

As an experiment, we tried to measure the roughness of dental roots and made measurements on ten teeth with the help of the light-slit microscope. The average roughness of our sampling was 29.6 μ. Individual roughness of teeth varied from 15 to 52.2 μ.

Molecular Specific Surface. The principle of this measurement is based on the adsorption of molecules of various gases on the surface of the object being examined. Adsorption must occur with total covering of the surface by a monomolecular layer. If we know the diameter of these molecules and the number of molecules adsorbed on the surface, the molecular specific surface can be computed.

During a study of the structure and porosity of the alveolar bone in normal cases and in periodontal diseases, we computed the specific surface of the crown and root of an incisor of a person about thirty years old. Results were as follows: for the crown, 1 gr of substance gives 0.45 m²; for the root, 1 gr of substance gives 6.5 m².

The procedure using nitrogen gas followed for these measurements was described by Brunauer (1943), Emmett (1945), and McBain (1932).

Volume of the Root

For this study the teeth can be considered amorphous bodies.

In the literature, we find few works dealing with this subject. Por (1948) studied the comparative volume of teeth of the left side of the jaw against teeth of the right side and reported a slightly higher volume in the left-side teeth. To calculate these volumes he devised an apparatus using mercury.

Muller (1959, 1963) studied the volume and surface area of roots and crowns and their significance in normal and pathological cases. A measuring device was also constructed by Zaray (1962) and then modified by Kutasi, Zaray and Kovacs, as cited by Zaray (1962).

Kovacs (1962) studied the volume of deciduous teeth and compared the results with the volume of deciduous teeeth which had fallen as a result of resorption. This gave him an idea of the quantitative importance of resorption. He also studied permanent maxillary and mandibular teeth. He computed the volumes of 1,432 samples and listed in a table the average volume for each type of human tooth. This table is reproduced below:

TABLE 6

VOLUME OF PERMANENT HUMAN TEETH
(Hungarian Population)

Teeth	Number of Teeth Studied		Mean Volume	
	Left Side	Right Side	Left Side	Right Side
Maxillary				
Central incisors	36	33	0.57	0.57
Lateral incisors	42	38	0.36	0.46
Canines	25	50	0.66	0.48
First premolars	42	40	0.58	0.61
Second premolars	46	44	0.45	0.44
First molars	37	38	1.35	1.33
Second molars	36	36	1.12	1.11
Third molars	44	48	0.78	0.66
Mandibular				
Central incisors	56	60	0.15	0.15
Lateral incisors	58	54	0.32	0.33
Canines	56	48	0.50	0.45
First premolars	62	58	0.42	0.40
Second premolars	52	42	0.52	0.55
First molars	48	50	1.28	1.25
Second molars	44	38	1.02	1.06
Third molars	35	36	1.05	0.91

SOURCE: Kovacs 1966.

In order to allow comparison between the volume of roots of human teeth and that of teeth of other species, we suggest the use of an index as follows:

$$\frac{\text{volume of root} \times 100}{\text{volume of crown}}$$

Computation of the volume of teeth is based on the principle of immersion of an object in a liquid, the volume of which is known. Por (1948) and Kovacs (1962, 1966) used mercury, whereas Muller (1959, 1963) used plain water.

Preparation of the teeth is very important, since any crack or canal can modify the results because the liquid penetrates into the tooth. To obviate this, the tooth should be examined with a magnifying glass and all possible holes and cracks should be closed with wax. We immersed our samples in hot paraffin, which penetrates all the holes, and, when cold, washed the surface with alcohol. Afterward, to ensure waterproof condition of the tooth, we painted it with nail polish. This is especially necessary when the tooth is to be immersed in water.

The difficulty lies in the fact that the root, in principle, should be separated from the tooth, which is not always possible. However, the root can be held in the water up to the level of the cementoenamel junction.

Buccolingual and Mesiodistal Diameters at Various Levels on the Root

It is advantageous to measure these diameters on the root because that part of the tooth is less subject to deterioration by decay and attrition than the crown. To overcome the difficulties encountered in measuring the crown diameters Goose (1963) in 1956 had already suggested that the buccolingual and mesiodistal diameters be measured at the level of the tooth neck, parallel to the usual mesiodistal diameter. We would recommend measurements at the following levels:

Single-rooted teeth

    1. cementoenamel junction on the crown;
    2. cementoenamel junction on the root;
    3. middle of the root.

Multirooted teeth

    1. cementoenamel junction on the crown;
    2. cementoenamel junction on the root;
    3. level of bifurcation—diameter of the tooth;
    4. level of bifurcation—diameter of each root;
    5. middle of root between bifurcation and apex.

The measurement procedure is the same as that followed to measure the diameter of the crown in the buccolingual and mesiodistal directions. The millimeter gauge can be used, as well as an instrument used in jewelry to measure precious stones, the millimeter gauge and estimator, which fits curved surfaces better and is accurate up to 0.05 mm.

Perimeter

It is common practice to use measurements made on teeth to give an idea of their morphological features. In this connection, most investigators give the mesiodistal and buccolingual diameters of the crown together with its height when they want to indicate its shape and size. However, the shape of a tooth is often rather complex and the same diameters can be found on teeth having widely different shapes and, consequently, sizes. This gave us the idea of measuring the perimeter of the crown, since this value indicates the actual size of the crown better than its diameters.

To get a complete idea of the size of the tooth, the perimeter of the roots should also be measured. This will help to register the differences between teeth of different eras or species. For instance, the teeth of the *Sinanthropus* mentioned by Weidenreich (1937) look much heavier than the teeth of people of present times. The differences can be clearly seen but no system up to now made it possible to register them.

Measurement of the perimeter of teeth are recommended at the following levels:

Single-rooted teeth
1. cementoenamel junction on the crown;
2. cementoenamel junction on the root;
3. middle of the root between the junction and apex.

Multirooted teeth
1. level of contact points (crown);
2. cementoenamel junction on the crown;
3. cementoenamel junction on the root;
4. level of bifurcation—whole tooth;
5. level of bifurcation—each root separately;
6. middle point between bifurcation and apex—each root.

We recommend measurement at the level of cementoenamel junction on the crown and on the root, since the perimeter at those two levels can be different. For instance, in human deciduous teeth or teeth of some zoological species, the thickness of enamel can make a difference in the two perimeters. In the case of fused roots, measurement of the perimeter of the whole root is still possible.

Several methods of measurement are possible. The simplest way is to encircle the tooth with metal wire, tighten the wire with pliers, cut it, and then measure it. If the wire can be pulled off easily without cutting it, one can measure it on a measuring cone like the one used in jewelry. The pliers can be replaced by a dentimeter in which the wire is inserted. One can use rings of varied diameters. One can use an improved dentimeter with measuring marks.

Root Shapes Examined in Cross Sections
This subject of root shapes has been included in our study because great differences between dental roots of similar or diverse species were noticed in the course of our research.

Generally, roots of the Carnivora are rather round or oval whereas those of the Omnivora are rather flat; those of the Herbivora look flatter still and show ridges and grooves. Differences are also found in roots of animals of the same species, and even between the roots of the same tooth. For instance, dental roots of gorillas are flatter than those of chimpanzees, especially the palatine roots of maxillary molars. Roots of human teeth are less flat than those of the hominoids. We also noticed that roots of supernumerary teeth are generally round or oval rather than flat.

The flat character of roots is significant because it is found in the direction of the applied forces. In human teeth, the mesial root of a molar is wider and flatter than the distal root.

All this led us to the study of transverse axes of flat or oval roots. For instance, on a cross section of a first or second human mandibular molar, it can be noticed that the axes of both roots converge toward the lingual side. To register these axes, we took photographs of cross sections of a certain number of roots and drew the transverse axes of the roots on the photographs. The angle shown at the meeting point of the buccal plane and the axes can also be measured. A diagram can be constructed in the same way as the root diagram mentioned before.

Distance between the Location of Apices of the Root
A few writers, such as Drennan (1928), de Terra (1905), and Pedersen (1949) measured the distance between the apices of some teeth, but only in particular cases. No mean value is given for a population.

The present study is limited to multirooted teeth. It consists in measuring the distance between the two apices in two-root teeth or in drawing and measuring the geometrical form of the apices in teeth having more than two roots.

Measurements can be made: (1) without taking into account the difference in level between the apices, in which case the millimeter gauge can be used; (2) taking this difference into account, in which case the sliding compasses will be used. This instrument was mentioned in an earlier section dealing with the topography of the bifurcation.

In multirooted teeth, angles formed by the apices are measured with a goniometer. To draw the geometrical figure formed by the apices in three-root teeth it is sufficient to measure one angle and the adjacent sides and then close the figure. In four-root teeth, two adjacent angles and the sides of those angles will be measured and the figure closed.

Apex Morphology
Great variability is found in the shape of the apex of teeth from man and zoological species. When studying this subject it was observed that there is indeed no typical shape for any species. Even in the same tooth the shapes of the various apices can be different. The greatest variability is found in the apex of fused roots. It can be said, however, that as a rule pointed apices are more frequently observed in the teeth of the Carnivora and that wide and flat apices are more often found in the teeth of the Herbivora.

We have tried to determine some sort of classification of apex shapes in the teeth of man and anthropoids. The data is given below.

Relationship between Peculiarities of the Root and Peculiarities of the Crown
Several writers have stated that there is a relationship between peculiarities or anomalies found on the crown and those found on the root; others, on the con-

trary, have said that there is no such relationship. In any case, it seems that this problem has never been thoroughly investigated; the morphology of teeth has not been studied from this point of view. By this we mean a systematic study of each part of the tooth on macrophotographs, involving dimensions and study of even small characteristics which could help decide with some certainty that a peculiar feature on the crown corresponds to one on the root and vice verse.

However, some writers have discussed the relationship that can exist between the crown and the root in relation to anomalies. Von Reckow, as mentioned in Brabant, Klees, and Werelds (1958), noticed in teeth with supernumerary roots an increase in the size of the crown or abnormal development of a cusp. Similarly, Meyer (1952) observed supernumerary cusps on the crowns of teeth having supernumerary roots. This relationship of dependence can also be inverted and one can say that since the crown is a primary developed body and the root a secondary developed body, when an anomaly in volume or shape of some importance is found in the crown it must be accompanied by a modification in the volume or shape of the root. On the other hand, De Jonge (1958) and Visser (1948) noticed that a Carabelli's cusp on the crown was accompanied by a longitudinal ridge in the root. The relationship between the morphology of the crown and that of the root was also mentioned by Aichel (1917) and de Terra (1905).

In the course of our own investigations we noticed that to anomalies of and variations in the roots also correspond peculiarities in the cementoenamel junction line. For instance, in the case of fused roots, the perimeter at the cementoenamel junction level is smaller than when the roots are normal; if there are supernumerary roots, the perimeter of the tooth at the junction level is larger; and a groove in the root very often corresponds to a small notch in the junction line.

We also studied some first and second maxillary premolars. Those which had supernumerary roots or fused supernumerary roots (three canals) also showed in nine cases out of ten some widening of the neck of the tooth on the buccal side. Knowing this, it is possible, when examining the mouths of patients, to diagnose three canals in a tooth when a widening in the neck of it is found on the buccal side.

Root Anomalies Related to Other Anomalies and Variations

We believe it would be of great interest to investigate the connection between some anomalies and variations of the roots and anomalies and malformations of the dentition. The following could be studied: anomalies of the root of a tooth in relation to anomalies of other teeth; anomalies of permanent teeth in relation to anomalies of deciduous teeth; anomalies or variations of roots in relation to malformations such as harelip and cleft palate. This problem has hardly been investigated.

Cheraskin and Langley (1956) have observed that to a three-root first mandibular molar corresponded two-root first and second mandibular premolars. We ourselves noticed that to a four-root second maxillary molar corresponded a three-root second maxillary premolar.

The connection between anomalies of deciduous teeth and anomalies of temporary teeth was dealt with by Brabant and Kovacs (1964) in relation to prismatism, and by Bruszt (1966), who observed that to a supernumerary deciduous tooth corresponded a permanent tooth with a very long root.

Observation of Teeth in Situ

This study helps us understand the teeth as they are considered in the jaw and in relation to their anatomic environment. Knowing the ontogenetic development of teeth and looking at their environment, we can more easily understand the peculiar shape of some roots.

Anatomic environment that has an influence on the development of the roots consists, for deciduous teeth, of the location of the germ of temporary teeth; for temporary teeth, of the nearness of nasal cavity and maxillary sinus, of the foramen mentalis, and of the dental canal. Generally, when the apex of mandibular molar roots shows a pronounced distal curving, one notices that the mandibular canal is very close by.

The in situ study of embedded teeth allows one to observe that their development depends greatly on anatomic environment and space available. The penetrative phase in the development of the root starts when the tooth hits an obstacle and the root continues to develop in accordance with local environment. Numerous unfavorable local conditions can explain the great morphologic variability of embedded teeth. In the embedded third mandibular molar, for instance, a very pronounced distal curvature of the root is often found which is caused by the obstacle constituted by the dental canal. It is also well known that nerves and blood vessels of the mandibular canal can be found between the roots of that third molar or be completely surrounded by them. This is explained by the fact that during the penetrative phase the root surrounds the nerves and mandibular vessels.

The same influences of environment are exerted on the development of supernumerary roots. In our collection of teeth we have eighteen first mandibular molars with such roots. In nearly all cases we observed the same morphologic peculiarity: the supernumerary root has started to develop in a distal direction and then, suddenly, curves toward the other root. The same thing was observed on a supernumerary root in a broken jaw coming from excavations. On that jaw we found that the obstacle causing the change in direction of the root was the internal oblique line of the mandible.

This study can be made with the help of X rays or on broken jaws from excavations.

Internal Morphology

When studying the internal morphology of the teeeth, the following can be examined: height of pulp chamber, morphology of pulp chamber floor, and location and shape of entrances to root canals.

It is well known that the *height of the pulp chamber* shows great variability, depending on the type of tooth, age, wear, decay, filling, and whether the tooth is deciduous or permanent. However, on rather intact material, a somewhat regular decrease in height can be observed from one tooth to its neighbor in the jaw. For instance, we have noticed on roentgenograms of human teeth from various eras that in deciduous teeth the height of the pulp chamber in the first molar is greater than in the second molar. In permanent teeth, on the contrary, the height of the pulp chamber increases from the first to the third molar.

This study is possible (*a*) on X rays; (*b*) on cross-sections, the tooth being cut at the level of the cementoenamel junction, which allows study of the floor of the pulp chamber; and (*c*) on longitudinal sections of the tooth cut at the bifurcation, which allows several measurements.

When we were studying the ontogenetic morphology of multirooted teeth, a ridge was observed in the interradicular area, where the transverse processes had met. This led us to examination of the morphology of the other side of this area, *the floor of the pulp chamber*. This study was made on macrophotographs. We observed a ridge on the pulp chamber floor between the entrances to the root canals, corresponding exactly to the outer crest. This ridge was also mentioned by Everett, Jump, and Holder (1958) in their study on the bifurcational ridge. This inner ridge was wider toward the mesial canal entrance than toward the distal one. Such difference in width was found in seventeen out of twenty cases. The ridge was more pronounced in the teeth of adults than in those of young individuals.

Studies of roots have been sparse in comparison to studies of crowns, but this presentation has indicated the range of possibilities and directions that such investigations might take.

ACKNOWLEDGMENTS

I would like to thank Professor L. Cahan, director of the Royal Museum of Central Africa, Tervuren (Belgium), and Professor M. Poll of the zoological department of the same museum, where I viewed samples.

REFERENCES

Aichel, O. 1917. Die Beurteilung des rezenten und prähistorischen Menschen nach der Zahnform. *Zeit. Morphol. Anthropol.* Vol. 20, no. 3.

Alexandersen, V. 1962. Root conditions in human lower canines with special regard to double-rooted canines. *Tandlaegebladet,* vol. 66.

Ballschmiede, G. 1922. Wurzellose Zähne. Med. diss., Greifswald.

Boyd, J. L., et al. 1958. A preliminary investigation of the support of partial dentures and its relationship to vertical loads. *Dent. Pract. Dent. Rec.*

Brabant, H. 1967. Paleostomatology. In *Diseases in antiquity,* ed. D. Brothwell and A. T. Sandison, chap. 45. Springfield, Ill.: Charles C. Thomas.

———. 1969a. Observations sur la denture des populations Mégalithiques. *Bull. GIRS,* no. 3–4.

Brabant, H. 1969b. Résorption dentaire. In *Encyclopédie médico-chirurg.-stomat.* In press.

Brabant, H.; Kless, L.; and Werelds, R. 1958. *Anomalies, mutilations et tumeurs des dents humaines,* vol. 1. Paris; J. Prélat.

Brabant, H., and Kovacs, I. 1961. Contribution à l'étude de la persistence du taurodontisme dans les races modernes et sa parenté possible avec la racine pyramidale des molaires. *Bull. GIRS,* no. 2–3.

———. 1964. Contribution à l'étude du taurodontisme des molaires temporaires. *Bull. GIRS,* no. 3–4.

Brabant, H., and Sahly, A. 1962. La paléostomatologie en Belgique et en France. *Acta Stom. Belgica,* vol. 59.

Broca, P. 1879. Instructions relatives à l'étude anthropologique du système dentaire. *Bull. Soc. Anthrop., Paris,* 2d ser., no. 3.

Brodie, A. G. 1934. The significance of tooth form. *Angle Orthod.,* vol. 4.

Brown, R. 1950. A method of measurement of root area. *J. Canad. Dent. Assoc.,* no. 16.

Brunauer, S. 1943. *The adsorption of gases and vapours.* Vol. 1, *Physical adsorption.* Princeton, N.J.: Princeton University Press.

Bruszt, P. 1966. Egy Különlegesen hosszu felsö közepsö metszöfog fejlödésének megfigyelése. *Fogorvosi Szemle,* no. 11.

Campbell, T. D. 1925. *Dentition and palate of the Australian aboriginal.* Adelaide: Hassel Press.

Carlsen, O. 1967. Odontogenetic morphology. *Särtryck Odont. Tidskr,* vol. 75.

———. 1968. The cervical enamel line mesially and distally on the human maxillary deciduous molars. *Acta Odont. Scand.,* vol. 26.

Charon, L. F. 1949. Recherches comparatives sur les mutilations dentaires. *Archives Stom.,* vol. 4.

Cheraskin, E., and Langley, L. L. 1956. Dynamics of oral diagnosis. Chicago: Year Book Publishers.

Dechaume, M. 1959. *Précis de stomatologie.* Paris: Masson et Cie.

De Jonge, Th. E. 1958. *Anatomie der Zähne.* Munich and Berlin: Zahn-, Mund-Kieferhkd., Verlag von Urban u. Schwarzenberg.

Demptster, W. T.; Adams, W. J.; Duddles, R. A.; and Arbor, A. 1963. Arrangement in the jaws of the roots of the teeth. *J. Amer. Dent. Assoc.,* no. 67.

Drennan, M. R. 1928. The dentition of a bushman tribe. *Ann. South African Mus.,* no. 24.

Emmett, P. H. 1945. *Ind. Eng. Chem.,* vol. 37.

Euler, H., and Brabant, H. 1954. A propos de l'apposition de cément sur l'émail des dents humaines. *Arch. Stom.,* no. 4.

Everett, F. G.; Jump, E. B.; and Holder, Th. D. 1958. The intermediate bifurcational ridge: A study of the morphology of the bifurcation of the lower first molar. *J. Dent. Res.,* vol. 37.

Frederiksen, G., and Hegdahl, T. 1963. Nivaforskjellen mellom bifurkaturen og emaljecementgrensen hos dens molaris inferior primus og dens molaris inferior secundus. *Den Norske Tannlaegeforenings Tidende,* vol. 73, no. 4.

Goose, D. H. 1963. Dental measurement in anthropological studies. In *Dental anthropology,* vol. 5. London and New York: Pergamon Press.

Gorjanovic-Kramberger, K. 1908. Ueber prismatische Molarwurzeln rezenter und diluvialer Menschen. *Anat. Anz.,* no. 32.

Herpin, A. 1928. *Les dents de l'homme,* vol. 1. Paris: Semaine Dentaire.

Jespen, A. 1963. Root surface measurement and a method for x-ray determination of root surface area. *Acta Odont. Scan.,* vol. 21, no. 1.

Jorgensen, D. K. 1950. Macroscopic observations on the formation of the subpulpal wall. *Odont. Tidskr.,* vol. 2.

———. 1956. *The deciduous dentition.* Copenhagen: Bianco Lunos Bogtrykkeri.

Keil, A. 1966. *Grundzüge der Odontologie.* Berlin: Gebr. Borntraeger.

Kerebel, B. 1964. Histologie du parodonte. *Encycl. médico-chirurg.-stomat.,* vol. 11.

Klees, L. 1956. Contribution radiographique et histologique à l'étude des canaux radiculaires et de leur traitement. *Arch. Stom.,* October 1955, January 1956, April 1956.

Kloehn, S. J. 1938. Significance of root form as determined by occlusal stress. *J. Amer. Dent. Assoc.* and *Dent. Cosmos.,* vol. 25.

Kovacs, D., and Kaan, M. 1966. Összehasonlito felületmérések természetes fogakon és lemezes fogpotlasokon. *Fogorvosi Szemle,* no. 2.

Kovacs, I. 1958. Les causes de l'incurvation des racines dentaires. *Rev. Belge Stom.* no. 55.

———. 1963. Contribution à l'étude de la morphologie ontogénétique des racines des dents humaines. *Bull. Gr. Int. Rech. Sc. Stom.,* no. 1.

———. 1964. Contribution à l'étude des rapports entre le développement et la morphologie des racines des dents humaines. *Bull. Gr. Int. Rech. Sc. Stom.,* no. 1.

———. 1967. Contribution to the ontogenetic morphology of roots of human teeth. *J. Dent. Res.,* supp. vol. 46, no. 5.

Kovacs, Z. 1962. Tejörlöfogak térfogatméretei. *Fogorvosi Szemle.,* vol. 55.

———. 1966. Marado fogak térfogatmérése. *Journée Stomat. Szeged.* no. 4.

McBain, J. W. 1932. *The sorption of gases and vapours by solids.* London: Routledge.

Massler, M., and Schour, I. 1941. Studies in tooth development: Theories of eruption. *Amer. J. Orth. Oral Surg.,* vol. 27.

Meyer, W. 1951. *Lehrbuch der normalen Histologie und Entwicklungsgeschichte der Zähne des Menschen.* Munich: Carl Hanser.

————. 1952. *Pathologie der Zähne und des Gebisses.* Munich and Berlin: Zahn-, Mund- u. Kieferhkd., Verlag von Urban u. Schwarzenberg.

Moeschler, P. 1968. L'extension interradiculaire de l'émail dentaire: Un essai d'interprétation. *Bull. GIRS,* no. 4.

Muhlreiter, E. 1920. Anatomie des menschlichen Gebisses, ed. Th. E. De Jonge Cohen, Leipzag: Arthur Felix.

Muller, J. J. 1959. Die Wurzeloberfläche menschlicher Zähne und ihre Bedeutung für Ersatzkonstruktionen im Belastungsbereich des normalen und pathologischen Parodontiums. *Schw. M.s.z.,* vol. 69, no. 2.

————. 1963. Die Gemessenen Kronen- und Wurzeloberflächen. Rapports et Comm. du XVIIe Congrès ARPA (Les Parodontopathies). Paris: Masson et Cie.

Noyes, F. B.; Schour, I.; and Noyes, H. J. 1943. *Dental histology and embryology.* Philadelphia: Lea and Febiger.

Orban, B. 1962. *Oral histology and embryology.* Saint Louis: Mosby.

Owen, R. 1874. *Odontography.* London: Baillière.

Pedersen, P. O. 1949. *The East Greenland Eskimo dentition.* Copenhagen: Bianco Lunos Bogtrykkeri.

Pedersen, P. O., and Thyssen, H. 1942. Den Cervicale Emaljerands Forløb Hos Eskimoer. *Odontologisk Tidskr.,* no. 5.

Por, L. 1948. Az emberi fogak térfogatai. *Fogorvosi Szemle,* no. 41.

Sakai, T. 1967. Morphologic study of the dentinoenamel junction of the mandibular first premolar. *J. Dent. Res.* no. 5, suppl.

Schroeder, B. 1926. Das Wurzelmerkmal. *Deutsche Monatschr. Zahnhkd.,* no. 44.

————. 1963. Zur entwicklungsmechanischen Erklärung des Achen-, Flächen-, und Winkelmarkmales. *Deutsche Zahn-, Mund- Kieferhkd.,* no. 40.

Shaw, J. C. C. M. 1928. Taurodont teeth in South African races. *J. Anat. Lond.,* no. 62.

Sicher, A., and Tandler, N. 1928. *Anatomie für Zahnärzte.* Berlin.

Siffre, A. 1921. La dent et la denture de l'homme. *C. R. Soc. Anthrop. Paris,* Dec. 15. Reprint.

Taviani, S. 1953. I denti dell'uomo. Milan: Casa Editrice Ambrosiana.

Terra, M. de. 1905. *Beiträge zu einer Odontographie der Menschenrassen.* Berlin: Berlinische Verlagsanstalt.

Tratman, F. K. 1950. A comparison of the teeth of people of Indi-European racial stock with the mongoloid racial stock. *Dent. Rec.*

Twiesselmann, F., and Brabant, H. 1960. Observations sur les dents et les maxillaires d'une population d'âge franc de Coxyde, Belgique. *Bull. Int. Rech. Sc. Stom.,* vol. 3.

Tylman, S. D., and Tylman, S. G. 1960. Theory and practice of crown and bridge prosthodontics. Saint Louis: Mosby.

Visser, J. B. 1949. Beitrag zur Kenntnis der Menschlichen Zahnwurzelformen. Inaug. diss., Zurich.

Watson, A. E., and Woods, E. C. 1926. Some irregularities of the enamel margin observed in human molars. *Brit. Dent. J.,* vol. 47.

Wegner, H. 1939. Neue klinische und histologische Untersuchungen an wurzellosen Zähnen. *Deutsche Zahnärtzt. Zeitschrift.,* vol. 3.

Weidenreich, F. 1937. The dentition of Sinanthropus Pekinensis. *Paleontol. Sinica,* n.s.D. no. 1, Peking.

Wiemer, A., and Lehmann, R. 1957. Prüfen und Messen technischer Oberflächen. *Technik.,* no. 7.

Zaray, E. 1962. Készülékek a fogak térfogatanak meghatarozasahoz. *Fogorvosi Szemle,* no. 10.

Zellner, R. 1957. Mitteilung über drei Fälle von familiärer genuiner Wurzelmissbildung des gesamten Gebisses. *Deutsche Zahn-, Mund- Kieferhkd.,* vol. 26.

13 Penetrance and Expressivity of Dental Traits

Albert A. Dahlberg

*Department of Anthropology and
Zoller Memorial Dental Clinic,
University of Chicago*

Many traits of the dentition are substantial and positive entities that can be described and measured. Their appearance (penetrance) and degree of expression have been the basis of most comparative dental studies and descriptions. These units have been valuable not only in the study of evolution and diversification but also in genetic and developmental problems; they also have the virtue of recording events that occurred during the developmental process and of portraying something of the phylogenetic past, thus permitting and inviting study of the intrinsic as well as the extrinsic nature of teeth.

Some dental traits have shortcomings and advantages that are not clearly understood. Research has made contributions to a better understanding, but there are many questions still to be answered. Why, for example, do some teeth lack structures or cusps common to others, and why are some seemingly only partially developed? Most traits vary from population to population in frequency of occurrence and in penetrance and expression. The hypoconulid, metacone, protostylid, and Carabelli's cusp are notably variable in these respects (fig. 1).

We speak of gradients of expressivity of form and size in meristic (repeated) series and explain some of these variants in terms of the field concept of development. This concept is helpful in viewing variation in the dentition, but we do not know exactly the mechanisms involved. Two examples, the protostylid and Carabelli's cusp, can be used as illustrations.

The protostylid, the cusp which occurs in some dentitions on the anterior part of the buccal surface of lower molars, has a range of expression through six

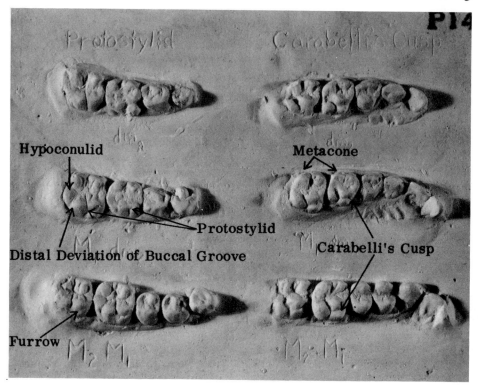

Fig. 1. The plaque shows six casts of posterior teeth. Lowers are pictured on the left and uppers on the right. The cusps are all large and fully expressed. The protostylid and Carabelli's cusp are seen on both deciduous and permanent molars. The pits, cusps, distal deviation of the buccal groove, and the furrow class of expression of the protostylid are well illustrated on the two models at lower left. The metacones and hypoconulids are well developed.

different classes. It may be represented as a pit, a furrow, a deviation of the buccal groove, an irregularity on the surface, a small cusp, or a large cusp. Likewise, the Carabelli's cusp of upper molars has many possible expressions from a smooth surface to a pit, furrow, double furrow, Y-groove formation, small cusp, and large cusps. These gradations can vary as a result of developmental factors, but they also show evidence of genetic control, although of a polygenic nature.

In a sense these different expressions are graded sequences, but it is impossible to give exact values of biological developmental distances between each step for statistical interpretations. Nevertheless it is useful and perhaps not unreasonable to ascribe a single unit value arbitrarily between these classes. Snyder et al. (1968) used this technique for a comparative study of dentition. Their scoring system indicated the affinities between the mestizos and Tarahumara of Mexico.

A consideration of some of the phenomena and characteristics of the development and structure of teeth gives insight into the penetrance and expressivity of tooth form and size. Developing teeth respond to body regulatory mechanisms from the early initial invagination of cells in morphodifferentiation to the final erupting process, but they increase in size only during the developing stage. Teeth have certain limits of variation, and their affinity to adjacent teeth is recognized by the gradations within the tooth groups. They have a morphological relationship with their corresponding members on the opposite side of the mouth. They are unique in chemical composition and in the calcification process, and the intricacies of the latter bear heavily on the problem of tooth form, expression, and penetrance of some substructures which cannot be observed or determined without sacrificing the tooth. The outline of the amelo-dentinal junction is an example.

Once the calcification of a crown is completed tooth form can be changed only by chemical or physical removal of substance, as in abrasion or wear. Bone, on the other hand, is responsive to pressures and environmental impacts which result at times in considerable remolding and new adaptation. The mandible, maxilla, and muscle attachments are subject to such possible changes throughout life. Dentin is viable, much like bone, but the crown is completely covered by the hard protective enamel. The nature of the dentin formation, developing inward toward the pulp, leaves the unchangeable outer form in direct permanent outline. Only the inner odontoblast cell-lined surface can remodel, by reactivation of these cells to form secondary dentin.

The outer enamel surface bears the characteristics with which the tooth meets the environment. The variations in surface contours determine its functional value. These qualities are modified in the development process by timing and peculiarities of the calcification sequences. Once any two or more cusps become united by calcification extension and fusion of the intervening areas, further separation of the cusps by the continuing multiplication of intervening cells is impossible. The relative size of the tooth in that dimension is finally determined. The completion of the enamel growth does involve limited additional variation owing to gradients in the process.

Pattern development in the embryonic stage of tooth development is progressive and is not established or developed at any one time; there is a gradual extension of development and calcification of different parts from the anterior part of the tooth to the posterior (Kraus 1962). Division and growth of cells is independent of the calcification process. Retardation of calcification by chemical or enzyme action would give time for growth and more cell divisions, which would result in a different ultimate morphology or expression. This is a likely answer to the question posed earlier regarding the varied expression of cusps, tooth parts, and proportions. Considerable support for such an explanation is given by recent advances in biochemical and developmental research.

In 1962 and 1968 I presented a hypothesis for explaining form, pattern, and size reductions in the dentition (Dahlberg 1968). To quote,

> It is entirely possible that the uniqueness and character of the process of development of teeth is responsible for a "freezing" of a stage in the differentiation of the tissues to produce a phenotype lacking elements that are late in forming. Delayed or accelerated initiation of the calcification process and tubule formation following the first alignment stage might well have an interceptive action of the distal parts of the final enamel crown form. . . . The calcifying process can effectively freeze the stage of pattern formation which has been achieved even though a very different phenotype could result if more opportunity for cellular development before calcification were given.

A bone can be calcified and later renew its growth in various dimensions, but a tooth cannot. New characterizations may be added to bone—brow ridges and adult facial features are familiar examples. But change in teeth must be accomplished before or during the calcification process by gradients in rate or extent of the process itself.

Butler (1967, and this volume) has demonstrated an important phase in the development of tooth size proportion and intercuspal distance in his studies of embryonic tooth germs. He showed that the distance between cusps was greater in proportion to the advance in calcification of the cusps. The cusps themselves were farther and farther apart until the stage when the calcification of the separate cusps finally made contact and produced a calcified bridge. Once the bridge is formed no further intercuspal growth is possible. The same process continues between these bridged cusps and other distal adjacent ones which started calcifying later in the sequence. Butler's contribution here is most significant: it is apparent that intercuspal tissue growth and rate of progress in formation of the calcified bridge are two major factors governing the intercuspal distance, and hence, the proportions and dimensions of pattern and occlusal surface size. The location, sequence, relationship, and timing of the original activity and other cusp-cell activity in the earliest stages are also governing factors.

One can see how an increase or retardation of intercuspal cell proliferation or a change in rate of calcification could alter the pattern size and proportion of the tooth. The dental difference between one genus and another is in many instances based on surface and cusp pattern proportions and size.

The work of Kraus (1962, 1965) has also contributed to understanding the intrinsic nature of cusps, which is important in considering penetrance of structures on tooth surfaces. He calls attention to some early calcifying areas that did not become cusps at all. What would their potential be in the presence of altered calcification-cell development timing ratios?

Korenhof's work (1960) is also noteworthy. His endocasts of the dentin-free crowns of von Koenigswald's collection give much information on the relationship between small early variations of the amelodentinal junction and the final outer cusp and crown form. Quite obvious from these and other studies of this type (Kraus 1952, Staley 1967) is the importance of growth gradients in the calcifying process itself. The difference between the amelo-dentinal pattern and the outer coronal pattern is considerable. A simple comparison quickly shows that growth is not uniform in rate or quantity in all parts of the enamel.

Let us return now to the partial expression of a feature or the penetrance and expressivity problem. It is recognized that there are also many small cusps that are in their ascendency (non- or preadaptive) and are not of any significant size. We do not necessarily think of them as incompletely expressed. They are not in the same category suggested for the partially expressed hypoconulid, hypocone, and so on. These latter structures, such as the five major cusps of lower molars, have a phylogenetic history and are a current exhibition of the genotype in man. We know what they are like in their fully expressed form.

The hypoconulid was referred to as varying greatly in expression from individual to individual and from tooth to tooth within the molar tooth group. It may be a well-developed cusp or any gradation from this to a mere ripple on the distal portion of an occlusal surface. Not infrequently a small bilateral discordance is evident in this cusp from one side to another. For the most part these variations are probably developmental because of the irregularity of occurrence and their degree. Environmental factors are assumed to be responsible for some variant expressions, but only to a limited degree. The subclinical and nonvisual expressions found on endocasts and at points beneath the often smooth outer enamel surface are of importance.

At this time there are no experimental data or other proofs that full fruition of a hypoconulid or other trait has been chemically intercepted, but, drawing from known and documented conditions that occur in biochemical tissue systems, one could assume that similar mechanisms could be operative in the dentition. Dr. Kollar's statements about the depressant action of beta-2-thienylalanine on tooth tissue development in tissue cultures are especially significant in this regard. Altered enzyme systems have been shown to produce biochemical blocks and to intercept or affect the intended course of development of an organ or part. Such incidents have been described in the literature (Wyngaarden 1962) as "inborn errors" and "inherited disorders" resulting from the change or loss of a single protein and its resulting enzyme in a biochemical sequence. It is necessary to recognize the possibility that such a gene-induced enzyme alteration could cause a growth or calcification change that might involve rates of timing, which would affect the original patterning and field.

The use of some dental traits in comparative and genetic studies has been based on their degree of expression. Modification of structure, whether by denial of full development or by increase or accentuation of ridges such as on the lingual surfaces of incisors, involves growth differentials which are in the main gene-controlled. A big problem is that dental traits are almost all polygenic, built over time by layers of many genes. Further analysis of traits and more biochemical, embryological, and pedigree studies are a likely source of answers to these problems of tooth form. Environmental impacts in the developmental process compete with the phylogenetically established and pleiotropically created units of dimension that are measurable and the nonmetrical characterizations such as shapes, pits, furrows, patterns, surfaces, crests, and color. That most tooth traits are continuous variables complicates certain avenues of solution. The intrinsic nature of penetrance and expression of dental traits is relevant to morphological problems.

REFERENCES

Butler, P. M. 1967. The prenatal development of the human first upper permanent molar. *Archs. Oral Biol.* 12:551–63.

Dahlberg, A. A. 1968. On the teeth of early sapiens. In *Evolution and hominisation,* 2d ed., ed. G. Kurth, pp. 273–80. Stuttgart: Gustav Fischer.

Korenhof, C. A. W. 1960. *Morphogenetical aspect of the human upper molar.* Utrecht: Uitgeversmaatschappij Neerlandia.

Kraus, B. S. 1952. Morphologic relationships between enamel and dentin surfaces of lower first molar teeth. *J. Dent. Res.* 31:248–56.

———. 1962. Areas of research in dental genetics. In *Genetics and dental health,* ed. C. J. Witkop, Jr., pp. 57–70. New York: McGraw-Hill.

Kraus, B. S., and Jordan, R. E. 1965. *The human dentition before birth.* Philadelphia: Lea Febinger.

Snyder, R. G.; Dahlberg, A. A.; Snow, C. C.; and Dahlberg, T. 1969. Trait analysis of the dentition of the Tarahumara Indians and mestizos of the Sierra Madre Occidental, Mexico. *Amer. J. Phys. Anthropol.,* vol. 31, no. 1.

Staley, R. 1967. A comparison of the dentin and enamel surfaces of human incisor teeth. M.A. thesis, University of Chicago.

Wyngaarden, J. B. 1962. Inherited disorders of metabolism. In *Genetics and dental health,* ed. C. J. Witkop, Jr., pp. 27–42. New York: McGraw-Hill.

14 The Inheritance of Tooth Size in British Families

D. H. Goose   *School of Dental Surgery,*
University of Liverpool, England

In the United Kingdom there has been a reduction in palate width in relatively recent times. For example, jaws of the Saxons in the sixth or seventh century were nearly all broad and well formed, whereas certain jaws in modern skulls (from the seventeenth to the nineteenth century) show narrowing. If the mean palate widths of these modern jaws are compared with medieval, Saxon, and Romano-British, all of which are rather similar, the amount of reduction is seen to be significant (table 1). Some recent measurements of Liverpool parents show that the trend to reduction has not been reversed and, in fact, may be continuing (table 2). Therefore it seems that somewhere around the sixteenth

TABLE 1

COMPARISONS BETWEEN MODERN PALATE WIDTHS AND MEDIEVAL, SAXON AND ROMANO-BRITISH COMBINED

Width	Sex	Difference (mm)	Degrees of Freedom	*t*	*P*
P^1–P^1	M	1.50	165	3.320	<0.01
	F	—	—[a]	—[a]	
M^1–M^1	M	1.10	126	2.017	<0.05
	F	1.55	78	1.992	<0.05[b]
M^2–M^2	M	2.56	240	6.243	<0.001
	F	2.31	130	4.848	<0.001

[a] Not possible to estimate because of small numbers.
[b] On the borderline.

TABLE 2
COMPARISON OF PALATE WIDTHS
(Male)

	N	$P^1–P^1$	N	$M^1–M^1$
Liverpool	41	35.89 ± 0.48	14	47.61 ± 0.84
Modern	29	36.19 ± 0.43	46	48.63 ± 0.44
Medieval	49	37.84 ± 0.31	19	50.27 ± 0.70
Saxon	43	38.04 ± 0.33	29	49.34 ± 0.52
Rom.-Brit.	46	37.20 ± 0.33	34	49.76 ± 0.52

or seventeenth century British jaws were becoming smaller, and since no particular changes in population occurred in this period it was probably an environmental dietary effect, doubtless mediated through genetic constitution. In fact, weight is given to this by the relative lack of attrition in modern skulls compared with earlier ones, indicating the change to a softer diet.

During the same period it is not easy to see any consistent change of size in teeth (table 3). However this is partly due to attrition in the early skulls, which makes any reduction in modern teeth difficult to detect.

TABLE 3
COMPARISONS OF UPPER TEETH
(Male)

	N	md 6	N	bl 6	N	Combined 4–7
Modern	65	10.49 ± 0.07	65	11.46 ± 0.07	33	33.11 ± 0.25
Medieval	51	10.15 ± 0.07	51	11.32 ± 0.08	41	31.87 ± 0.20
Saxon	54	10.39 ± 0.07	55	11.59 ± 0.07	50	32.59 ± 0.18
Rom.-Brit.	58	10.39 ± 0.07	57	11.69 ± 0.07	48	32.54 ± 0.20

Recently Lavelle (1968) found in his series of Saxon teeth that the molars were smaller, but the premolars, canines, and incisors were greater than a living sample of orthodontic patients in the midlands. Owing to the difficulties both of the representativeness of the different samples and the effects of attrition it may never be possible to know exactly what changes have taken place in teeth during historical periods. Neither is it possible to say how much genetic factors, on one hand, or environmental factors on the other are playing a part in these changes in jaws and teeth. Consequently it was felt that a study of living families might throw more light on the mechanisms involved. There have, in fact, been rather few family studies on this subject, but one can mention the interesting early work of Hohl (1934) and Martin (1934), and more recently Garn and his colleagues (1964–67), Lewis and Grainger (1967) and Goose (1967).

Material and Method

In the study to be described 123 families (including 17 from earlier study, Goose 1967) were involved, being selected by reference to school lists of fourteen- to fifteen-year-old children. Those parents who agreed to cooperate and who had most of their own teeth were visited at a suitable time in their own homes and dental impressions in alginate were taken of the father, mother, and children over fourteen years of age. The impressions were cast without delay in Kaffir D dental stone and measurements were made with specially sharpened callipers to 0.1 mm. Double determinations revealed very small errors of measurements, normally $\frac{S_i}{M}$ % less than 1 %.

Results

The resemblance between human relatives may be expressed as a correlation coefficient—for example, Pearson and Lee (1903) found it to be, between parents and offspring, 0.51 for stature; Penrose (1949) found it to be 0.49 for intelligence; and Holt (1961), 0.50 for dermal ridge counts. However, it is probably better to use heritability, as it is more common in animal studies and has a more identifiable meaning. Before proceeding further, however, it will be well to mention that no evidence of assortative mating was seen, the father/mother correlations not being significantly different from zero. The heritability (h^2) is equal to the ratio of the additive genetic variance to the phenotypic variance and can be calculated from the offspring/parent regression or offspring/midparent regression, as these are uncomplicated by dominance and interaction variances. It is better to use the father than the mother, since there may be nongenetic maternal factors. Since many posterior teeth had been lost in the parents, this study has concentrated on the maxillary incisors and canines.

Table 4 shows the findings in the material described and it is as well to point out that the heritability depends on the population studied only and therefore cannot necessarily be presumed to belong to other populations with different environmental conditions, gene frequencies, and so on. The sexes are separated

TABLE 4

HERITABILITY OF TOOTH WIDTHS

	N	First Incisor	N	Second Incisor	N	Combined
Father/son	58	0.98 ± 0.13	51	0.64 ± 0.11	56	0.54 ± 0.18
Mother/daughter	58	1.39[a]	53	0.63 ± 0.27	64	0.59 ± 0.22

[a] S.E. not possible.

at first in case there are substantial differences, and it is clear that for these anterior teeth the heritabilities are rather high, which indicates that environmental factors do not play a prominent role in the size of these teeth as measured mesiodistally. The midparent figures agree in confirming this and suggest that the teeth developing in a relatively protected area are not much influenced by environmental factors (table 5). This is not, of course, to say other measurements would not produce different results, and it is known, for example, that fluoride may modify tooth morphology (Paynter and Grainger 1956, Moller 1967, and Wallenius 1959).

TABLE 5
HERITABILITY OF TOOTH WIDTHS
(Offspring/Midparent)

First incisor	59	1.10 ± 0.11
Second incisor	46	0.73 ± 0.15
Canine	62	0.62 ± 0.13

Discussion

Fisher (1918) has shown that 0.5 is the theoretical value of the correlation coefficients between parents and children in the case of multifactorial inheritance with genes having small and additive effects without dominance (expected value of midparent/child correlation = 0.71). In the present data table 6 shows that none depart significantly from 0.5 at the 0.05 level. In table 7 the levels for I^2 and C for midparent/son appear low and do, in fact, differ significantly from the theoretical figure of 0.71, although none of the others do. Thus it is probable that this type of inheritance is involved.

TABLE 6
PARENT/OFFSPRING CORRELATIONS FOR MESIODISTAL DIAMETERS
OF MAXILLARY INCISORS AND CANINE

	I^1		I^2		C	
	N	r	N	r	N	r
Father/daughter	60	0.48	55	0.54	58	0.52
Mother/son	64	0.52	58	0.34	61	0.37
Mother/daughter	58	0.56	53	0.27	64	0.28
Father/son	58	0.45	51	0.42	56	0.32

Garn et al. (1965) have suggested that sex linkage may play a part in tooth size following their study of sib/sib correlations, and Lewis and Grainger

TABLE 7

Midparent Offspring Correlations for Mesiodistal Diameters
of Maxillary Incisors and Canine

	I^1		I^2		C	
	N	r	N	r	N	r
Midparent/son	42	0.72	31	0.45	42	0.39
Midparent/daughter	43	0.65	32	0.63	42	0.62

(1967) partly confirmed this in their study of parent/offspring pairs. The theoretical correlations relating to one pair of sex linked genes are as follows (Maynard-Smith, Penrose, and Smith 1961):

$$\text{Father/daughter and mother/son} = 0.71$$
$$\text{Mother/daughter} = 0.50$$
$$\text{Father/son} = 0$$

In table 6, although father/daughter values are high, father/son do not in any way tend toward their theoretical value of 0; for example, its lowest value of 0.32, for the canine, is not significantly different from the father/daughter value of 0.52. In the case of sibs the theoretical values for one pair of sex linked genes are sister/sister 0.75; brother/brother 0.50, and sister/brother 0.35. Reference to table 8 shows that only for I^2 is the correct order realized and only one correlation (brother/sister for I^2) is significantly different from 0.5 at 0.05 level. Thus it does not seem that sex linkage plays a part in the present data.

TABLE 8

Sib Correlations for Mesiodistal Diameters
of Maxillary Incisors and Canine

	I^1		I^2		C	
	N	r	N	r	N	r
Sister/sister[a]	21	0.48	21	0.53	13	0.28
Brother/brother[b]	16	0.60	17	0.44	14	0.52
Sister/brother	31	0.37	29	0.11	25	0.44

[a] Twelve from orthodontic department.
[b] Seven from orthodontic department.

Garn et al. (1967) also postulated a genetic control for canine sexual dimorphism showing that this effect "spilled over" into the immediately adjacent teeth, and table 9 shows the present data. Although P^1 for children is rather low in this case the percentage difference is higher otherwise for I^2 than I^1 and

TABLE 9
Percentage of Sex Difference in Mesiodistal
Crown Widths of Maxillary Teeth

	I[1]	I[2]	C	P[1]	P[2]
Parents	3.4	4.5	6.4	4.3	3.4
Children	5.6	5.8	5.8	2.7	2.7

P[1] than P[2], thus confirming their findings. Garn et al. (1965) also calculated the correlation coefficients between the canine and adjacent teeth in sibships which they found higher for I[1] and P[1]. In the present data only nine complete sib pairs were available, unfortunately, but the values confirm their hypothesis, being I[1]C = 0.09, I[2]C = 0.57, P[1]C = 0.89, P[2]C = 0.79.

It has been shown that the heritabilities of tooth size are high and therefore environment does not play much part, but previous investigators have commented on differences between the generations for tooth size (Garn, Lewis, and Walenga 1968, Goose 1967, and Hanna 1963). In the present data the results for mesiodistal dimensions are given in table 10. In all cases the offspring are

TABLE 10
Differences between Generations for Mesiodistal Diameters
of Maxillary Incisors and Canine (mm)

	Father/Son			Mother/Daughter		
	N	Diff.	S.E.	N	Diff.	S.E.
I[1]	58	0.25 ± 0.08		58	0.26 ± 0.07	
I[2]	51	0.26 ± 0.08		53	0.20 ± 0.09[a]	
C	56	0.19 ± 0.06		64	0.23 ± 0.06	

[a] $p < 0.01$, except here, where it is < 0.05.

significantly larger than their parents. Goose (1967) suggested that this difference might be dietary, owing to the effect of welfare foods which the children had in Britain (but their parents did not). Alternatively it could be simply due to approximal attrition in the older generation, making their teeth effectively smaller. In order to try to distinguish between these hypotheses the bucco-lingual dimensions of the premolars and molars were measured, these being relatively unaffected by attrition in modern populations. Unfortunately only first premolars and first molars were present in sufficient numbers to measure, but these are given in table 11 and it will be observed that all these were significant except P[1] for father/son at 0.05 level; thus the dietary hypothesis seems to be the likely one.

TABLE 11

DIFFERENCES BETWEEN GENERATIONS FOR BUCCOLINGUAL CROWN WIDTHS
OF MAXILLARY FIRST PREMOLARS (P^1) AND FIRST MOLARS (M^1)
(mm)

	Father/Son			Mother/Daughter		
	N	Diff.	S.E.	N	Diff.	S.E.
P^1	41	0.03 ± 0.10[a]		40	0.23 ± 0.09	
M^1	23	0.22 ± 0.09		17	0.32 ± 0.14	

[a] $P < 0.05$, except here, where it is not significant.

Summary

Upper alginate impressions were taken of the jaws of members of 123 families in the Liverpool area and measurements made on the models obtained from them. From these were calculated heritabilities and correlation coefficients of mesiodistal widths of the incisors and canines of the right side.

The heritabilities were high, indicating little environmental influence, and the parent/offspring correlations did not differ significantly from 0.5, being therefore compatible with a hypothesis of multifactoral inheritance with genes of small and additive effect but without dominance.

There was no definite evidence that sex-linked genes played a part in the inheritance of mesiodistal tooth width of these teeth, but there was evidence that the canine showed the most difference between sexes and that this effect "spilled over" into the adjacent teeth.

A generation difference existed both in mesiodistal and buccolingual dimensions, the children showing larger values than the parents.

ACKNOWLEDGMENTS

I would like to thank Professor C. A. Clarke of the department of medicine, University of Liverpool, for his part in making this study possible under the auspices of the Nuffield unit of medical genetics, and for his considerable advice and encouragement. I would like to thank Professor A. B. Semple, medical officer of health, and Mr. C. P. R. Clarke, director of education of the City of Liverpool, for their help in the administration of this scheme. My thanks are also due to all the families who kindly consented to the invasion of the privacy of their homes. Finally I wish to thank Mr. D. E. J. Bowden for the collection of the data and Mrs. N. Carruthers and Mrs. D. Davie for their unfailing assistance with the numerous calculations and abundant clerical work.

REFERENCES

Fisher, R. A. 1918. *Trans. Roy. Soc. Edinb.* 52:399.

Garn, S. M.; Lewis, A. B.; and Kerewsky, R. S. 1964. *J. Dent. Res.* 43:306.

————. 1965. *J. Dent. Res.* 44:439.

————. 1966. *J. Dent. Res.* 45:1819.

Garn, S. M.; Lewis, A. B.; Kerewsky, R. S.; and Jegart, K. 1965. *J. Dent. Res.* 44:476.

Garn, S. M.; Lewis, A. B.; Swindler, D. R.; and Kerewsky, R. S. 1967. *J. Dent. Res.* 46:963.

Garn, S. M.; Lewis, A. B.; and Walenga, A. 1968. *J. Dent. Res.* 47:503.

Goose, D. H. 1967. *J. Dent. Res.* 46:959 (suppl.).

Hanna, B. L.; Turner, M. E.; and Hughes, R. D. 1963. *J. Dent. Res.* 42:1322.

Hohl, F. 1934. Die Vererbung der Eckzahngrosse. Inaug. diss., Gottingen.

Holt, S. B. 1961. In *Recent advances in human genetics,* ed. L. S. Penrose. London: J. and A. Churchill.

Lavelle, C. L. B. 1968. *J. Dent. Res.* 47:811.

Lewis, D. W., and Grainger, R. M. 1967. *Arch. Oral Biol.* 12:539.

Martin, W. 1934. Über die Vererbung der Schneidzahngrosse. Inaug. diss., Gottingen.

Maynard-Smith, S.; Penrose, L. S.; and Smith, C. A. B. 1961. *Mathematical tables for research workers in human genetics.* London: J. and A. Churchill.

Moller, I. J. 1967. *J. Dent. Res.* 46:933.

Paynter, K. J., and Grainger, R. M. 1956. *J. Canad. Dent. Assoc.* 22:519.

Pearson, K., and Lee, A. 1903. *Biometrika* 2:357.

Penrose, L. S. 1949. *The biology of mental defect.* London: Sidgwick and Jackson.

Wallenius, B. 1959. *Odont. Revy.* 10:76.

15

The Dentition of
the Afghan Tajik

A. D. Beynon   *Department of Oral Anatomy, Dental School,*
University of Newcastle upon Tyne, England

The general course of human evolution has been known for many years, and new fossil evidence is constantly being discovered confirming and completing the predicted evolutionary sequence. One major problem in human evolution is still obscure, and that is the question of origin, both in terms of space and time, of the living races of man. One school of thought proposes a comparatively recent origin, from a common basal *sapiens* stock, and the other, exemplified by Coon (1962), suggests that each race is of considerable antiquity, arising nearer half a million years ago; furthermore, Coon proposes that each race evolved from the *Homo erectus* to the *sapiens* stage independently in different parts of the world.

Western Asia has a special significance in the evolution of modern mammalian species owing to its unique geographic position, linking Europe, Africa, and Asia, and its changing climate during and following the Pleistocene. It is a contact zone between three major faunal areas—the India/Indochina (Oriental), Africa (Ethiopian), and Europe/Asia (Palearctic). During the Pleistocene it was subjected to alternating cold moist and warm dry climatic conditions which were sufficiently challenging to provide a powerful evolutionary stimulus to the development of many new species, including man. Coon (1962) has proposed an origin for the Caucasoid race within this area, although, as yet, no human remains before the *sapiens* stage (which includes some of the oldest material known) have been discovered in this area.

More recently, Western Asia has played a central role in the evolution of human civilization, for it was here, during the post-Pleistocene (Recent) period, that the conjunction of climatic and ecological factors occurred which

271

enabled, or perhaps forced, man to develop the techniques of agriculture (Clark 1962). This birth of farming, which was essential for the development of large static communities within which cultural specialization could occur, began about eight thousand years ago in the area extending from Palestine through Syria and Iraq to Iran. Dahlberg (1960) has reported on the dentition of early agriculturalist human remains discovered near Jarmo, Iraq, but few dental studies have been carried out on the teeth of modern inhabitants of Western Asia, who are probably descended from the early pioneer farmers.

The significance of dental morphological characteristics has been recognized in evolutionary and ethnographic studies for many years. Gregory (1916) first described the lower molar pattern of Dryopithecus, which was an early primate widely distributed throughout Europe and Africa during the Miocene epoch. The mandibular molars are characterized by five cusps—mesiolingual, mesiobuccal, distobuccal, distolingual, and distal—and the mesiolingual cusp and the distobuccal cusp are in broad contact, separating the mesiobuccal and distolingual cusps. Viewed from the lingual side, the lingual fissure forms a Y shape (fig. 1a). Gregory later showed that this pattern is characteristic of the lower molars of Simiidae and Hominidae. However, during the course of evolution, this basic pattern has been modified, particularly in man, to whom

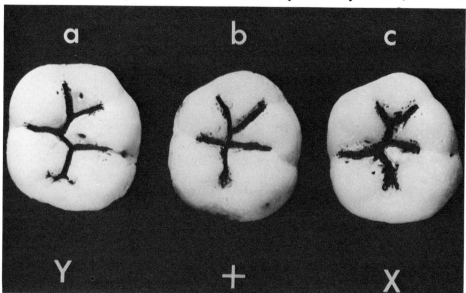

Fig. 1. Specimens of three five-cusped mandibular left first molars, showing changes in their cuspal relationships: (a) the original Dryopithecus pattern, with the mesiolingual cusp in broad contact with the distobuccal cusp; (b) and (c) changes through point contact of the four central cusps (+) to a reversed relationship (×) with the mesiobuccal cusp in contact with the distolingual cusp.

this discussion is subsequently limited. The degree of modification varies in individual teeth within the molar series—and indeed varies within individuals and ethnic groups.

The pattern consists of two components—cusp number and cuspal relationships. The pattern may be modified by a reduction in the number of cusps from five to four, or the cuspal relationships may be altered; that is, the mesiolingual/distobuccal cusp contact may be lost (fig. 1*b*, *c*).

Hellman (1928) classified these various modifications into a series progressing from primitive to modified forms. Although he treated the two components together, he regarded the cuspal relationship as the more conservative feature. This assumption was not challenged for a number of years, and most subsequent authors followed his original classification.

However, in 1955, Jørgensen (1955) questioned this observation when he pointed out that the two components can, and do, vary independently of one another, and he concluded that these elements should be treated separately. He studied the lower molar morphology of recent Danes and Dutchmen and compared his results with published work on a variety of different ethnic groups, which was then analyzed according to his own views. Jørgensen plotted his results in the form of a correlation diagram with the percentage frequency of Y pattern as the ordinate, and percentage frequency of five cusps as the abscissa. He found that individual molar teeth from each of the three major ethnic groups occupied specific areas (fig. 2). Although differences between racial groups have been recognized for many years, Jørgensen's treatment and graphic presentation of his results clearly distinguish the three major racial groups.

This characterization is of considerable value in comparative racial studies and has been utilized in this study to determine the ethnic relationships of the Afghan Tajiks. The Tajiks are widely distributed in the eastern sector of Western Asia, occupying large areas in eastern Iran, southern USSR, and Afghanistan (Brice 1966, Stamp 1962).

During the summer of 1965, I participated in an expedition to the Upper Panjshir valley in northeastern Afghanistan, where a dental morphological survey was carried out on thirty-three Tajik males in the village of Kaujon, which is situated at an approximate altitude of 9,000 feet. The Tajik economy depends upon subsistence cereal cultivation and semicommercial pastoralization; both of which are limited by the short growing season and the long, cold winters (Horsley 1968).

Materials and Methods

Thirty-three Tajik males were available for examination. The age of the subjects ranged from seven to sixty years. This figure represented most of the male

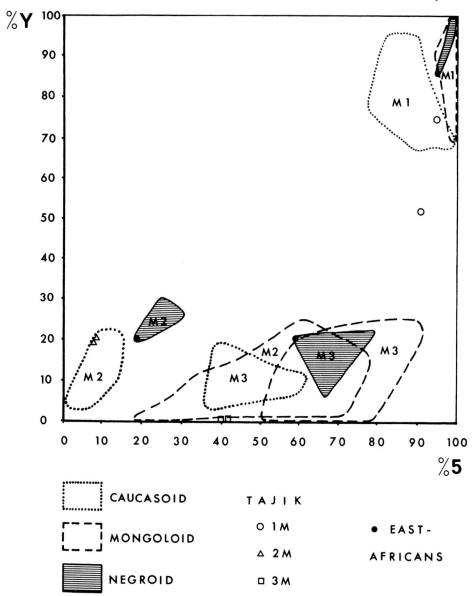

Fig. 2. Correlation diagram (after Jørgensen 1955, including results from East Africans, Chagula 1960) showing the percentage frequency of expression of each Dryopithecus pattern component—Y-fissure pattern, and five cusps—in different human populations, and the relationship of each Tajik molar (right and left sides) to these population distributions.

inhabitants, although it was not possible to establish with certainty the total population of the village. The women, living in a strict Moslem community, were not available for dental examinations.

A number of morphological characteristics were studied by direct visual observation in the mouth. There were no facilities for taking dental impressions and preparing study models.

1. *Mandibular molars*
   a) Dryopithecus pattern (cusp number and relationships)
   b) Tooth size:
       (1) The mesiodistal diameter (length) was measured between the contact points.
       (2) The buccolingual diameter (width) was the larger dimension measured in this direction.
2. *Frequency of specialized morphological characters*
   a) Carabelli's tubercle
   c) Shovel-shaped incisors

Results

In some cases, teeth were not present owing to extraction or noneruption, or teeth were present, but severe attrition, particularly in older subjects, had resulted in obliteration of occlusal morphological details. The numbers of teeth studied are summarized in table 1.

In the first mandibular molar there was found to be a major difference in frequency of Dryopithecus pattern representation in the right and left sides. The Y pattern was altered to a greater extent than the cusp number, which was the more conservative feature, since five cusps were found in over 90% of the teeth examined.

In the second mandibular molar, both components were modified to a much greater degree, both features being found in less than a quarter of the specimens. In this tooth, however, the Y pattern rather than the cusp number was the more conservative feature.

In the third molar the Y pattern was completely lost, whereas the five-cusped form had increased in frequency relative to the second molar. These results are shown in table 1, and are plotted in diagrammatic form in figure 2.

The size of the mandibular molar teeth was found to vary within fairly wide limits, the first molar teeth being the largest in both dimensions. The second molar tooth was the shortest in length, although in width larger than the third molar, which was intermediate in length between the first and third molars. Mean dimensions and standard deviations are shown in table 2.

The frequency of expression of shovel-shaped incisors was very low. In only one case (3%) was a strong shovel shape found, and only four others showed indications of slight shoveling. This total comprised only 15% of the population. Severe attrition in older subjects made identification of Carabelli's tu-

TABLE 1

Frequency of Different Cuspal Relations and Numbers of Cusps on Lower Molars of
34 Tajik Males Aged 7 to 65 Years

	M₃ Sin.	M₂ Sin.	M₁ Sin.	M₁ Dex.	M₂ Dex.	M₃ Dex.
Total sample of teeth	20	27	29	30	26	16
Total teeth with pattern visible	17	25	23	20	26	15
Y pattern	5 (29.4%)	5 (20.0%)	12 (52.2%)	15 (75.0%)	5 (19.3%)	4 (26.7%)
+ pattern	12 (70.6%)	5 (20.0%)	6 (26.1%)	4 (20.0%)	10 (38.3%)	11 (73.3%)
× pattern		15 (60.0%)	5 (21.7%)	1 (5.0%)	11 (42.3%)	
Three cusps		1 (4.0%)				
Four cusps	10 (58.8%)	22 (88.0%)	2 (8.7%)	1 (5.0%)	24 (92.4%)	9 (60.0%)
Five cusps	7 (41.2%)	2 (8.0%)	21 (91.3%)	19 (95.0%)	2 (7.6%)	6 (40.0%)

bercle difficult; although indications ranging from double deep grooves to separate cusps were found in fourteen (41%) of the subjects.

TABLE 2
MEAN SIZES OF LOWER MOLAR TEETH, LEFT AND RIGHT COMBINED (in mm)

Tooth	N	Mesiodistal Length	Buccolingual Width
M_1	40	10.9 ± 0.73	10.4 ± 0.54
M_2	35	10.3 ± 0.59	10.0 ± 0.47
M_3	20	10.6 ± 0.68	9.9 ± 0.46

Discussion

Although the study was carried out on a comparatively small number of individuals, the numbers presented include more than half of the male population of an isolated and self-contained community; and it is considered that a representative cross section has been obtained. However, the fact that the sample is of males only should be considered when assessing the results.

The pattern of modification of both components of the Dryopithecus pattern is typical; the first molar is most conservative, the second molar is most highly modified, and the third molar is intermediate in degree of modification. However, when the results are compared with other studies graphically in the form of a correlation diagram (fig. 2) (after Jørgensen 1955), several outstanding similarities with and differences from other groups are apparent. The general pattern of distribution corresponds much more closely to the typical Caucasoid pattern than to either the Mongoloid or the Negroid groups; although the degree of correlation varies with each tooth, and indeed the degree of modification of each component varies with individual teeth.

Jørgensen commented upon the variation in expression of each component of the Dryopithecus pattern in teeth from right and left sides, and this variation was also found in the present study, being most marked in the first molar, although the variation affected the cusp relations (Y pattern) to a much greater degree than cusp number. The modification of the cusp relationship is more marked than in any other Caucasoid populations so far studied, although the cusp number is relatively conservative. The second molar, although considerably modified, is relatively conservative. The third molar, however, is the most modified, showing a reduced frequency of five cusps and in particular a total absence of Y-pattern cuspal relationships.

Most of the previous studies were carried out on mixed male and female samples, and it is possible that the present findings reflect a sex difference in

Dryopithecus pattern expression. However, recent studies on Japanese children have demonstrated no sex differences in pattern frequency in first and second molars (Matsuda 1961) and deciduous molars (Hattori 1968).

The purely Caucasoid character of the Tajik dentition suggested by the molar morphology is supported by the very low frequencies of shovel-shaped incisors, which characterize Mongoloids (Hrdlicka 1920), and the comparatively high frequencies of Carabelli's tubercle, which is characteristic of Caucasoids (Dahlberg 1963).

These findings of a highly developed Caucasoid dentition in living inhabitants of Western Asia give support to the suggestion that the Caucasoids originated in this region. There is no direct evidence to support the hypothesis that the Caucasoid race evolved separately from the *erectus* to the *sapiens* in Asia, and the confirmation or rebuttal of this theory awaits the discovery of earlier hominid remains. However, the morphological differences which exist between the living races suggest that the separation and isolation necessary to produce these differences must have occurred a considerable time ago. The morphological changes which have occurred are essentially reflections of environmental adaptation, and it is not unreasonable to suppose that a race, once differentiated, which remained comparatively isolated within the original initiating environment, should continue to evolve further along the path of racial subspeciation. These ideas are highly speculative and much further work remains to be done on modern inhabitants of Western Asia to confirm this suggestion.

Another interesting feature of the Tajik dentition is the unusually small mesiodistal length of the molar teeth, when compared with other studies (Scott and Symons 1961, Sicher 1965) (table 3). Numerous investigators (Garn et al. 1965, Lunt 1967) have demonstrated that males have significantly larger teeth than females; and it is probable that in a mixed Tajik sample, the differences in tooth size would be even greater. Possible explanations for this reduction in molar size are related to diet and masticatory function.

In European populations, there appears to have been an increase in molar size from both Anglo-Saxon (Lavelle 1968), and medieval times (Lunt 1967) to the present. Lunt (1969) has provided a possible explanation for this increase in molar size in recent times, which is contrary to the observed evolutionary trend toward molar reduction, by tentatively attributing this to improved dietary conditions. Barnet (1957) has reviewed the recent increase in height and weight of European children and has concluded that this is due to improved nutrition, although improved medical care may also have played an important part. The Tajiks live at near subsistence levels in an extremely harsh and limiting environment, where they are completely isolated by snowdrifts for four

TABLE 3

MEAN MESIODISTAL LOWER MOLAR TOOTH SIZES OF VARIOUS ETHNIC GROUPS
(in mm)

Tooth	Tajik[a]	American White[b]	American White[c]	Lapp[a,c]	Eskimo[c]	Pecos Indian[c]	Java-nese[a,c]	Aborig-inal[c]	Bantu[c]	Bushman[c]
M_1	10.9	11.5	11.2	11.0	11.8	12.0	11.5	12.3	11.0	10.9
M_2	10.3	10.7	10.7	10.5	11.4	11.4	10.9	12.5	11.0	10.6
M_3	10.6	—	10.7	9.9	11.4	11.1	10.9	11.9	11.1	9.9

[a] Males only. All other measurements are from mixed samples.
[b] Sicher 1965.
[c] Results of several studies summarized in Scott and Symons 1961.

months during the winter. The people are short in stature, although they did not appear to be suffering from any obvious nutritional deficiencies. It is accordingly possible that the small size of the molar teeth is a consequence of continuing nutritional insufficiency.

Another possible explanation of the reduction in molar size is related to altered masticatory function extending over thousands of years. During the course of human evolution, there has been a progressive reduction in tooth size (with the exceptions noted above), which has been attributed to a reduction in masticatory function, consequent upon changes in diet and methods of food preparation. It is probable that Tajiks have been agriculturalists, although simple ones, depending for their economy on the cultivation of cereal foods for thousands of years; and it may be that this dietary change has reduced the functional demands upon the masticatory apparatus leading to a reduction in molar tooth size.

Another unusual finding was that the third molar, although comparatively small, was larger than the second molar. This feature has not been reported in other studies, where the third molar is always the smallest molar tooth. Dahlberg (1961) has shown that mandibular molars possessing five cusps tend to be larger than those with only four cusps. In this group, approximately 40% of the third molars possessed five cusps, whereas less than 10% of the second molars had five cusps. However, this does not provide an adequate examination of this finding, since in most populations (see fig. 2), with the possible exception of some Mongoloid groups, the third molar usually has a higher frequency of five cusped forms than the second molar. This curious characteristic of the Tijak molars may also be a reflection of altered masticatory function extending over a long period.

These findings of a highly modified Caucasoid dentition in a remote community of primitive agriculturalists living in Western Asia today are of considerable interest, and further studies are needed to clarify the significance of these observations.

Conclusions

1. A dental morphological survey was carried out on thirty-three Tajik males resident in the Upper Panjshir valley in northeast Afghanistan.
2. The morphological characters studied were:
   a) Mandibular molars
      (1) Frequency of occurrence of Dryopithecus pattern components
      (2) Mesiodistal and buccolingual dimensions
   b) Maxillary dentition

(1) frequencies of occurrence of both Carabelli's tubercle and shovel-shaped incisors
3. The mandibular molars were found to be highly modified in both components of the Dryopithecus pattern, and were also small in size. The crown morphology was characteristic of peoples of the Caucasoid race, an observation confirmed by the frequencies of occurrence of both Carabelli's tubercle and shovel-shaped incisors.
4. These dental morphological findings suggest that the Tajiks are a highly evolved Caucasian people in a physical if not a social context.

ACKNOWLEDGMENTS

I would like to express my appreciation to Professor C. H. Tonge for his encouragement and assistance in this project. I would like to thank the research staff of the Turner Dental School, Manchester, and in particular Professor J. L. Hardwick and Dr. P. Holloway, for their assistance in the planning of this study. I would also like to thank Proctor and Gamble Ltd. for their financial assistance, and Miss L. Noble-Nesbitt for typing this manuscript. This study was carried out during my tenure as a senior research associate supported by the Medical Research Council.

REFERENCES
Barnett, A. 1957. *The human species*. Harmondsworth, England: Penguin Books.
Brice, W. C. 1966. *South-west Asia*. London: University of London Press.
Chagula, W. K. 1960. The cusps on the mandibular first molars of East Africans. *Amer. J. Phys. Anthrop.* 18:83–90.
Clark, G. 1962. *World prehistory: An outline*. Cambridge: at the University Press.
Coons, C. S. 1962. *The origin of races*. London: Jonathan Cape.
Dahlberg, A. A. 1960. The dentition of the first agriculturalists (Jarmo, Iraq). *Amer. J. Phys. Anthrop.* 18:243–56.
———. 1961. Relationship of tooth size to cusp number and groove conformation of occlusal surface patterns of lower molar teeth. *J. Dent. Res.* 40:34–38.
———. 1963. Analysis of the American Indian dentition. In *Dental anthropology*, ed. D. R. Brothwell, 5:161. London and New York: Pergamon Press.
Garn, S. M.; Lewis, A. B.; Kerewsky, R. S.; and Jegart, K. 1965. Sex differences in intraindividual tooth-size communalities. *J. Dent. Res.* 44:476–79.
Gregory, W. K. 1916. Studies on the evolution of the Primates. *Bull. Amer. Mus. Nat. Hist.* 35:239.
Hattori, R. 1968. A morphological study on the groove of the occlusal surface in deciduous molar teeth: Aichi-gakuin. *J. Dent. Sci.* 6:39–55.
Hellman, M. 1928. Racial characters in human dentition. *Proc. Amer. Philos. Soc.* 67:157.

Horsley, H. 1968. A survey of land use in the Upper Panjshir valley. In *Environmental research in the Samir Valley of the Hindu Kush, Afghanistan,* ed. A. James, 8:1–9. University of Newcastle upon Tyne.

Hrdlicka, A. 1920. Shovel shaped teeth. *Amer. J. Phys. Anthrop.* 3:429.

Jørgensen, K. D. 1955. The Dryopithecus pattern in recent Danes and Dutchmen. *J. Dent. Res.* 34:195–208.

Lavelle, C. L. B. 1968. Anglo-Saxon and modern British teeth. *J. Dent. Res.* 47:811–15.

Lunt, D. A. 1967. Odontometric study of medieval Danes. *J. Dent. Res.* 46:918–22.

———. 1969. *Acta Odont. Scand.,* suppl. (In press).

Matsuda, T. 1961. Studies on the Dryopithecus pattern of the Japanese residing in Hokuriku district. *Folia Anat. Japonica* 37:317–30.

Scott, J. H., and Symons, N. B. B. 1961. *Introduction to dental anatomy.* 3d ed. Edinburgh and London: E. and S. Livingstone.

Sicher, H. 1965. *Oral anatomy.* 4th ed. Saint Louis: C. V. Mosby Co.

Stamp, D. 1962. *Asia: A regional and economic geography.* London: Methuen.

16 The Human Dentition during the Megalithic Era

Hyacinth E. Brabant *Université Libre de Bruxelles, Belgium*

Introduction

Several previous essays on the dentition of Neolithic man in Europe have been devoted to comparisons with dentition in the preceding and the following eras. They have contributed to understanding the problems of the evolution of the dentition in recent times (Brabant 1962, 1968, 1969; Brabant and Moeschler 1970; Brabant, Sahly, and Bouyssou 1961). Dental morphological studies have contributed to knowledge of the Neolithic civilizations, among which the Megalithic is one of the most interesting and an important source of material. The purpose of this chapter is to compare the dental morphological data of the Megalithic era with those of other eras. Such a study must include a very large number of teeth in order to give substance to the low-frequency traits.

In a former essay titled "Comparison of the Characteristics and Anomalies of the Deciduous and the Permanent Dentition" (Brabant 1967), many areas of investigation were suggested and many questions were left unanswered. I therefore decided to check the former conclusions by examining a new and important collection of teeth from the Megalithic era of France. Special attention was paid not only to the permanent dentition but also to the temporary dentition, which is often neglected in such investigations. In this essay, only a limited number of important morphological characteristics will be considered.

Material and Methods

The dental remains from the Megalithic era that were examined come from various regions of France and are housed primarily in the Institut de paleontologie humaine in Paris. These materials are related to an era spreading from approximately 2500 to 1000 B.C. A total of 7,986 teeth were studied, 1,117 temporary and 6,869 permanent teeth (table 1). The teeth were examined according to the same methods used in former investigations. Only unworn or

TABLE 1

NUMBERS OF TEMPORARY AND PERMANENT TEETH OF FRENCH MEGALITHIC EPOCH

Origin	Department in France	Temporary Teeth	Permanent Teeth	Total
Dolmens of Monpalais	Deux-Sèvres	110	114	224
Dolmen of Manthelan	Indre-et-Loire	42	610	652
Dolmen of Sublaines	Indre-et-Loire	457	2,369	2,826
Dolmen of Puechcamp	Aveyron	106	1,034	1,140
Dolmen of Bennac	Aveyron	296	2,006	2,302
Dolmen of Vezinies and La Bergerie	Aveyron	79	521	600
Dolmens of Les Marais, Poulines, and Barbigault	Loir-et-Cher	27	215	242
Total		1,117	6,869	7,986

slightly worn teeth were used in making measurements. The most important normal and abnormal morphological characteristics were noted (Brabant 1962; Brabant, Sahly, and Bouyssou 1961; Brabant and Twiesselmann 1967).

Results of the Observations

Permanent Teeth

Crown-Size. The numbers in the groups varied between 50 and 150. Table 2 shows the mesiodistal and the buccolingual sizes of the crowns. It is interest-

TABLE 2

MESIODISTAL CROWN SIZE OF PERMANENT TEETH OF THE MEGALITHIC EPOCH (in mm)

Teeth	Monpalais	Manthelan	Sublaines	Bennac	Average
Upper central incisor	8.27	8.68	8.65	8.22	8.45
Upper lateral incisor	6.83	7.08	6.60	6.80	6.82
Upper canine	7.53	8.02	7.67	7.71	7.73
Upper first premolar	6.89	7.09	6.67	6.73	6.84
Upper second premolar	7.01	6.58	6.72	6.55	6.71
Upper first molar	10.41	10.93	10.16	10.66	10.54
Upper second molar	9.88	9.98	9.45	9.52	9.71
Upper third molar	9.63	9.97	8.17	8.77	9.13
Lower central incisor	5.81	5.36	4.95	5.03	5.28
Lower lateral incisor	5.98	5.94	5.91	5.78	5.90
Lower canine	6.85	7.26	6.87	6.66	6.91
Lower first premolar	6.92	6.83	6.77	6.91	6.85
Lower second premolar	7.17	7.66	7.08	7.28	7.29
Lower first molar	10.95	11.34	11.33	10.97	11.24
Lower second molar	10.01	10.79	9.96	10.12	10.22
Lower third molar	10.48	10.84	10.27	10.22	10.45

ing to note that the size of the teeth coming from the various dolmens are very nearly the same.

If a comparison is made between the teeth of the Belgian-French Neolithic period and those of the Middle Ages (tables 3 and 5), one notices that they are almost identical. The size of the teeth in western Europe did not change since the Neolithic period, except for a slight reduction in size of molars (Brabant 1968). The same is true for the upper Paleolithic (tables 3 and 5). One notices a slight reduction in the size of the premolars and some molars, which confirms previous observations (Brabant and Twiesselmann 1964).

TABLE 3

COMPARISON OF THE AVERAGE OF MESIODISTAL CROWN SIZE OF MEGALITHIC PERMANENT TEETH WITH THE TEETH OF OTHER EPOCHS

Teeth	Upper Paleolithic[a]	French Neolithic[b]	Belgian Neolithic[c]	Megalithic	Middle Ages[d]
Upper central incisor	8.33	8.47	8.33	8.45	8.30
Upper lateral incisor	6.39	6.75	6.51	6.82	6.43
Upper canine	7.81	7.63	7.55	7.73	7.60
Upper first premolar	6.66	6.78	6.58	6.84	6.47
Upper second premolar	6.51	7.20	6.37	6.71	6.33
Upper first molar	10.61	11.11	10.21	10.54	10.00
Upper second molar	9.98	10.84	9.79	9.71	8.86
Upper third molar	9.34	——	8.36	9.13	8.32
Lower central incisor	5.09	5.78	5.20	5.28	5.07
Lower lateral incisor	5.79	5.98	5.71	5.90	5.73
Lower canine	7.05	6.84	6.65	6.91	6.63
Lower first premolar	6.87	7.24	6.52	6.85	6.42
Lower second premolar	7.09	7.88	6.66	7.29	6.56
Lower first molar	11.37	11.27	10.82	11.14	10.72
Lower second molar	11.05	10.69	9.85	10.22	9.96
Lower third molar	11.08	——	9.91	10.45	9.97

[a] Brabant 1970.
[b] Brabant, Sahly, and Bouyssou 1961.
[c] Brabant 1962.
[d] Brabant and Twiesselmann 1967.

Characteristics of Tooth Shape. The shovel-shaped incisor was frequently observed (fig. 1). The frequency of this shovel shape in central and lateral incisors at different periods can be noted in table 6. This table shows the relative concordance of the frequency of the various forms of shovel-shaped teeth during the Neolithic and the Megalithic eras. Between 40 and 60% of the individuals had no shovel-shaped teeth. This table shows, also, that in these populations the shovel shape was more pronounced in the lateral than in the central incisor.

TABLE 4

BUCCOLINGUAL CROWN SIZE OF PERMANENT TEETH OF THE MEGALITHIC EPOCH

Teeth	Monpalais	Manthelan	Sublaines	Bennac	Average
Upper central incisor	7.08	7.08	7.12	7.02	7.07
Upper lateral incisor	6.62	6.76	6.61	6.34	6.58
Upper canine	7.98	8.32	8.27	8.28	8.21
Upper first premolar	9.12	9.42	8.75	8.81	9.02
Upper second premolar	8.10	8.83	9.05	8.77	8.68
Upper first molar	12.21	11.79	11.25	11.13	11.59
Upper second molar	11.73	11.32	11.44	10.93	11.35
Upper third molar	10.94	10.66	10.85	10.76	10.80
Lower central incisor	6.21	6.11	5.80	5.92	6.01
Lower lateral incisor	6.62	6.38	6.18	6.32	6.37
Lower canine	7.81	8.18	7.75	7.75	7.87
Lower first premolar	7.10	7.46	7.53	7.34	7.35
Lower second premolar	7.26	8.18	8.28	7.90	7.90
Lower first molar	10.23	10.53	10.72	10.41	10.47
Lower second molar	9.28	10.18	9.63	9.33	9.60
Lower third molar	10.02	10.12	9.45	9.88	9.86

TABLE 5

COMPARISON OF THE AVERAGE OF BUCCOLINGUAL CROWN SIZE OF MEGALITHIC PERMANENT TEETH WITH THE TEETH OF OTHER EPOCHS

Teeth	Upper Paleolithic[a]	French Neolithic[b]	Belgian Neolithic[c]	Megalithic	Middle Ages[d]
Upper central incisor	7.30	7.28	7.28	7.07	7.10
Upper lateral incisor	6.49	6.51	6.30	6.58	6.21
Upper canine	8.60	8.24	8.29	8.21	8.33
Upper first premolar	9.24	9.29	8.48	9.02	8.59
Upper second premolar	9.58	7.88	8.83	8.68	8.81
Upper first molar	11.99	10.35	11.32	11.59	11.22
Upper second molar	11.80	9.61	10.74	11.35	10.65
Upper third molar	11.59	——	9.98	10.80	10.13
Lower central incisor	6.12	6.13	5.89	6.01	5.96
Lower lateral incisor	6.56	6.68	6.31	6.37	6.26
Lower canine	8.18	7.89	7.72	7.87	7.77
Lower first premolar	8.14	6.93	7.38	7.35	7.32
Lower second premolar	8.40	7.14	8.11	7.90	7.86
Lower first molar	11.10	10.12	10.17	10.47	10.28
Lower second molar	10.93	9.89	9.82	9.60	9.72
Lower third molar	10.56	——	9.51	9.86	9.46

[a] Brabant 1970.
[b] Brabant, Sahly, and Bouyssou 1961.
[c] Brabant 1962.
[d] Brabant and Twiesselmann 1967.

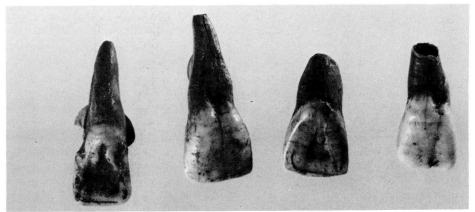

Fig. 1. Incisor teeth of the Megalithic era with shovel-shaped lingual surfaces.

TABLE 6

DISTRIBUTION OF SHOVEL-SHAPED INCISORS IN EUROPEAN NEOLITHIC
POPULATIONS: COMPARISON WITH MODERN WHITE POPULATIONS

Origin	Degree	Median Incisor	Lateral Incisor
French Neolithic[a]	Shovel	4.2	7.4
	Moderate	25.2	30.4
	Trace	13.7	12.1
	No shovel	56.8	50.0
Belgian Neolithic[b]	Shovel	3.7	9.6
	Moderate	——	——
	Trace	——	——
	No shovel	——	——
Swiss Neolithic[c]	Shovel	2.1	12.4
	Moderate	18.5	34.6
	Trace	17.6	13.9
	No shovel	61.6	38.9
French Megalithic[d]	Shovel	5.4	13.2
	Moderate	25.4	33.9
	Trace	11.0	9.4
	No shovel	58.0	43.3
Belgian Middle Ages[d]	Shovel	2.7	8.0
	Moderate	16.5	20.3
	Trace	21.2	24.0
	No shovel	59.5	48.0
American white modern[e]	Shovel	1.4	1.4
	Moderate	5.2– 7.6	7.4– 8.8
	Trace	21.8–24.5	30.0–36.4
	No shovel	66.5	50.0–59.6

[a] Brabant, Sahly, and Bouyssou 1961.
[b] Brabant 1962.
[c] Brabant and Moeschler 1971.
[d] Brabant and Twiesselmann 1964.
[e] Hrdlicka 1920.

These observations confirm previous findings (Brabant 1967) and are in accord with those of Carbonell (in Brothwell 1963). According to the latter author, 1–5% well-marked shovel-shaped central upper incisors and 55–70% without shovel shape are found in modern white populations, the remaining being moderate or discrete forms.

Among the upper lateral incisors in the present Neolithic studies, 1–5% show a well-marked shovel shape also, and 40–60% were without that shape, the remaining being moderate or discrete. On the contrary, in Mongoloid populations, about 80–95% of the incisors are shovel shaped and 4–20% show none of the trait (table 3; Carbonell 1963).

In Neolithic and Megalithic populations, the rate is higher than in modern white populations; 5% for central incisors and 7–13% for lateral incisors with well-marked shovel shape; 38–60% of central or lateral incisors were not shovel shaped. This confirms the reduction of the frequency of the shovel-shaped tooth in western Europe since the Neolithic era (Brabant 1967).

Coronal-radicular Groove. It is during the Megalithic period that the coronal-radicular groove seems to have been the most frequent (about 12–21% for the two upper incisors, as against 8–13% in other groups) (fig. 2, table 7). The significance of this groove is not known. It is often associated with the shovel-shaped tooth and is more frequent in the lateral than in the

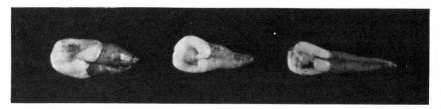

Fig. 2. Illustration of coronal radicular grooves on upper incisors (Megalithic).

TABLE 7

FREQUENCIES OF CORONAL-RADICULAR GROOVE

Orgin	Median Incisor	Lateral Incisor
French Neolithic (Les Matelles)[a]	2.4	10.7
Swiss Neolithic[b]	4.6	8.6
Belgian Neolithic[c]	1.8	6.3
French Megalithic	5.1–6.9	7.2–14.2[d]

[a] Brabant, Sahly, and Bouyssou 1961.
[b] Brabant and Moeschler 1971.
[c] Unpublished.
[d] According to the dolmen (Brabant 1969).

central incisor. Perhaps it may indicate a tendency for root division, or a genetic pecularity.

Peg-shaped Upper Lateral Incisor. Peg-shaped upper lateral incisors were not observed. The few peg-shaped teeth that were collected were supernumerary. The frequency of peg-shaped lateral incisors found in modern populations is about 0.9–2.8% (Meskin and Gorlin 1963).

The large *lingual tubercle* (fig. 3) was observed twice. It was associated

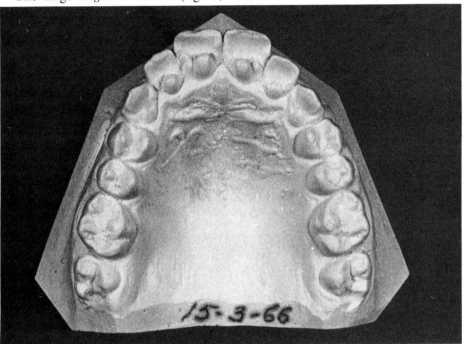

Fig. 3. Lingual tubercles on upper central and lateral incisors (Delforge and Libotte).

with shovel-shaped teeth, but can exist independently. Carbonell (1963) stated that "the association of shovel-shape with a lingual tubercle in modern man is infrequent."

Lingual Pit. A pit on the lingual surface of the central incisor was observed three times at the Matelles and five times in the entire collection of teeth from the Megalithic era.

The number of the cusps of the upper molars has been reduced since the Neolithic era (table 8). This reduction is moderate for the first molar, but well marked on the second and the third. It is the third molar that most frequently presents only three cusps. In previous papers, attention was called to this reduction of the cusps during the Paleolithic era (Brabant 1970).

TABLE 8

FREQUENCIES OF THE CUSPS IN THE UPPER PERMANENT MOLARS

Origin	Teeth	Four Cusps	Three to Four Cusps	Three Cusps
European Neolithic[a]	First molar	100.0	——	——
Megalithic Puechcamp	" "	100.0	——	——
Megalithic Manthelan	" "	98.0	2.0	——
Megalithic Sublaines	" "	100.0	——	——
Middle Ages[b]	" "	100.0	——	——
European modern[c]	" "	90.0	9.5	0.5
European Neolithic[a]	Second molar	70.0	20.0	10.0
Megalithic Puechcamp	" "	75.8	13.7	10.3
Megalithic Manthelan	" "	62.0	28.0	10.0
Megalithic Sublaines	" "	75.0	21.8	3.1
Middle Ages[b]	" "	36.8	47.3	15.7
European modern[c]	" "	38.0	32.0	30.0
European Neolithic[a]	Third molar	30.0	25.0	45.0
Megalithic Puechcamp	" "	25.6	35.8	38.4
Megalithic Manthelan	" "	22.3	23.3	53.4
Megalithic Sublaines	" "	37.5	37.5	25.0
Middle Ages[b]	" "	0.0	62.5	37.5
European modern[c]	" "	17.0	29.0	54.0

[a] Brabant and Twiesselmann 1964. Mean levels.
[b] Merovingiens of Sublaines, France; Brabant and Cordier (unpublished).
[c] Brabant and Twiesselmann 1964. Mean levels.

The reduction of the number of the cusps is also noticed on the lower molars, since the Neolithic and even earlier. This reduction is moderate for the first molar, more marked for the two others. It is interesting to note that the third molar is occasionally less reduced than the second. This observation confirms earlier findings (Brabant and Twiesselman 1964).

Table 9 shows the distinct evolution of the pattern Y5 toward the Y4, Y3, +5 and +4 patterns between the Neolithic and the present era.

The frequency of the *tubercle of Carabelli* in various human groups is shown in table 10. It shows that important variations do not exist in the frequency of this characteristic during the Neolithic period in Europe. The significance of this tubercle is not understood.

The tubercle of Bolk is far less frequent than the tubercle of Carabelli. Table 11 shows no significant variation in frequency in the various human groups during the Neolithic, the Megalithic, the Middle Ages, and the modern era.

TABLE 9

OCCLUSAL PATTERNS IN THE LOWER PERMANENT MOLARS

Origin	Teeth	Y6	Y5	+5	Y4	+4	Y3 or Less
European Neolithic[a]	First molar	0.6	89.0	8.0	2.3	0.0	0.0
Megalithic Bennac	" "	0.0	69.1	16.5	14.0	0.0	0.0
Megalithic Manthelan	" "	2.0	72.3	14.0	1.6	0.0	0.0
Megalithic Sublaines	" "	2.3	78.5	16.5	2.5	0.0	0.0
Middle Ages[b]	" "	0.0	38.4	46.1	7.6	7.6	0.0
European modern[c]	" "	0.3	67.2	11.0	17.5	4.0	0.0
European Neolithic[a]	Second molar	0.0	0.0	2.4	9.4	88.0	0.0
Megalithic Bennac	" "	0.0	4.4	4.4	25.5	65.5	0.0
Megalithic Manthelan	" "	0.0	3.3	3.3	12.3	81.4	0.0
Megalithic Sublaines	" "	0.0	0.0	2.2	13.6	84.0	0.0
Middle Ages[b]	" "	0.0	8.2	0.0	16.6	66.6	8.3
European modern[c]	" "	0.0	6.0	2.5	3.5	88.0	0.0
European Neolithic[a]	Third molar	0.0	10.0	5.0	23.0	61.0	1.0
Megalithic Bennac	" "	0.0	21.5	28.4	10.0	38.5	1.5
Megalithic Manthelan	" "	0.0	10.6	39.0	7.0	41.0	2.3
Megalithic Sublaines	" "	0.0	23.3	12.3	6.6	56.6	1.0
Middle Ages[b]	" "	0.0	40.0	20.0	3.4	36.4	0.0
European modern[c]	" "	0.0	13.0	39.0	16.5	30.5	0.9

[a] Brabant 1968.
[b] Merovingiens of Sublaines; Brabant and Cordier (unpublished).
[c] Brabant and Twiesselmann 1964. Mean levels.

TABLE 10

PERCENTAGE DISTRIBUTION OF CARABELLI'S TUBERCLE
(Upper Molars)

Origin	M₁			
	0	Pit	Groove	Tubercle
Belgian Neolithic[a]	76.0	9.0	11.5	3.5
French Neolithic[b]	—	—	—	5.1
Megalithic Sublaines	78.0	8.0	12.0	2.0
Megalithic Vezinies	72.9	7.6	5.2	9.3
Megalithic Bennac	72.4	7.6	18.5	1.5
Middle Ages[c]	61.4	9.3	17.3	12.0
American white Modern[d]	15.0	22.2	62.7	
	M₂			
Belgian Neolithic[a]	—	—	—	—
French Neolithic[b]	—	—	—	—

TABLE 10—cont.

Megalithic Sublaines	100.0	0.0	0.0	0.0
Megalithic Vezinies	100.0	0.0	0.0	0.0
Megalithic Bennac	100.0	0.0	0.0	0.0
Middle Ages[c]	—	—	—	—
American white Modern[d]	61.0	16.0	23.0	

	M_3			
Belgian Neolithic[a]	—	—	—	—
French Neolithic[b]	—	—	—	—
Megalithic Sublaines	100.0	0.0	0.0	0.0
Megalithic Vezinies	97.5	0.0	0.0	2.4
Megalithic Bennac	100.0	0.0	0.0	0.0
Middle Ages[c]	—	—	—	—
American white Modern[d]	92.8	7.1	0.0	

[a] Brabant (Unpublished).
[b] Brabant, Sahly, and Bouyssou 1961.
[c] Brabant and Twiesselmann 1967.
[d] Dahlberg 1963.

Temporary Teeth

Crown Size. Table 12 shows the mesiodistal and buccolingual measurements of the crowns of temporary teeth of four dolmens. The averages are almost identical for the Paleolithic, the Neolithic, and the Middle Ages. In the deciduous teeth also there has been no apparent reduction of the crown size since the Neolithic era.

Variation in Shape. The literature on the temporary dentition is limited, especially as far as the shovel-shaped trait is concerned. Table 13 shows that the shovel shape is less marked and less frequent in the temporary dentition in present-day Europe. No other variation of shape has been observed.

Taurodontism did not exist in any molar, although it has been observed in other series of teeth to a frequency of about 1%.

Number of Cusps. Distribution of differing numbers of cusps in upper and lower molars is represented in tables 14 and 15. There have been few modifications in these teeth since the Neolithic era, except for the second upper molar, which tends, to a certain degree, to lose its hypocone.

Summary

In this study, I examined approximately 8,000 teeth from the Megalithic era (2500–1000 B.C.), coming from France. The purpose was to investigate the essential characteristics of the crowns of these teeth as well as the frequency of variations and then to make comparisons.

TABLE 11

PERCENTAGE DISTRIBUTION OF BOLK'S TUBERCLE
(Lower Molars)

Origin	M_1			
	0	Pit	Groove	Tubercle
Belgian Neolithic[a]	100.0	0.0	0.0	0.0
French Neolithic[b]	100.0	0.0	0.0	0.0
French Megalithic	100.0	0.0	0.0	0.0
Middle Ages[c]	100.0	0.0	0.0	0.0
American white Modern[d]	26.0	68.0	6.0	
	M_2			
Belgian Neolithic[a]	100.0	0.0	0.0	0.0
French Neolithic[b]	100.0	0.0	0.0	0.0
French Megalithic	100.0	0.0	0.0	0.0
Middle Ages[c]	94.0	3.9	1.1	0.9
American white Modern[d]	52.5	30.0	17.5	
	M_3			
Belgian Neolithic[a]	96.6	2.0	0.0	1.2
French Neolithic[b]	98.0	0.0	1.2	0.7
French Megalithic	89.0	3.0	2.6	5.3
Middle Ages[c]	96.0	2.0	1.1	0.9
American white Modern[d]	71.4	28.6	0.0	0.0

[a] Brabant (Unpublished).
[b] Brabant, Sahly, and Bouyssou 1961.
[c] Brabant and Twiesselmann 1967.
[d] Dahlberg 1963.

Concerning the permanent teeth, it was noticed that:

1. The crown sizes are the same as those of the teeth of the Neolithic era and of the Middle Ages that were previously examined. No important variation of tooth size occurred except for an occasional moderate reduction in the premolars and molars.

2. The shovel-shaped incisor shows the same frequency in various groups of Neolithic teeth examined. The lateral incisor showed a shovel shape more often than the central. The frequency of the shovel-shaped incisor diminished after the Neolithic era.

TABLE 12

COMPARISON OF CROWN SIZE OF UPPER PALEOLITHIC, NEOLITHIC, MEGALITHIC AND
MIDDLE AGES TEMPORARY TEETH

	Mesiodistal Size				
Teeth	Upper Paleolithic[a]	French and Belgian Neolithic[b]	Swiss Neolithic[c]	Megalithic	Middle Ages[d]
Upper median incisor	7.00	——	6.63	6.75	6.30
Upper lateral incisor	6.10	——	5.18	5.67	5.20
Upper canine	7.30	——	6.77	6.89	6.80
Upper first molar	9.00	7.46	7.12	7.13	7.10
Upper second molar	9.83	9.02	9.09	8.92	9.00
Lower median incisor	4.65	——	3.91	4.05	4.00
Lower lateral incisor	5.00	——	4.69	4.85	4.60
Lower canine	——	——	6.03	5.79	5.90
Lower first molar	9.11	8.39	8.24	8.49	8.00
Lower second molar	10.14	10.43	9.90	10.12	9.90

	Buccolingual Size				
Teeth	Upper Paleolithic[a]	French and Belgian Neolithic[b]	Swiss Neolithic[c]	Megalithic	Middle Ages[d]
Upper median incisor	6.95	——	5.10	5.34	5.00
Upper lateral incisor	6.50	——	4.85	5.10	4.90
Upper canine	6.50	——	6.34	6.25	6.00
Upper first molar	6.35(?)	8.91	8.20	8.52	8.40
Upper second molar	6.76(?)	10.17	9.47	9.86	9.80
Lower median incisor	5.50	——	3.78	3.83	3.70
Lower lateral incisor	6.50	——	4.47	4.41	4.20
Lower canine	——	——	5.77	5.45	5.50
Lower first molar	7.43	7.31	7.16	6.98	7.00
Lower second molar	9.92	9.52	8.83	9.02	8.80

[a] Matiegka (Quoted according to Brabant 1970).
[b] Brabant 1962, 1965.
[c] Brabant and Moeschler 1970.
[d] Mydlarz 1964.

3. The coronal-radicular groove is frequent in the incisor of the Megalithic era (about 12–20%).

4. The peg-shaped lateral incisor was not encountered in the numerous incisors from the Megalithic era that were examined. The infrequent peg-shaped teeth found in that era were supernumerary. The frequency of the peg-shaped tooth has, therefore, increased since the Neolithic.

TABLE 13
FREQUENCIES OF SHOVEL-SHAPED TEMPORARY MEDIAN INCISORS

Origin	Shovel	Moderate	Trace	No Shovel
Belgian and Swiss Neolithic[a]	0	0.0	4.5	95.5
French Megalithic	0	3.4	7.2	89.3
American white[b]	0	0.0	50.0	50.0
Modern Belgian[c]	0	1.2	14.0	84.7
American Negro[b]	0	10.0	10.0	80.0
Japanese[b]	0	76.6	23.4	0.0

[a] Unpublished.
[b] Hanihara 1963.
[c] Brabant 1965.

TABLE 14
FREQUENCIES OF CUSPS IN TEMPORARY UPPER MOLARS

Origin	Teeth	Four Cusps	Three Cusps	Two Cusps
French Megalithic	First molar	0.0	29.5	71.5
Modern white[a]	" "	0.0	40.0	60.0
Modern Polish[b]	" "	0.0	31.0	69.0
Modern Japanese[a]	" "	20.1	64.6	15.2
French Megalithic	Second molar	99.0	1.0	——
Medieval Danish[c]	" "	100.0	0.0	——
Medieval Belgian[d]	" "	98.0	1.9	——
Modern white[a]	" "	73.7	26.3	——
Modern Japanese[a]	" "	70.7	29.3	——

[a] Hanihara 1963.
[b] Szlachetko 1959.
[c] Jørgensen 1956.
[d] Brabant 1965.

TABLE 15
FREQUENCIES OF CUSPS IN TEMPORARY LOWER MOLARS

Origin	Teeth	Six Cusps	Five Cusps	Four to Five Cusps	Four Cusps
Megalithic	First molar	——	——	48.5	51.5
Medieval Danish[a]	" "	——	——	47.7	52.2
Medieval Belgian[b]	" "	——	——	29.0	71.0
Modern[a]	" "	——	——	44.8	55.1
Megalithic	Second molar	2.5	97.5	——	——
Medieval Danish[a]	" "	2.7	97.1	——	——
Medieval Belgian[b]	" "	——	100.0	——	——
Modern[a,b]	" "	2.2	93.7	4.0	——

[a] Jorgensen 1956.
[b] Brabant 1965.

5. A few cases of lingual tubercle have been observed. Generally, but not always, they are associated with the shovel-shaped trait. In addition some cases of a lingual pit of the central incisor were found.

6. The number of cusps of the molars tends to decrease after the Neolithic era: to a lesser extent on the first molars, more frequently on the third and second lower molars. At the same time, there is a tendency toward a simplification of the outline of the grooves. This evolution is relatively fast.

7. The study of the tubercles of Bolk and Carabelli did not furnish significant results.

In the temporary teeth, it has been noticed that:

1. There has been no important reduction in the crown size since the Neolithic period.

2. The shovel-shaped incisor is less frequent and its shape is less marked than in the permanent teeth.

3. The number of the cusps has undergone few changes since the Neolithic era, except on the second upper molar, which tends to lose its hypocone.

4. Taurodontism was not observed in either temporary or permanent teeth.

REFERENCES

Brabant, H. 1962. Contribution à l'étude de la paléopathologie des dents et des maxillaires: La denture en Belgique à l'époque néolithique. *Bull. Inst. Roy. Sc. Nat. Belg.* 38:1–32.

————. 1965. Observations sur l'évolution de la denture temporaire humaine en Europe occidentale. *Bull. Group. Int. Rech. Sc. Stom.* 8:235–302.

————. 1967. Comparison of the characteristics and anomalies of the deciduous and the permanent dentition. *J. Dent. Res.* 46:897–902.

————. 1968. La denture humaine à l'époque néolithique. *Bull. Soc. Roy. Anthrop. Préhist. Belg.* 79:105–20.

————. 1969. Observations sur les dents des populations mégalithiques d'Europe occidentale. *Bull. Group. Int. Rech. Sc. Stom.* 12:429–60.

————. 1970. La denture de l'homme du Paléolithique supérieur européen. In *L'homme de Cro-Magnon, 1868–1968: Anthropologie et archéologie,* ed. G. Camps and G. Olivier. Paris: Editions Arts et Metiers Graphiques.

Brabant, H., and Moeschler, A. 1971. Etude des dents trouvées dans les cimetières néolithiques de Barmaz I, Barmaz II, et Chamblandes, canton de Vaud, Suisse. *Arch. Suisses Anthropol. Gen.* In press.

Brabant, H.; Sahly, A.; and Bouyssou, M. 1961. Etude des dents préhistoriques de la station archéologique des Matelles, département de l'Hérault, France. *Bull. Group Int. Rech. Sc. Stom.* 4:382–448.

Brabant, H., and Twiesselmann, F. 1964. Observations sur l'évolution de la denture permanente humaine en Europe occidentale. *Bull. Group. Int. Rech. Sc. Stom.* 7:11–84.

————. 1967. Nouvelles observations sur la denture d'une population ancienne d'âge franc de Coxyde, Belgique. *Bull. Group. Int. Rech. Sc. Stom.* 10:5–180.

Brothwell, D. 1963. *Dental anthropology.* London: Pergamon Press.

Carbonell, V. 1963. Variations in the frequency of shovel-shaped incisors in different populations. In *Dental anthropology,* ed. D. Brothwell. London: Pergamon Press.

Dahlberg, A. A. 1963. Analysis of the American Indian dentition. In *Dental anthropology,* ed. D. Brothwell. London: Pergamon Press.

Hanihara, K. 1963. Crown characters of the deciduous dentition of the Japanese-American Hybrids. In *Dental anthropology,* ed. D. Brothwell. London: Pergamon Press.

Hrdlicka, A. 1920. Shovel-shaped teeth. *Amer. J. Phys. Anthrop.* 3:429–65.

Jørgensen, D. K. 1956. *The deciduous dentition: A descriptive and comparative anatomical study.* Copenhagen: Bianco Lunos Bogtrykkeri.

Meskin, L. H., and Corlin, R. J. 1963. Agenesis and peg-shaped permanent maxillary lateral incisors. *J. Dent. Res.* 42:1476–79.

Mydlarz, A. 1964. Observations sur les dimensions des dents temporaires d'âge médiéval. *Bull. Group. Int. Rech. Sc. Stom.* 7:121–41.

Szlachetko, K. 1959. Investigations on the morphology of the human deciduous dentition. *Acta Fac. Rerum Nat. Univ. Comenianae.* 3:247–79.

17 A Cinefluorographic Study of Feeding in the American Opossum, *Didelphis marsupialis*

Karen Hiiemae — *Anatomy Department, Guy's Hospital Medical School, University of London;*
Museum of Comparative Zoology, Harvard University
The Nuffield Institute for Medical Research, Oxford University

A. W. Crompton — *Museum of Comparative Zoology, Department of Biology, Harvard University;*

Introduction and Review of the Literature

The feeding behavior of the American opossum, *Didelphis marsupialis*, has been examined using a combination of cinephotography, radiography, and cinefluorography. For this study *Didelphis* has been taken as exemplifying the primitive mammalian condition of the jaw apparatus. This view has been based not only on the general similarities between the jaws of the opossum and many primitive Cretaceous mammals such as *Alphadon* and *Simolestes*, but also on the anatomy of the muscles of mastication (Hiiemae and Jenkins 1969), their comparative anatomy (Barghusen 1968), and the morphology of the teeth (Crompton and Hiiemae 1970). There were, therefore, two purposes to this study: first, to examine feeding mechanisms and behavior in a primitive generalized mammal and, second, to use that information to interpret the evolution of dental function in the early mammals. The results of the general investigation into feeding behavior and mandibular movements are given in this paper. The analysis of the chewing cycle and its power stroke has been correlated with the form and function of the tribosphenic molar and discussed elsewhere (Crompton and Hiiemae 1970).

As far as we are aware, there has been no previous analysis of masticatory movement or feeding behavior in the opossum or any other primitive mammal. Hartman (1952) gives some general observations in his account of the biology of *Didelphis*. Using 16 mm monochrome cinefilm, Patterson (1956) recorded the behavior of a single specimen of *Solenodon* feeding on newborn mice. No detailed analysis was possible. Cinefluorography has been used to examine feeding behavior in a number of highly specialized mammals: the rabbit

(Ardran, Kemp, and Ride 1958); the rat (Hiiemae and Ardran 1968); and the wallaby (Ride, personal communication).

Materials and Methods

For this and subsequent investigations, a colony of *Didelphis* was established at the Peabody Museum of Natural History at Yale University. The animals were obtained by trapping in the Branford-Hamden areas of Connecticut. In southern New England the opossum has become a garbage scavenger and local pest, and there was no difficulty in trapping considerable numbers of specimens. No attempt was made to establish a breeding colony.

The behavior of the opossum at rest, during normal activity, and in feeding has been studied by direct observation, cinephotography, and cinefluorography as well as by conventional radiography. In the early stages of this investigation invaluable help and advice was given by Dr. G. M. Ardran of the Nuffield Institute for Medical Research, University of Oxford. Dr. Ardran very kindly made the conventional radiographs used in this study.

The apparatus used has been described elsewhere (Crompton 1968; Crompton and Hiiemae 1969a, 1970). The behavior of the animals during fluoroscopy was monitored by a closed-circuit television system and recorded as required on videotape. Sequences of ingestion, mastication, and deglutition were recorded on 16 mm cinefilm at camera speeds of 30 and 60 frames per sec in the lateral and dorsoventral projections.

If the normal feed was withheld before recording, the opossums were found to feed readily under the experimental conditions; so no training period was necessary. Animals were fed condensed milk, a proprietary brand of canned dog food (minced meat, offal, cereals, and vitamins), chicken gizzard, whole chicken legs or wings, and toffee. Since the milk and dog food were not radio-opaque, barium sulphate was added in some cases. To increase the accuracy with which the films could be analyzed, steel "friction grip" pins[1] were inserted into the dentary on each side anteriorinferior to the canine alveolus in three animals, under Nembutal anesthesia. No differences were observed in the behavior of the marked and unmarked animals.

Both the video tape and the cinerecordings were analyzed. Video tapes were replayed at normal and reduced speeds to give general behavioral information, but they are unsatisfactory for detailed analyses of movement. The cinefilms were examined on a variable-speed analyzing projector at speeds ranging from 16 to 2 frames per sec. The arrangement of the apparatus imposes certain limitations on the analysis. To avoid overheating the X-ray tube with the high

---

[1] Unitek Ltd., California.

milliamperage required for cinefluorography, there is an automatic cutout after 20 sec, followed by a short pause. In practice this means that a complete sequence of ingestion, mastication, and deglutition cannot be filmed without interruption. This does not constitute a problem when examining the path of jaw movement during a single cycle, but it limits the numbers of cycles that can be examined sequentially. The small samples used in the compilation of table 1 reflect the number of cycles completed during a given 20 sec. A second limitation on behavioral analysis is the difficulty of obtaining sequences in which the animal is accurately in plane for most or all of the available 20 sec. Of the 2,500 ft of film used during this study, rather less than 5% could be used for detailed analysis. This was examined in two ways: the recorded movements of the lower jaw relative to the upper jaw and snout were plotted by projecting each frame of a sequence individually, then tracing the salient features and reference points. Successive tracings were then superimposed to give the path of movement of the lower jaw, the food, or the tongue relative to the reference points. In a few cases the cervical spine was used as the main reference point so that relative movements of the cranium and lower jaw could be plotted. The pattern and rhythm of movement during ingestion, mastication, and deglutition were examined by counting the number of frames (on film taken at 60 frames per sec) required for each stroke of each cycle. The gape at which each cycle commenced was measured by tracing the profile of the occlusal surfaces of upper and lower molars and measuring the angle between them. These results are shown in table 1 and samples are illustrated graphically in figures 7 and 11.

The results of this study are illustrated by single frames from the cinephotographic and cinefluorographic studies, by conventional radiographs, and by montages of tracings from the single-frame analysis. Cinephotographic and cinefluorographic recordings showing typical sequences of the full range of feeding behavior have been combined on a 16 mm cinefilm entitled *Feeding in the American Opossum*.

Observations and Discussion

The opossum is, by comparison with both the rabbit (Ardran, Kemp, and Ride 1958) and the rat (Hiiemae and Ardran 1968), a slow feeder. This has made it possible to record all the intermediate positions of the jaws during the execution of any mandibular movement by using film taken at a camera speed of 60 frames per sec. All jaw movement in *Didelphis* was found to be cyclical. The duration and amplitude of the cycle depend on the feeding activity in progress and also on the consistency of the food. The number of cycles involved in the ingestion or mastication of food depends on its bulk and consistency. The observations made in this study are described under three main

TABLE 1
DURATION OF MASTICATORY CYCLE

Behavior	Food		Prepartory Stroke		Power Stroke		Recovery Stroke		Total Cycle		Degree of Gape	
			Mean	S.D.	Mean	S.D.	Mean	S.D.	Mean	S.D.	Mean	S.D.
Lapping/licking	Milk	(34)	2.1	0.3	2.9	0.6	7.6	0.7	12.9	0.8	6.0[a]	1.5
Puncture-crushing	Chicken leg or wing	(14)	7.2	0.9	6.1	1.6	11.7	2.2	25.0	4.0	29	4.9
	" " "	(10)	7.5	1.2	5.2	0.4	12.4	3.2	24.9	3.3	33.5	10.7
	Chicken gizzard	(14)	8.3	0.6	5.0	0.8	16.1	1.1	29.5	1.5	38.7	4.7
	"	(14)	6.8	0.9	6.0	0.6	16.8	2.3	29.5	2.8	28.0	5.0
Shearing mastication	Dog food	(10)	6.6	0.6	5.0	0.0	11.6	1.6	23.2	2.1	24.8	4.2
	" "	(14)	5.5	0.7	4.6	0.6	9.8	1.5	19.9	1.6	20.7	5.1
	" "	(14)	5.4	1.9	4.7	0.7	11.1	1.3	21.4	2.5	19.7	5.0
	Chicken leg or wing	(18)	6.2	1.1	5.0	1.0	11.4	2.5	22.0	3.6	25.3	4.1
	" " "	(14)	7.4	1.1	5.8	1.5	11.3	4.2	24.5	5.9	24.5	3.3
	Chicken gizzard	(12)	7.7	1.5	8.0	2.7	20.8	3.9	36.5	5.8	26.4	9.1
	"	(13)	6.5	0.5	5.6	0.8	15.9	1.3	28.0	1.6	24.2	2.1
	"	(19)	5.4	1.2	5.4	1.3	9.7	1.6	20.5	3.9	22.3	6.3

NOTE: The mean duration and its standard deviation are given in frame of film recorded at 60 frames per sec for the preparatary, power, and recovery strokes as well as the total cycle when *Didelphis* was feeding on the foods shown. The mean and standard deviation for the gape in each case are also shown. The figures in parentheses are the number of cycles counted in each sample.
[a] Mean of 12, not 34 cycles.

headings: first, a brief account of *feeding behavior* based on the direct visual, cinephotographic, and video-tape studies; second, a detailed account of the *rest position,* followed by the *mandibular movements in feeding,* namely *ingestion, food transference, mastication,* and finally *deglutition and regurgitation.*

Feeding Behavior

The opossum is a voracious and undiscriminating feeder, given to aggressive oral display when disturbed. The jaw apparatus is used as a weapon and can inflict severe damage. During temporary emergency double-caging at Yale some weaker animals underwent savage maulings amounting to nonfatal cannibalism; the limbs and feet were most often mauled. Female lactating opossums were observed to attack their young, causing fatal wounds or suffocation. In all these types of aggressive behavior the canines and premolars were used as slashing instruments. The violence with which the animal uses its teeth and jaws even in the feral state is reflected in the number of adult animals having fractured canines when trapped. Of twenty-four specimens trapped in 1967/68, four had broken lower canines and two had broken upper canines leaving only residual stumps.

On being presented with food, the hungry opossum immediately begins to feed and will consume a considerable quantity before pausing. There is, in these circumstances, no preliminary inspection of the food, although cursory examination may follow the first feeding bout. A partially satisfied animal is more selective and inspects the food before continuing. This inspection sometimes results in rejection, the animal curling up and ignoring its environment. This is typical postprandial behavior. *Didelphis* is occasionally coprophiliac, as was seen when the regular morning feed was delayed for experimental purposes.

The posture adopted during feeding depends on whether the forefeet are required to hold or steady the food. The animal normally adopts a semisquatting position using all four feet for support. The head is lowered to the food during ingestion and moved away and elevated during mastication. During the ingestion of some foods, notably those which are in unfixed containers or are of large bulk, the forefoot and, where necessary, the snout are used to control the position of the food or dish. One forefoot only is used, the right and left alternating with a changeover at the completion of a sequence of mastication.

Ingestion

Fluids are ingested by a combination of lapping and licking. While lapping the tongue sweeps through the liquid only and does not come into contact with the container, whereas in licking the liquid is removed from the bottom or sides of the container by the tongue. Once the process has commenced, it may continue without interruption for several seconds or until all the fluid has been ingested. "Mushy" or semisolid foods are ingested either by licking, if presented as scattered particles or small lumps, or by a process best described as "shoveling." In the second case the animal thrusts its lower jaw into the food mass, using it much like a shovel, separates a large lump, and then retreats from the food with the lump grasped between the upper anterior teeth and the tongue and lower anterior teeth. The incisors have been observed to function as more than a grasping organ only when soft food was presented on a metal spoon. In this case the upper incisors were used to scrape the food from the spoon.

In ingesting tough food, feeding behavior varied with size rather than consistency. Small lumps such as chicken gizzards or chicken hearts are grasped between the anterior teeth and then rapidly transferred to the molar region for mastication. Larger objects such as chicken wings or legs are inserted through the side of the mouth while being grasped with one forefoot and either held against the floor or more commonly carried to the mouth with the digits gripping one end. The opossum then begins to bite vigorously and rhythemically to separate a portion of the food. The head is moved sharply away from the food as the forelimb pulls it laterally, thereby assisting in tearing the food apart as the teeth come into occlusion. (The way the opossum ingests a chicken wing can be likened to the way children eat stick candy. The cheek teeth are used to crush the end of the sweet, while the hand controls its position and pulls it away from the mouth.)

Ingestion of tough bulky food and all mastication takes place on one side of the mouth only and is continued on that side for a variable number of cycles, with occasional pauses for the animal to adjust its grip on the food. The number of cycles on each side of the jaw during ingestion and the subsequent mastication of a piece of chicken leg were counted from a dorsoventral cinerecording. The results in one case are shown in chart 1. In this case the right side was predominant; at other times the left side may be favored. Since there is no observable pattern in the distribution and numbers of cycles occurring on either side in any given animal or between animals, no statistical analysis has been attempted. When the shift from one side to the other actually occurs, the food undergoing ingestion is dropped from the mouth and picked up by opposite forefoot. This may necessitate its being pushed in front or below the head toward the other side by the forefoot or the snout. Alternatively it may be passed from hand to hand (fig. 1).

In additon to gripping the food, the forefoot is used to control the position of large lumps between the cheek teeth. This was observed during the phase in which food such as a chicken gizzard is being transferred from the incisal area

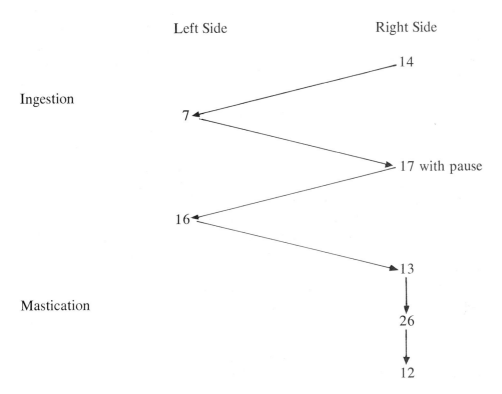

Chart 1. Numbers of biting and chewing cycles carried out on each side of the mouth during the ingestion and mastication of a piece of chicken leg.

to the cheek teeth for mastication. With small or medium-sized bites, the tongue can be seen to control the position of the food. Much of the bulk of larger objects protrudes outside the mouth and the tongue alone appears to be ineffective. In these cases, as when a whole chicken gizzard is about to be chewed, the forefoot on the active side moves to assist in positioning the material between the molars on that side.

At no time in this study have the anterior teeth been observed to cut food. There is, therefore, no parallel in *Didelphis* for the incising action of these teeth described in man or other specialized mammals. This is not surprising in view of the small size of these teeth and their low crown height in vivo. Figure 2*a* shows the palatal view of a plaster cast of a synthetic rubber impression of the palate of *Didelphis* taken immediately post-mortem; the incisors are very short and stumpy when compared with their appearance in a prepared skull (fig. 2*b*). The anterior teeth, canines and incisors, are routinely used in holding food. Turnbull (1968, personal communication) suggests that the incisors may be

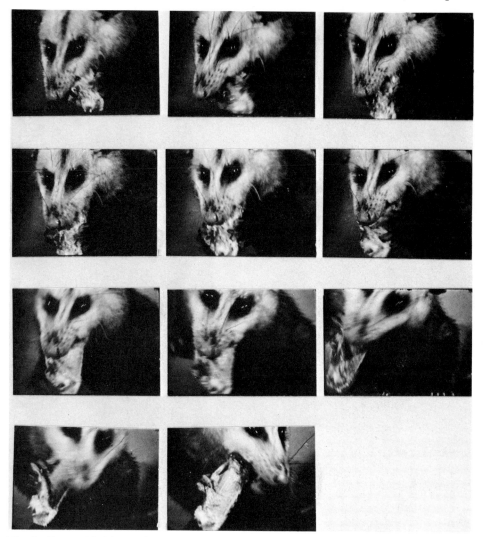

Fig. 1. Every third frame from a cinephotographic recording taken at 60 frames per sec, showing an opossum ingesting a chicken leg. This sequence shows the use of the forefeet in transferring the food from one side of the mouth to the other.

used for opening bird's eggs, on which the opossum is reputed to feed in the wild.

Mastication

Once food has been ingested and transferred to the molar region of the mouth cavity, it is rhythmically chewed until reduced sufficiently for bolus formation and deglutition. As has been stated above, mastication in *Didelphis* takes place

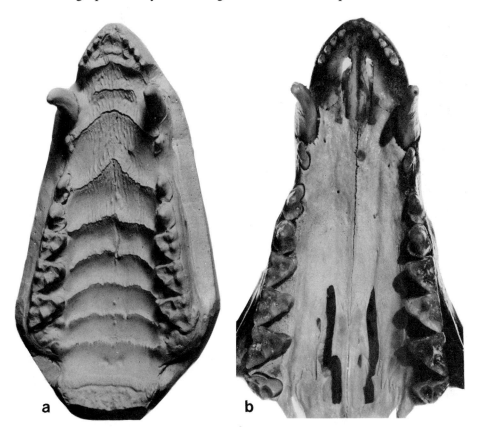

Fig. 2. (*a*) A cast taken from an impression of the palate in a specimen of *Didelphis* immediately post-mortem to show the height of the teeth and the palatal rugae as in life; (*b*) The same view of a prepared skull.

on only one side of the mouth at any one time, and the head is usually held up but tilted toward the active side. This means that to obtain accurately positioned dorsoventral radiographs, the tube-intensifier arm has to be rotated about 20° from the vertical. The shift of the food from one side to the other normally occurs intraorally except when large masses are involved and the forelimbs are utilized (see above). The time taken to triturate is correlated with the consistency of the food. Of the foods used in this study, chicken gizzard and toffee required the most chewing and not, as might have been expected, the whole chicken leg or wing. The explanation for this is the initial trituration the food undergoes during ingestion. Whatever the consistency of the food supplied, it is chewed by repeated cyclical movements of the jaw, tongue, and, in some cases, the cranium. The only variations in the pattern of mastication were found to be in the duration of each chewing cycle, both absolutely and in each of the three constituent strokes. There was no observable variation in the direction of movement.

Chewed food is swallowed toward the end of any bout of masticatory activity. A single large bite will be chewed and then swallowed before ingestion recommences. This is the normal pattern for solid material. The continuous sequence of ingestion observed for liquids is associated with more frequent deglutition. Three or more collections of fluid may be passed during ingestion with no observable interruption of the ingestive rhythm. An unexpected finding was that *Didelphis* frequently regurgitates a bolus for retrituration. This occurs primarily when material of mixed consistency, such as chicken leg or wing, has been eaten, but this has been observed with other tough foods.

The Rest Position

The jaw apparatus of *Didelphis* is rarely at rest except, presumably, when the animal is asleep. This assumption is difficult to verify, as the opossum sleeps in a curled-up position with the snout buried in its abdominal fur. When the animal is awake and inactive, the mandible is frequently held in "centric relation" (see Crompton and Hiiemae 1970) and with the teeth slightly apart, leaving a freeway space. This is comparable to the "rest position" described for man and other mammals. However, video tape and cinerecordings show that even in this position there are slight vertical movements of the lower jaw. These are of very small amplitude and appear linked with spasmodic dilation of the nares and haphazard movements of the tongue. The depth of the freeway space therefore fluctuates between 1 and about 3 mm (as seen in lateral-projection cinerecordings).

The rest position in *Didelphis* corresponds to that generally accepted for man and other mammals as regards the mediolateral position of the lower jaw (centric relation), but lies within a range of vertical positions. In view of this it is perhaps best regarded as falling within a "postural area" as suggested by Bowman and Ford (1968) for the rest position in man.

Mandibular Movements in Feeding

All mandibular movements in *Didelphis* observed during feeding are rhythmic and cyclical. The cycle consists of three basic movements: an upstroke, an occlusal phase, and a downstroke. These movements are normally termed the "preparatory," "power," and "recovery" strokes (Hiiemae 1967; Hiiemae and Ardran 1968; Crompton and Hiiemae 1969a, 1970). Although applicable to the chewing cycle in *Didelphis*, this nomenclature is not entirely applicable to the comparable movements of the jaw observed during ingestion. The movement patterns occurring during the various stages in the feeding cycle are discussed below.

Ingestion

There are two basic types of ingestion in *Didelphis,* depending on whether the food is passed into the mouth through the anterior or the premolar-molar region. In the latter case the movements involved are those of mastication. Ingestion through the front of the mouth involves movements which conform to the basic three-stroke cycle: an upstroke, a "near occlusion" phase (the power stroke), and a downstroke. However, since these movements are used to allow the tongue to move extraorally and also to position the (upper) anterior teeth to act as a gripping organ, the "near occlusion" phase is the least important in terms of function.

During all ingestion through the front of the mouth, the downstroke (recovery stroke) is used for collecting the food. This movement consists of two phases with an interrupt: an initial slight opening in which the tongue is protruded, a pause followed by a rapid further opening, and then movement into the upstroke. During the upstroke (preparatory stroke) food is transferred into the oral cavity.

In ingestion through the front of the mouth, the tongue is the most active part of the jaw apparatus as it collects the food (with or without the aid of the anterior teeth) and then transfers it into and through the oral cavity. This movement of food by the tongue depends on the passage of a series of contraction "waves" along its length, which form a series of "crests" and "troughs." Food is collected in a "trough" and its (anteroposterior) position is controlled by the adjacent crests. As the wave of contraction passes down the tongue, the "trough" appears to move distally, carrying the food with it. When soft foods and liquids are being ingested, they move smoothly backward but particles of harder material appear to 'bounce.' This effect may be produced by intermittent contact with the very pronounced ridgelike palatal rugae seen in this animal (fig. 2a). The same pattern of tongue activity is an integral part of the chewing cycle in *Didelphis* and is also involved in deglutition.

Licking and Lapping. Lapping is observed only when the animal is drinking, but licking is used in several types of behavior. Both lapping and licking are extremely rapid activities involving a limited range of vertical movement in each cycle. The number of cycles involved in a licking or lapping sequence were counted and range up to fifty-five without pause or until the food supply is exhausted.

The cycle commences with a downstroke. This is shown in figure 3a, b, where tracings of seven consecutive frames taken from a cinerecording of licking taken

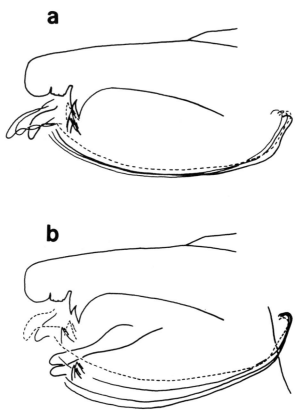

Fig. 3. A montage from single-frame tracings of a single licking cycle in *Didelphis*. The movements of the tongue during the last stages of the downstroke are shown in *a* and of the jaw and tongue during the upstroke in *b*. The last frame in fig. 3*a* is the first frame (*dotted line*) in fig. 3*b*.

at 60 frames per sec are shown superimposed. The last frame in figure 3*a* is the first in 3*b*. (For convenience the figure has been prepared with the long axis of the head horizontal rather than nearly vertical as actually occurs.) The first phase of the downward movement of the jaw is shown in 3*a*. From the rest position the mandible is dropped until the tip of the lower canine lies just below that of the upper. This represents a gape of about 6° measured between the molar occlusal surfaces. Coincident with the completion of this slight movement, the tip of the tongue is rapidly protruded. No further significant movement of the jaw occurs until the tongue has completed the collection of the food.

Once protruded, the tip of the tongue moves round the food, separating a portion where necessary or simply positioning the material ready for ingestion. These movements produce changes in the tongue's profile (fig. 3*b*). Finally, with the correct positioning of the tongue relative to the food, the jaw is moved sharply downward and the food is slipped onto the tip of the tongue, which then starts to retract (fig. 3b). At this point the downstroke continues and is rapidly completed. The jaw then moves sharply upward to the rest position as the food is carried into the oral cavity.

The pattern of movement immediately following the ingestion of food by licking depends on its consistency. If it is liquid, the period of the "near occlusion" phase or third stroke of the cycle is used to transfer the material toward the epiglottis, where it is collected. If a small particle of mushy or even fairly hard material has been ingested, the jaw is elevated to about the rest position while the food is passed by the tongue to the canine-premolar region. A transference cycle follows (see below).

The mandibular and tongue movements of lapping are similar to those of licking, but their relative timing is slightly different. The events of the first phase of the downstroke are the same. During the pause the tip of the tongue protrudes into the liquid and then begins to flick backward; the mouth may then be opened farther. The tongue now begins to move rapidly forward through the liquid and then upward as it is very sharply withdrawn. This last forward and upward movement produces a ripple in the surface of the liquid and is the point at which a small volume is "captured" on the surface of the tongue. As the tongue begins to retract, the lower jaw moves into the upstroke, which is rapidly completed. The ingested liquid is now moved distally on the tongue as the jaw is held in the "near occlusion" position, and the liquid is transferred to the molar region. A further cycle then commences which may be either licking or lapping in type.

Grasping and Shoveling. The mechanism by which semisolid or solid food is grasped or "shoveled" into the mouth is basically simple, but both the timing and the overall duration of the cycle are much more variable than for other modes of ingestion. The positioning and picking up of a discrete lump of hard food such as chicken gizzard or chicken heart is rapidly accomplished, but the separation of a lump from soft material such as dog food takes longer.

The usual pattern of jaw and tongue movement is as follows: the lower jaw is depressed and the tongue protruded; the food is licked and its position adjusted by the tongue; a further depression of the jaw follows as the upper anterior teeth, particularly the canines, are plunged into the material. The lower jaw then moves into the upstroke, which continues until the food is firmly gripped between upper and lower anterior teeth or the upper teeth and the tongue. No jaw movement occurs as the head is moved away from the food. This position corresponds with the "near occlusion" phase, although the vertical position of the mandibular depends on the dimensions of the bite. Tooth-food-tooth or tooth-food-tongue contact is maintained until the commencement of the next cycle, when the food is transferred distally from the canine to the molar region of the mouth.

Food Transference. All food ingested through the front of the mouth has to be passed distally to the molar region before mastication can commence. During mastication the anteromedial direction of the power stroke results in the forward shift of the food from the molars toward the premolars. The food has to be passed back to the molars in preparation for the next power stroke. A similar situation arises when hard, tough food such as a chicken wing is being ingested by mastication. If, owing to the remaining bulk of material outside the mouth, the tongue alone cannot implement the distal transfer of the food, the forefoot is used to lift the material from the premolar region and reposition it. Otherwise all food is repositioned within the oral cavity by a combination of jaw and tongue movement.

Broadly, intraoral food transference occurs in three situations: a rapid distal shift of liquid toward the epiglottis; the movement of soft material in bulk from the incisor-canine to the premolar-molar region of the mouth; and a shift from the premolar-molar region to the back of the molar series. The last occurs in every masticatory cycle. The second and third types are illustrated in figure 4a, b, c, d. In figure 4a a large mass of dog food is shown grasped between the anterior teeth (first frame, dotted line). As the jaw is depressed (next two frames) the bite is moved downward and slightly backward; during the following upstroke (fig. 4b) the food is carried upward and backward to bring it into the molar region. A power stroke usually follows to complete the food transference and mastication commences. The changing profile of the tongue during food transference is shown in figure 2c, d. A large bite extends from the canines to the premolars (dotted line, first frame), the jaw is slightly dropped and the tongue protruded; the tip of the tongue is then moved over the lower anterior teeth while the jaw is held in the slightly open position. This tongue movement occurs in most cases, but invariably when the food is at all sticky, and presumably serves to adjust the position of the bite on its surface. After this pause for adjustment the downstroke is resumed, the jaw opening widely as the tongue retracts carrying the food distally to the molar region (fig. 4d). Transference is completed in the early part of the upstroke and a power stroke follows.

During mastication, food is transferred during the recovery and preparatory strokes (fig. 5a, b). As the lower jaw moves downward, the bite is collected on the tongue and carried downward and slightly backward as the tongue forms a trough in the molar region. Further backward and upward shift of the bite occurs during the first half of the recovery stroke, bringing the food into position on the surfaces of the lower molars in preparation for the power stroke.

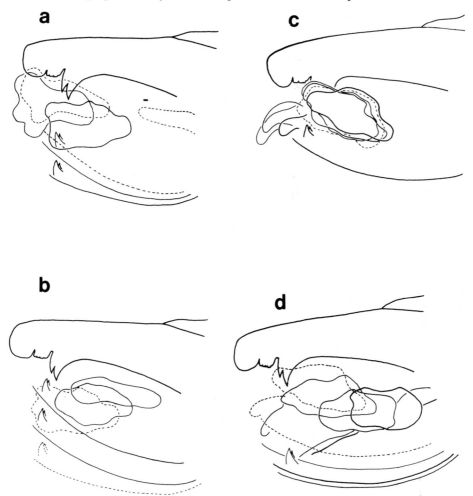

Fig. 4. Montages showing stages in food transference. Figure 4*a* and *b* show the successive positions of the jaw and the food (figure 4*c* and *d* also show the tongue profile. The tracing of the first frame in each sequence is shown with a dotted line.

Mastication

After ingestion and transference to the molar region, food is chewed until it is sufficiently reduced for bolus formation. In *Didelphis* food is chewed in two stages: it is initially pulped by a process best described as "puncture-crushing," in which the cusps of the teeth are plunged into the food without coming into occlusion. This is followed by a tooth-tooth contact in which molar surfaces are sheared across each other (Crompton and Hiiemae 1969*a*, *b*; 1970). The

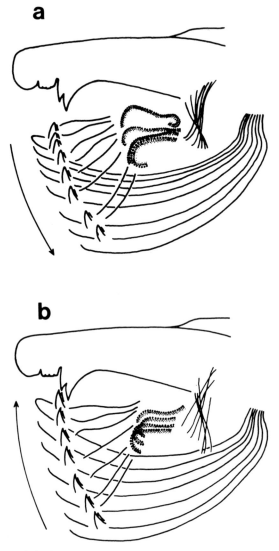

Fig. 5. The movements of the lower jaw, tongue, and food during the recovery stroke (*a*) and the following preparatory stroke (*b*). (*Reproduced by kind permission of the Linnaean Society of London.*)

duration of each of these activities is correlated with the consistency of the food. Soft material such as the dog food used in this study required little pulping, whereas more than 50% of the total time chewing chicken gizzard was spent in puncture-crushing. In effect the jaw movements used to ingest chicken leg or wing are probably the same as those used in the puncture-crushing phase of mastication. Radiologically the two are indistinguishable. The direction of jaw movement in the preparatory and recovery strokes in puncture-crushing and shearing is the same but they vary somewhat in amplitude and duration. This will be discussed below.

All chewing in *Didelphis* depends on the repetition of a basic chewing cycle. This consists of three strokes: preparatory, power, and recovery, which are distinguished by the different directions in which the jaw moves in each stroke. A full description of the chewing cycle has been given elsewhere and correlated with the morphology of the molars in *Didelphis* (Crompton and Hiiemae 1970). These findings are briefly reviewed here as a basis for observations on masticatory behavior.

A cycle begins at the position of maximum gape, or the maximally depressed position of the jaw. The jaw then moves upward and laterally toward the active side until tooth-food-tooth or tooth-tooth contact is achieved; this is the point of completion of the preparatory stroke. The preparatory stroke is followed by the power stroke, during which the lower jaw moves upward, medially, and finally slightly forward to a position where the syndesmosis lies just to the active side of the midline. The final recovery stroke, which follows the power stroke, is a simple vertical movement during which the mandible is depressed. During mastication, asymmetric and independent movements of the active and balancing sides occur and are mediated by the symphyseal joint or syndesmosis. Figure 6a shows the chewing cycle as seen in lateral-projection radiographs. The movement of the syndesmosis can be clearly seen in the dorsoventral projection (fig. 6b).

During the analysis of the movements of the two halves of the jaw in a single masticatory cycle, three impressions were gained: first, that there was a correlation between the overall duration of a cycle and the consistency of the food; second, that the duration of a cycle, the size of the gape, and the consistency of the food are all related; and third, that the constituent strokes in each cycle occupied a constant percentage of the total cycle time. To examine these observations, the time-relations between the strokes of the cycle, its total duration, and the size of the gape when animals were feeding on dog food, chicken wing or leg, and chicken gizzard have been determined.

Counts were made of the number of frames of 16 mm film taken at 60 frames per sec required to complete each stroke. The criteria used to define the beginning and the end of each stroke in lateral-projection cinerecordings were as follows: the preparatory stroke begins at the point of maximum gape for the cycle and was considered complete when no freeway space was visible between the teeth or when tooth-food-tooth contact was achieved. The power stroke continues from this point until the teeth come out of occlusion or tooth-food-tooth contact is broken. The recovery stroke begins at this point and continues

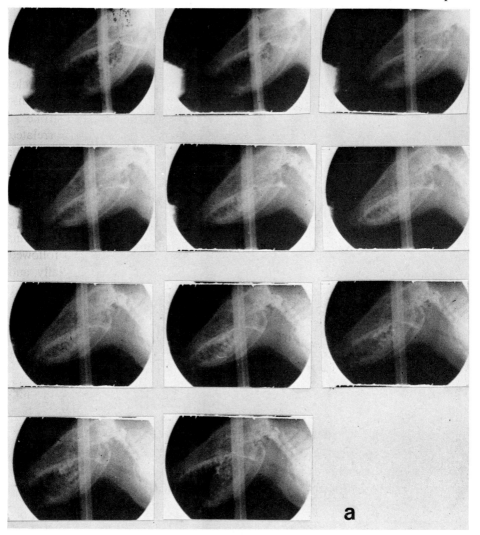

Fig. 6. Cinefluorographic recordings of the chewing cycle in *Didelphis* taken at 6 frames per sec.
    Series a shows the cycle in lateral projection when the animal was masticating (shearing) dog food. Frames 1 to 6 show the preparatory stroke, frames 7 to 12 the power stroke, and frames 13 to 21 the recovery stroke.

to maximum gape. "Turning points" between strokes were found by overshooting one or two frames and counting back. Counts were made of successive cycles within single 20-sec recording periods. The mean duration and standard deviation, measured in frames, of each stroke and of the total cycle are shown

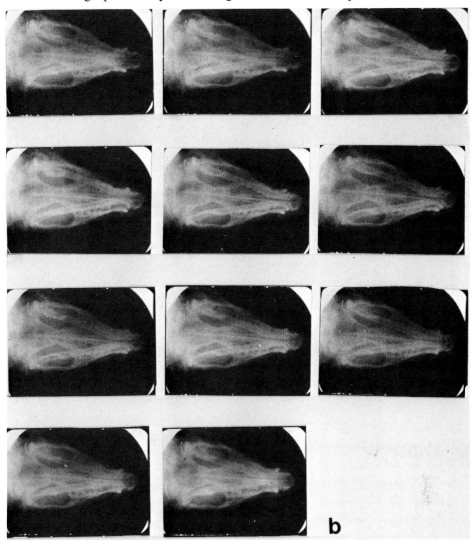

Series b shows every third frame in a dorsoventral recording of the cycle when the animal was shearing chicken gizzard. Frames 1 to 7 show the preparatory stroke, frames 8 to 16 the power stroke, and frames 16 to 31 the recovery stroke. Note the changing dimensions of the mandibular syndesmosis and the Bennett movement of the condyles.

in table 1. The duration of each stroke calculated as a percentage of the total cycle time and the mean duration for each stroke in puncture-crushing and shearing mastication are shown in table 2. In addition, the gape at which each successive cycle began was measured and the mean and standard deviation were

TABLE 2
DURATION OF MASTICATORY STROKES AS PERCENTAGE OF TOTAL CYCLE TIME

Behavior	Food	Preparatory Stroke Mean	Preparatory Stroke % T.C.	Power Stroke Mean	Power Stroke % T.C.	Recovery Stroke Mean	Recovery Stroke % T.C.	Total Cycle Mean	Degree of Gape S.D.	Degree of Gape Mean
Lapping/licking	Milk	2.1	16	2.9	24	7.6	59	12.9	6.0	1.5
Puncture-crushing	Chicken leg or wing (14)	7.2	29	6.1	24	11.7	47	25.0	29.0	4.9
	" " " (10)	7.5	30	5.2	21	12.4	49	24.9	33.5	10.7
	Chicken gizzard (14)	8.3	29	5.0	17	16.1	54	29.5	38.7	4.7
	" " (14)	6.8	23	6.0	20	16.8	57	29.5	28.0	5.0
	Overall mean % duration	27.7 ± 2.7%		21.0 ± 2.5%		51.7 ± 3.8%		100%	Mean gape 32.2°	
Shearing mastication	Dog food (10)	6.6	29	5.0	21	11.6	50	23.2	24.8	4.2
	" " (14)	5.5	28	4.6	22	9.8	50	19.9	20.7	5.1
	" " (14)	5.4	26	4.7	22	11.1	52	21.4	19.7	5.0
	Chicken leg or wing (18)	6.2	28	5.0	22	11.4	50	22.0	25.3	4.1
	" " " (14)	7.4	30	5.8	24	11.3	46	24.5	24.5	3.3
	Chicken gizzard (12)	7.7	21	8.0	22	20.8	55	36.5	26.4	9.1
	" " (13)	6.5	23	5.6	20	15.9	57	28.0	24.2	2.1
	" " (9)	5.4	26	5.4	26	9.7	47	20.5	22.3	6.3
	Overall mean % duration	26.0 ± 2.9%		22.4 ± 1.7%		51.0 ± 3.4%		100%	Mean gape 23.5°	

NOTE: The mean values for the duration of the masticatory strokes shown in table 1 are expressed as a percentage of total cycle time. The overall mean figures for each stroke in puncture-crushing and shearing mastication and the grand means for the gapes are also shown.

calculated. The actual rather than the mean figures obtained in the count were used to draw figures 7 and 12, where the cycles have been plotted as gape against time in frames for a real time period of 2 sec.

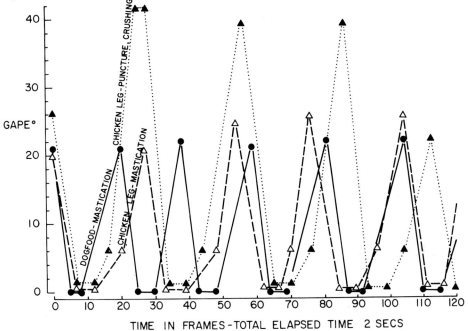

Fig. 7. The movement of the lower jaw during puncture-crushing and shearing mastication for chicken leg and dog food respectively. The number of frames of film (taken at 60 frames per sec) required for the completion of each movement has been plotted against the size of the gape at the beginning of each cycle and during the recovery stroke.

In figure 7 the movement of the lower jaw (as seen in lateral projection) in 120 frames of cinerecording or 2 secs real time has been plotted for sequences of dog-food mastication and for chicken leg or wing. This clearly shows the rhymthmicity of jaw movement in *Didelphis*. The simplest pattern is seen in dog-food mastication: a rapid preparatory stroke is followed by a slightly slower recovery stroke. In all cases the movement bringing the jaw down to the gape in readiness for the next cycle is much slower than the return upward stroke. (Note that the "peaks" in the figure correspond to "maximal gapes" between cycles.) The asymmetry in the rate of vertical movement in the preparatory and recovery strokes seen in the figure becomes more exaggerated with the tougher foods. Instead of an almost smooth downward movement, the recovery stroke occurs in two phases. During the first half (in the first five to seven frames showing the stroke) the jaw opens only to about 6°, that is, with the canine tips overlapping, the large movement bringing the jaw down to a gape of 20° occurs very rapidly in the second phase. The time, both absolutely and as a percentage of the total cycle time, taken to bring the jaw down to a gape of about 6° in licking and lapping is within the same range of time as in the first phase of the recovery stroke of mastication (tables 1 and 2). This slow first stage depends on jaw movement only, the second stage almost always involves cranial movement as well (see "The Mechanism of the Gape", below).

Figure 7 also illustrates graphically, in two cases over 4–5 cycles, an observation better substantiated in table 1, namely that the overall duration of the cycle and the size of the gape are much the same in true cutting mastication regardless of the initial consistency of the food. The exception to this, mastication of chicken gizzard (tables 1 and 2), is distinguished not by a larger gape but by a longer recovery stroke, which therefore increases the overall duration of the cycle. In figure 8 mean total cycle time has been plotted against mean gape for each of the cases shown in table 1. The standard deviations have also been plotted. Taken as a whole, the variation in gape during any sequence is greater than the variation in the cycle times. The extremely large standard deviations observed in one case of puncture-crushing (chicken leg) and of mastication (gizzard) are partly explained by interruptions in the normal rhythm owing to manual repositioning of the food. This usually involves a smaller than average gape with a much longer than usual recovery stroke. However, as this is normal behavior, these particular cycles were not excluded from the count. As mastication proceeds, the size of the gape normally diminishes. This effect is particularly marked in puncture-crushing. Figure 8 shows the small range of variation in gape and cycle time during mastication of dog-food, chicken wing or leg, and one case of chicken gizzard. This result suggests that the effect of the long period of preliminary puncture-crushing observed for tough food is to reduce its consistency to a pulp similar to dog food. Once this has been achieved the standard pattern of mastication ensues.

The third impression gained from the first analysis (Crompton and Hiiemae 1969a, 1970), that each stroke takes a fairly constant proportion of the total cycle time, has proved correct. The mean and standard deviations for the percentage duration of each stroke in each example of puncture-crushing and normal mastication show a close correspondence (table 2). However, when the duration of each cycle is expressed as a percentage of the total cycle time, the correspondence becomes even more apparent. In puncture-crushing the mean and standard deviations for the percentage duration of each of the three strokes are: the preparatory stroke $27.7 \pm 2.7\%$, the power stroke $21.0 \pm 2.5\%$, and the recovery stroke $57.7 \pm 3.8\%$. In shearing mastication they are $26.0 \pm 2.9\%$, $22.4 \pm 1.7\%$, and $51.0 \pm 3.4\%$ respectively. Therefore, irrespective

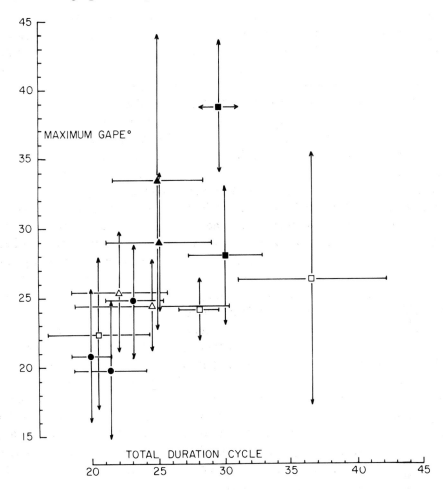

Fig. 8. The mean and one standard deviation of the gape plotted against the mean and one standard deviation of the total duration of the chewing cycle in mastication for each sample in tables 1 and 2. The symbols are as follows: *Puncture-crushing:* chicken wing or leg: ▲; chicken gizzard: ■; *Shearing:* dog food: ●; chicken wing or leg: △; chicken gizzard: □.

of the type of mastication in progress, the relative duration of each stroke remains virtually constant. If the power stroke is taken as unity, the ratio of their percentage durations becomes 1.3:1.0:2.4 for both types of mastication. Therefore the power stroke is the shortest stroke in the cycle, the preparatory stroke is slightly longer, and the recovery stroke is longer than the first two strokes taken together.

If the percentage durations of the three strokes of lapping-licking (the upstroke, near-occlusion phase, and downstroke) are also expressed as a ratio, this becomes 0.7:1.0:2.4. The relative increase in the duration of the recovery stroke, with a corresponding diminution of the preparatory stroke in lapping-licking, can be explained by the pause during the downstroke in which the tongue movements of ingestion occur. Even in licking cycles the percentage duration of the "near occlusion" phase corresponds to that of a normal power stroke.

These observations appear to have the corollary that if the recovery stroke is twice as long as the preparatory stroke, the possible rate of jaw opening is half that of jaw closing. This is not, in fact, true. A minor point, demonstrated in figure 7, is that the actual distance moved in the two strokes may be different, as in the first cycle shown for puncture-crushing. The cycle commenced at a gape of 26° and terminated at a gape of 41°. Similarly, the last cycle began at a gape of 39° and finished with a gape of 21°. This is due to the convention adopted here and in Hiiemae and Ardran (1968) that the cycle should be re-garded as commencing with the jaw in the depressed position. Figure 7 also shows, for both dog food and chicken wing or leg mastication, that the gapes are often comparable, so that the lower jaw moves much the same distance in both strokes. The recovery stroke is very much longer than the preparatory stroke because the jaw moves very slowly downward through the first 6° of gape. Further movement is then rapid and at essentially the same rate as the re-turn upward movement (fig. 5a, b). The finding that the power stroke has vir-tually the same absolute as well as percentage duration in both puncture-crushing and shearing suggests that its timing is not governed by either the consistency of the food or the occlusion.

These observations imply either a functional or a physiological explanation, a problem which will be examined further in the discussion. The observed vari-ation in jaw movement over similar percentage time suggests that a control mechanism must be sought.

The Mechanism of the Gape. Didelphis can open its mouth as much as 53° between its upper and lower molar surfaces (fig. 9 and table 3), but gapes within the range of 20–40° are usually associated with the various phases of mastication and of 3–10° with licking and lapping. Single-frame analysis of the cinefluorographic recordings has shown that small gapes up to about 15° are produced by mandibular depression alone but that larger gapes result from a combination of mandibular depression and cranial extension on the atlanto-occipital joint.

Figure 11 is a montage of five successive frames from a sequence of dog-food mastication in which the cervical vertebrae have been taken as the fixed reference points. The first frame shows the mouth open to a gape of about 15°

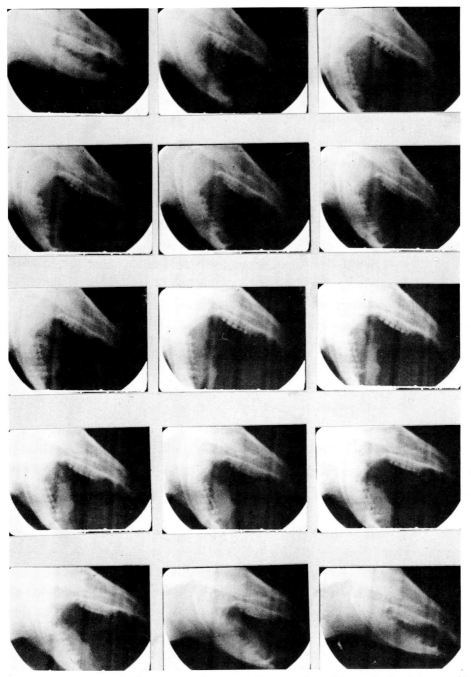

Fig. 9. Every third frame from a cinefluorographic recording of regurgitation taken at 60 frames per sec, showing both the size of the gape reached and the time for which it is held.

TABLE 3

GAPE DIMENSIONS

Food	Largest	Smallest	Mean	Standard Deviation
Milk	9°	3°	6.0°	1.5°
Dog food	38°	23°	29.5°	3.8°
Chicken wing or leg	40°	21°	33°	7.9°
Chicken gizzard	45°	31°	39.3°	5.6°

Note: Gapes in Regurgitation: 53°, 50°, 51°.

Measurements of the gape were taken from twelve successive masticatory cycles between upper and lower molar surfaces when feeding on various types of food. Recordings other than those used for table 1 were analyzed. These values were used to draw fig. 10, and those for chicken wing or leg and chicken gizzard include both puncture-crushing and shearing.

produced by simple mandibular depression. From this point, a slight downward movement of both the cranium and the lower jaw occurs while the same degree of gape is maintained. During the next three frames the mandible is held in this depressed position while the cranium and upper jaw are extended by movement at the atlanto-occipital joint until the final gape is attained. In the actual recordings the head appears to be "cranked up" on the neck.

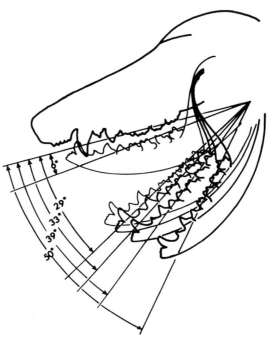

Fig. 10. The mean gapes reached when lapping (6°), masticating dog food (29°), chicken wing or leg (33°), and chicken gizzard (39°) and for one case of regurgitation (50°) drawn as seen in lateral projection radiographs.

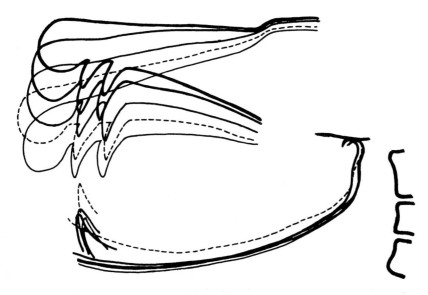

Fig. 11. Montage of five successive tracings of mouth opening in mastication using the cervical vertebrae as the fixed points.

The figure illustrates one particular case of jaw opening produced by a combination of active mandibular depression followed by passive movement at the squamodentary joint as the cranium is extended. Although the completion of mandibular depression preceded cranial extension in this case, facilitating its illustration, this is by no means always so. The first stages of the elevation of the upper jaw may begin as the lower jaw approaches its maximally depressed position and then continue as the jaw is held more or less stationary.

These observations suggest that large gapes in other animals may be produced by a similar mechanism. The use of cranial extension rather than further mandibular depression to enlarge the gape might be explained by the limited range over which the depressor muscles can act. If mandibular depression in *Didelphis* is produced primarily by the actions of the digastric, mylohyoid, and geniohyoid pulling the body of the jaw down toward the hyoid (see Hiiemae and Jenkins 1969), the need for cranial extension to enlarge the gape can be explained. For the anterior suprahyoid muscles listed above to be effective the hyoid must be fixed by the posterior suprahyoid and the infrahyoid musculature. The extent to which the hyoid can be retracted toward the vertebral column is limited not only by the muscles and soft tissues themselves but also by the need to maintain the airway. Once the digastric, mylohyoid, and geniohyoid have achieved maximal contraction, no further mandibular depression can occur. It follows that any further increase in the gape must depend on an upward movement of the cranium away from the lower jaw.

During simple mandibular depression in the recovery stroke, the movement is entirely vertical and the mandibular condyles rotate on the glenoid fossae of the squamosals. As cranial extension proceeds the reverse must occur: the glenoids rotating around the condyles. There is, however, a definite postglenoid flange in *Didelphis* extending down to the upper part of the condylar neck on the posteromedial aspect. Even allowing for the thick articular surfaces covering both the condyle and the fossa (Hiiemae, unpublished), this flange would prevent a gape, however produced, of more than 40° or so by impinging on the condylar neck. However, the mediolateral position of the condyles on the glenoid fossae does not remain constant (Crompton and Hiiemae 1969a, 1970). At the beginning of the preparatory stroke or in some cases during it, the condyles of both sides move laterally across the fossae in a simple Bennett movement. Since the widest gapes are reached at the junction of recovery and preparatory strokes in *Didelphis*, a simultaneous lateral shift of the condyles would prevent contact between the postglenoid flange and the condylar neck because the flange would then lie to the medial of the thickened posterolateral ridge on the neck of the condyle. It has not been possible to test this hypothesis using the cinefluorographic recordings because the movements of the condyle can be clearly seen only in the dorsoventral and the gape in the lateral projection. In view of the large gapes recorded, particularly in regurgitation (fig. 9), and the recorded Bennett shift of the condyles, synchronization of the sideslip with the final stages of cranial extension would explain how these gapes can occur without, apparently, interference from contact between the condylar neck and postglenoid flange.

Deglutition and Regurgitation

Deglutition marks the completion of a chewing sequence in *Didelphis*. When the opossum is feeding on solids, they are ingested in single "bite" units and then masticated, with the gradual formation of a bolus which is then passed. In lapping or licking of liquids, fluid from several laps accumulates on the dorsum of the tongue and is then passed with a single swallowing movement. This involves virtually no interruption of the lapping rhythm: three or more such fluid boli will be passed over a total of fifty or so lapping cycles. The passage of boli derived from solid food is, however, associated with a distinct change in the rhythm of the chewing cycle.

A bolus begins to form soon after the onset of shearing mastication. As the food is progressively reduced, the bolus gradually enlarges, coming to lie in very close relation to the epiglottis. As the last particles of food remaining in the molar region are sheared and reduced, a change in the rhythm of the chewing cycle occurs, presaging deglutition. Figure 12, prepared in the same way as figure 7, illustrates the progressive reduction in the gape and increase in the duration of the chewing cycles immediately before deglutition. The bolus is passed during the recovery stroke of a cycle of increased duration. This begins with a small gape (6° and 5° in the cases illustrated in figure 12) and a preparatory stroke of normal duration. The power stroke is lengthened, and during

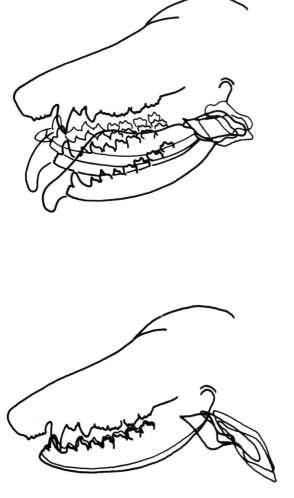

Fig. 12. A montage of tracings from a cinerecording of deglutition taken at 60 frames per sec, showing every second frame.

this time the position of the bolus on the dorsum of the tongue is adjusted in preparation for its passage. The recovery stroke begins slowly with a slight opening of the jaw (figure 12). This position is held momentarily, after which the jaw is very slightly elevated as the bolus is passed toward the esophagus and then depressed to the rest position. The recovery stroke then proceeds

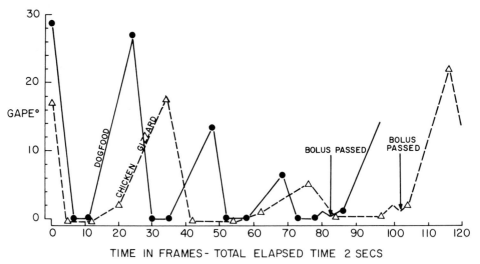

Fig. 13. The movements of the lower jaw over the last three masticatory cycles before deglutition showing the dimunition of the gape and the elongated recovery stroke in which swallowing occurs. The key is the same as for figure 7.

normally. Movement of the bolus into and down the esophagus is initially very slow and it remains visible just below the epiglottis for a considerable period before being carried down toward the stomach.

Mention has already been made of the indiscriminate and voracious feeding behavior of *Didelphis*. A similar comment can be made about the opossum's masticatory behavior when it is hungry and feeding on tough foods. In these circumstances, food is sometimes rapidly chewed and then swallowed only to be regurgitated for further chewing. This type of behavior was observed when animals were feeding on both chicken wing or leg and on chicken gizzard. A bolus was swallowed and almost immediately regurgitated. To do this, the animal ceases all other activity, usually ingestion, and then holds a very wide gape with its head bent well down so that the open mouth faces the ground. The tongue is pulled well forward and the hyoid elevated. The bolus, visible beyond the epiglottis, is then moved forward over the dorsum of the tongue and then falls through the mouth until it is caught as the jaw is elevated. Figure 9 shows stages in this process taken from the cinerecording used in the demonstration film (see section on materials and methods). In that case, the first attempt to regurgitate the bolus was unsuccessful; the stills are taken from the second attempt. Regurgitation, as can be seen from figure 9 and from table 3, involves the widest of all recorded gapes, reaching as much as 53° in one case. Once the bolus has been returned to the mouth, the food is remasticated until it is of suitable consistency and then reswallowed. Although on one occasion it was possible to identify discrete slivers of bone in a regurgitated bolus in a recording, it has not been possible to examine one more closely. Regurgitation is unpredictable and consequently difficult to record. Although antiperistalsis and regurgitation of the stomach contents is a well-known pathological phenomenon in man and forms a well-recognized part of masticatory activity in ruminants, it has not, as far as we are aware, been reported in other mammals. In *Didelphis* the bolus is regurgitated from the upper part of the esophagus, almost immediately after its deglutition. This suggests that receptors in the mucous membrane of the region "trigger" the process. This does not explain, however, the initial passage of an unsuitable bolus. In man, the oral mucous membrane covering the margins of the oropharynx is well supplied with touch and pressure receptors (Kawamura 1964). These are regarded as forming a protective ring preventing the further passage of foreign bodies and unsuitable material into the esophagus or trachea. Without evidence as to the existence or position of comparable receptors in *Didelphis*, an explanation of the initiation and mechanism of regurgitation cannot be provided.

Observations and Summary

Feeding behavior and the mandibular movements of feeding in *Didelphis* have been described for the various stages of the sequence ingestion-mastication-deglutition. These observations are summarized in table 4, in which the movements of the lower jaw, tongue, and food during the three stages of the masticatory cycle are shown.

Analysis of the rhythm of crushing-puncturing and shearing mastication has shown that: the power stroke is of approximately the same absolute as well as relative duration in all cases; the preparatory and recovery strokes vary considerably in their absolute duration but occupy a constant percentage of the total cycle time; and there is a distinctive modification of the normal cycle rhythm in deglutition. Measurements of the gape have shown that there is no correlation between the number of degrees of gape and the length of the cycle, but that gapes over 35° tend to be associated with puncture-crushing and gapes of 18–26° with shearing mastication. Very large gapes over 45° have been recorded in regurgitation.

TABLE 4
MOVEMENTS OF JAW AND TONGUE DURING MASTICATORY CYCLE

Activity	Preparatory Stroke		Power Stroke		Recovery Stroke	
	Jaw	Tongue	Jaw	Tongue	Jaw	Tongue
Mastication						
Puncture-crushing and shearing	Moves upward and laterally	Carries food upward and backward	Moves upward, medially, and forward	Controls position of food with cheek	Moves downward, initially slowly for tough foods	Collects food and moves it downward and backward
Ingestion						
Licking/lapping	Very rapid movement upward	Tongue retracts carrying liquid	No movement, teeth in occlusion or near occlusion	Tongue transfers liquid distally	Jaw moves downward—pause—jaw rapidly depressed	Tongue protruded, flicked through liquid
Grasping/shoveling	Moves upward until bite is grasped	Tongue moves to control position of bite	Head retracted from food. No observable jaw activity	—	Jaw depressed; upper jaw plunged into food mass—pause—slight downward movement	Tongue moves to control food
Food transference	Jaw upward	Tongue carries food upward and backward	Moves into power stroke or equivalent	—	Jaw depressed —pause— jaw sharply depressed	Tongue usually protruded, position of food adjusted; food carried downward and backward

General Discussion

The opossum is an extremely primitive mammal. It is reported to be omnivorous in the feral state, feeding on carrion, bird's eggs, grubs, fruit, and so on, but the changing ecology of the northeastern United States, resulting from a spreading suburbanization, has probably provided an easily obtained and plentiful new source of food—domestic garbage. This may, to some extent, explain the success and spread of *Didelphis* in New England and upper New York State.

Unlike the rabbit and the rat, the only other animals whose feeding behavior has been examined cinefluorographically, the opossum has no obvious adaptive specializations of the teeth and jaws. Detailed comparisons between two mammals of rodent habit and *Didelphis* would therefore have little value and will not be attempted. The observations reported in this paper do, however, raise a number of more general questions.

Tough or hard foods presented in large bulk are ingested through the side of the mouth by a process identical to mastication, hence the use of the term "ingestion by mastication." Although this is familiar behavior in carnivores, it has not previously been documented in a very primitive and generalized mammal. Tough or hard foods, whatever their bulk, are chewed by a combination of puncture-crushing and shearing cycles. The use of the premolars and molars in these two ways, pulping and slicing, must be reflected in the wear faceting visible on their occlusal surfaces. This has proved to be the case in *Didelphis* (Crompton and Hiiemae 1969*b*, 1970). Although the teeth are used differently in the two types of mastication, the general pattern of movement is the same. Such differences as are present are of degree, specifically in the gape reached between cycles. These observations raise a number of questions: (*a*) Is the pattern of movment of the masticatory cycle intrinsic or acquired? (*b*) Are the variations in the pattern of movement due to feedback based on the nature of the food? (*c*) Are they purely a function of the biomechanics of the system? (*d*) What is the significance of the variation in the gape, other than to assist in regurgitation? These problems cannot be solved with the techniques now available to us but should be briefly discussed.

The information available on the control of mastication has been obtained from two sources. The control of mastication has been examined by neurophysiological techniques in cats, with particular reference to the receptor system present in the mammalian oral cavity and to the reflex control of jaw movement. The available data have been extensively reviewed (Kawamura 1964), but while discussing the role of the various types of receptors in the jaw apparatus little information has been gained as to the control of normal feeding movements. As this study and others (Ardran, Kemp, and Ride 1958; Hiiemae and Ardran 1968) have shown, lapping, licking, and chewing are rhythmic processes. The reflex behavior experimentally elicited in a decerebrate cat is rarely so. However, recent work has indicated that rhythmic responses analogous to lapping can be obtained by suitable stimulation of some oral sites (Thexton 1969). Behavior strictly analogous to normal masticatory movements has not been elicited.

The second source of information on the mechanisms and control of feeding behavior is human studies, many with a clinical dental bias. Man is not a satisfactory experimental animal (Møller 1966). However, "unconscious" chewing, seen for example in the chewing of gum, is certainly rhythmic and cyclical. This suggests that the jaw movements of lapping and licking and of puncture-crushing and shearing mastication can all be regarded as having a similar wave-form varying in its wavelength and amplitude. Ingestion, such as grasping, shoveling, and licking, even in this study is irregular and discontinuous and does not, therefore, conform to this pattern. It would seem likely that once a mammalian jaw apparatus had evolved, a basic pattern of jaw movement in chewing also developed and has persisted. Such differences as can readily be discerned between the various groups of mammals (Crompton and Hiiemae 1969b) can be explained by alterations in the direction or amplitude of the strokes of the cycle.

The evidence obtained in this study would suggest that whether the pattern of masticatory movement is the result of a rhythm intrinsic to the central nervous system or whether it is based on chains of reflexes, local factors such as the physiology of the muscles and the nature of the food will regulate its timing. The powerful adductor jaw musculature in *Didelphis* (Hiiemae and Jenkins 1969), as in most mammals, acts to elevate the jaw and provides the force used in triturating the food. The smooth upward movement seen in the preparatory stroke and the medial, forward, and upward movement of the power stroke in shearing can be attributed to the action of the adductor musculature. The question remains of which muscles act to depress the jaw and why this should begin very slowly (in the recovery stroke). The lateral pterygoid and the digastric, with or without the assistance of the remaining hyoid musculature, have been regarded as prime movers in mandibular depression (Kawamura 1964). Downward movement of the lower jaw cannot, however, occur without synergistic relaxation of the adductors. It is possible that part of the slow first stage of recovery stroke may represent the period in which the adductor muscles begin to relax after the powerful upward movement of the power stroke and the mandibular depressors become effective in overcoming the inertia of the system.

The influence of the consistency of the food on the pattern of movement is seen in the increased gapes observed for puncture-crushing as compared with shearing mastication. The similarity in the duration of the upstroke from a gape of 20° and one of 40° suggests that in the latter case the jaw is moving rather more rapidly. This may in itself greatly enhance the puncturing effect and explain why the larger gapes occur. *Didelphis* is not the only mammal in which cranial movement contributes to the production of a gape. Similar observations have been made in man, although the maximum degree of opening in man is very much less than the 53° recorded in *Didelphis*.

In conclusion, it should be stated that this type of behavioral study can provide information on the manner in which an animal, in this case the opossum, ingests, chews, and swallows its food and on the frequency and amplitude of the movements involved. The evidence obtained here suggests that the central nervous system controls the basic pattern of movement which is probably regulated by local factors. To confirm this, physiological experiments correlating experimental studies with normal behavioral data are required.

ACKNOWLEDGMENTS

This study has been made possible by the award of National Institutes of Health, United States Public Health Service research grant DE 02648-01.

We should like to express our very deep appreciation of the great assistance given to us by Dr. G. M. Ardran of the Nuffield Institute for Medical Research, University of Oxford, during the early stages of this investigation. In addition, our thanks are due to Dr. J. W. Osborn and Dr. A. Thexton for reading the manuscript and for much helpful criticism, to Miss Margaret Newton and Mrs. Louise Holtzinger for clerical assistance, and to Miss Diane Barker, Mrs. Rosanne Rowen, and Mr. A. Coleman for help in preparing the figures.

REFERENCES

Ardran, G. M.; Kemp, F. H.; and Ride, W. D. C. 1958. A radiographic analysis of mastication and swallowing in the domestic rabbit *Oryctolagus caninulus* L. *Proc. Zool. Soc. Lond.* 130:257–74.

Barghusen, H. R. 1968. The lower jaw of cynodonts (Reptilia, Therapsida) and the evolutionary origin of mammal-like adductor musculature. *Postilla* 116:1–49.

Bowman, A. J., and Ford, F. W. 1968. A method for relating electromyographic recordings to mandibular movement. *J. Dent. Res.* 47, no. 6 (suppl.):972.

Crompton, A. W. 1968. Studying function by x-ray. *Discovery, Peabody Mus.* 3:23–32.

Crompton, A. W., and Hiiemae, K. 1969a. Functional occlusion in tribosphenic molars. *Nature* 222:678–79.

———. 1969b. How mammalian molars work. *Discovery, Peabody Mus.* 5:23–34.

————. 1970. Molar occlusion and mandibular movements during occlusion in the American opossum, *Didelphis marsupialis*. *Zool. J. Linn. Soc.* 49:21–47.

Hartman, C. G. 1952. *Possums*. Austin: University of Texas Press.

Hiiemae, K. M. 1967. Masticatory function in the mammals. *J. Dent. Res.* 46: 883–93.

Hiiemae, K., and Ardran, G. M. 1968. A cineradiographic study of feeding in *Rattus norvegicus*. *J. Zool. Lond.* 154:139–54.

Hiiemae, K., and Jenkins, F. A. 1969. The anatomy and internal architecture of the muscles of mastication in the American opossum, *Didelphis marsupialis*. *Postilla*, no. 140.

Kawamura, Y. 1964. Recent concepts of the physiology of mastication. In *Advances of oral biology*, vol. 1, ed. P. H. Staple. London: Academic Press.

Møller, G. 1966. The chewing apparatus: An electromyograph study of the action of the muscles of mastication and its correlation to facial morphology. *Acta Physiol. Scand.* 69, suppl. 280.

Patterson, B. 1956. Early cretaceous mammals and the evolution of mammalian molar teeth. *Fieldiana Geol.* 13:1–105.

Thexton, A. T. 1969. Characteristics of the jaw opening reflex in the cat. *J. Physiol.* 201:67–68P.

Turnbull, W. D. 1970. The mammalian masticatory apparatus. *Fieldiana Geol.* 18, no. 2:149–356.

Contributors

G. R. BAIRD
  Zoller Memorial Dental Clinic
  University of Chicago
  950 East 59th Street
  Chicago, Illinois 60637

A. D. G. BEYNON
  Department of Oral Anatomy
  The University of Newcastle
    upon Tyne
  Sutherland Dental School
  Northumberland Road
  Newcastle upon Tyne 1, England

A. BOYDE
  Department of Anatomy
  University College, London
  Gower Street
  London, W. C. 1., England

H. BRABANT
  Université Libre de Bruxelles
  Clinique Stomatologique
  Rue Haute, 322
  Bruxelles 1, Le, Belgium

P. M. BUTLER
  Department of Zoology
  Royal Holloway College
  (University of London)
  "Alderhurst" Bakeham Lane
  Englefield Green, Surrey, England

W. A. CLEMENS
  Department of Paleontology
  University of California
    at Berkeley
  Berkeley, California 94720

A. W. CROMPTON
  Museum of Comparative Zoology
    and Department of Biology
  The Agassiz Museum
  Harvard University
  Cambridge, Massachusetts 02138

A. A. DAHLBERG
  Department of Anthropology and
    Zoller Memorial Dental Clinic
  University of Chicago
  1126 East 59th Street
  Chicago, Illinois 60637

D. H. GOOSE
  School of Dental Surgery
  The University of Liverpool
  Pembroke Place
  P. O. Box 147
  Liverpool, L69 3BX, England

P. HERSHKOVITZ
  Research Curator, Mammal
    Division
  Field Museum of Natural History
  Roosevelt Road at Lake Shore
    Drive.
  Chicago, Illinois 60605

K. HIIEMAE
  Department of Anatomy

Guy's Hospital Medical School
London, England
Museum of Comparative Zoology,
Harvard University
Cambridge, Massachusetts 02138

E. J. KOLLAR
Department of Anatomy
University of Chicago
Chicago, Illinois 60637

I. KOVACS
132, avenue du parc
Bruxelles 6, Le, Belgium

W. A. MILLER
Department of Oral Biology
School of Dentistry
State University of New York
at Buffalo
4510 Main Street
Buffalo, New York 14226

D. F. G. POOLE
Medical Research Council
Dental Research Unit
Lower Mauldin Street

Bristol 1, England

E. L. SIMONS
Peabody Museum of Natural
History
Yale University
New Haven, Connecticut 06520

M. V. STACK
University of Bristol
Dental School
Lower Mauldin Street
Bristol 1, England

C. H. TONGE
The University of Newcastle
upon Tyne
Sutherland Dental School
Northumberland Road
Newcastle upon·Tyne 1, England

W. D. TURNBULL
Field Museum of Natural History
Roosevelt Road at Lake Shore
Drive
Chicago, Illinois 60605
The Dental School

Author Index

Subject Index

Abrasion, 182, 258
Acellular cement, 91
Adapids, 129
Aegialodon, 184
Aegyptopithecus zeuxis, 193, 194, 198, 200, 201, 202, 203
Aeolopithecus chirobates, 193, 194, 201
Afghan Tajiks, 273
Age: chronological, 60; fetal, 60; threshold, 60
Alaspis, 69
Allometry, 4, 7
Alouatta, 112
Alphadon, 190, 299; didelphoid, 152
Alveolar: bone, 38; resorption, 212
Amblystoma, 46
Ameloblasts, 17, 74, 82, 86
Amelodentinal junction, 74, 82, 259
Amino acids, 75
Amphipithecus, 202, 203
Amphitherium, 121
Amphybia, 17, 46, 54, 72, 73, 75
Anaptomoiphus, 121
Anomalies, 219, 220, 224, 225, 250
Anterior accessory cusp, 128
Anthropoids, 193, 196, 197, 230, 244, 249
Antigens, graft, 54
Antiperistalsis, 329
Apatite crystallites, 77
Apical foramen, 50
Apidium: moustafai, 193–96; *phiomense*, 193, 195–98
Apterodon, 203
Arachnids, 185
Arthrodira, 71
Artiodactyla, 84, 85, 88, 91, 152
Aspidin, 70

Atlanto-occipital joint, 324
Attrition, 275

Babyrousa babyrussa, 90
Bats, 112, 115
Bennett movement, 317, 326
Beta-2-thienylalanine, 17–19, 27, 54, 261
Bifurcation, root, 225, 226, 228, 231, 247, 248
Bilophodonty, 130
Biochemical block, 261
Biosynthetic mechanisms, 27
Biting, 305
Blastocyst, 47
Bolk, tubercle of, 290, 293, 296
Bone, 56, 66
Brachyteles, 127
Bradypus tridactylus, 91
Buccal groove, 258

Caenomeryx, 129
Calcification, 6, 8, 9, 12, 13, 34, 259, 260; degrees of, 8; pulpal, 89
Calcitonin, 56
Callicebus, 112, 123, 125; *torquatus*, 97, 103, 105, 107
Callimico goeldii, 132
Callithricidae, 96, 97
Callithrix, 98, 115
Canine teeth, 98, 99, 115
Caniniform teeth, 98, 182
Caninization, 32, 96–99
Carabelli's cusp, 250, 257, 258, 275, 278, 281, 290, 296
Carnivora, 85, 88, 102, 151, 211, 236, 239, 241, 244, 248, 249
Carpolestidae, 98

341